Dermatology
in Clinical Practice

Zohra Zaidi · Sean W. Lanigan

Dermatology in Clinical Practice

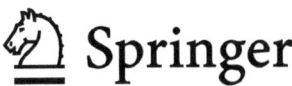 Springer

Authors
Dr. Zohra Zaidi
7 B 9th Zamzama St.
Karachi-74400
Clifton
Pakistan
zohrazaidi@hotmail.com

Dr. Sean W. Lanigan
Consultant Dermatologist,
Birmingham
United Kingdom

ISBN 978-1-84882-861-2   ISBN 978-1-84882-862-9 (eBook)

DOI 10.1007/978-1-84882-862-9

Springer Dordrecht Heidelberg London New York

Library of Congress Control Number: 2009938034

Cover design: eStudio Calamar Figueres/Berlin

Printed on acid-free paper

Springer is part of Springer Science+Business Media (www.springer.com)

Preface

Books on dermatology are either focused for medical students or for students of dermatology. A general practitioner sees a lot of skin patients; about 17% of their patients are related to skin disease. We therefore decided to write a book that should meet the needs of a general practitioner.

To make the book helpful for the primary care physician, we have focused more on common skin problems and have discussed the diagnosis and treatment of these disorders in depth to help the general practitioner in diagnosing and treating them. The chapter on the management of skin diseases also gives the details of topical, systemic, and the physical modalities used in treating skin disease. Uncommon skin diseases are only mentioned where required. The chapter on cutaneous manifestations of systemic diseases will help the general practitioner to correlate the cutaneous signs of the common medical problems seen by them. Emphasis is laid on the bacterial, fungal, and parasitic disorders that are prevalent in tropical countries. We have included the common diseases of other continents, as the general practitioner especially of developed countries has patients from all over the world.

Congenital and hereditary disorders are discussed with the corresponding chapters, which makes it easier for the reader to remember. A number of practical points are included with each subject, and history of dermatology is included where appropriate to make the subject interesting to read.

The general practitioner refers a number of cases to the dermatology clinic for dermatological procedures such as phototherapy, cryosurgery, and lasers. These procedures are included in the appendix at the end of the book. This will help the practitioner to have a basic knowledge about the procedure to be performed on their patients.

Skin rashes are often an enigma for beginners; a little insight into the subject with a clear understanding can make the rash so simple to diagnose. We have tried to make this book simple, practical, and easy to use. We hope that general practitioners find it helpful; it could also be of interest and benefit to medical students.

Karachi, Pakistan   Dr. Zohra Zaidi
Birmingham, UK   Dr. Sean W. Lanigan

Acknowledgments

The authors thank the following consultants for contributing their photographs to the book: Dr. Badr Dhanani, Consultant Dermatologist, Institute of Skin Diseases, Karachi, Pakistan, Dr. Khalid Hussain, Consultant Dermatologist, Lincoln County Hospital, Lincoln, UK, Dr. Naseema Kapadia, Consultant Dermatologist, Aga Khan University, Karachi, Pakistan, Dr. Aziz Khan, Consultant Dermatologist, Dow Institute of Health Sciences, Karachi, Pakistan, Dr. Daulat Pinjani, Consultant Dermatologist, Institute of Skin Diseases, Karachi, Pakistan, Surgeon Captain Rehanuddin, Head, Department of Dermatology, PNS Shifa, Karachi, Pakistan, Dr. Zarnaz Wahid, Professor of Dermatology, Dow Institute of Health Sciences, Karachi, Pakistan, and Dr. Shernaz Walton, Consultant Dermatologist, Hull and East Yorkshire Hospital NHS Trust, UK and Esen Rizvi for graphics.

Contents

Morning Prayer of Maimonides

O God let my mind be clear and enlightened. By the bedside of the patient let no alien thought deflect it. Let everything that experience and scholarships have taught me, be present in me, and my mind hinders not in my tranquil work. For great and noble are those scientific judgments, that serve the purpose of preserving health and lives of thy creatures.

Keep far from me the delusions that I can accomplish all things. Give me the strength, the will and the opportunity to amplify my knowledge more and more. Today I can disclose things in my knowledge, which yesterday I would have not dreamt of; for the art is great, but the human mind presses on untiringly.

In the patient let me see only the man. Thou, All-Bountiful One, have chosen me to watch over life and death of thy creatures. I prepare myself now for my calling. Stand Thou by me in this great task, so that it may prosper. For without Thine aid man prospers not even in the smallest things.

Maimonides (1135–1204)

Moses Maimonides was one of the greatest Jewish scholars of all times. He was a rabbi, physician and philosopher. Maimonides was the first person to write the systematic review of all Jewish law. Maimonides was trained as a physician in Spain. He wrote a number of books on medicine, ethics and on aphorisms. His treatises became influential for generation of physicians. Maimonides was a physician to Sultan Saladin, after his death he continued to be a physician to the royal family. When Almohades from Africa conquered Cordoba and threatened the Jewish community, Maimonides' family choose exile

Chapter 1
Skin: Structure and Function

Skin is the largest organ of the body, covering an area of 1.7 m^2; it weighs about 15% of the total body weight. The skin protects us against the external environment. The thickness, pigmentation, and distribution of the appendages of the skin vary in different parts of the body, depending upon the function and needs of the area.

1.1 Structure

The skin consists of the epidermis, dermis, and beneath it is the subcutaneous layer.

1.1.1 Epidermis

The epidermis consists of many cells, about 95% are keratinocytes, and the other prominent cells are melanocytes, Langerhans cells, and Merkels cells. The epidermis does not have any blood vessels; it obtains its nutrients from the blood vessels of the dermis diffusing through the dermoepidermal junction (Fig. 1.1).

Z. Zaidi, S. W. Lanigan, *Dermatology in Clinical Practice*,
DOI: 10.1007/978-1-84882-862-9_1,
© Springer-Verlag London Limited 2010

EPIDERMIS

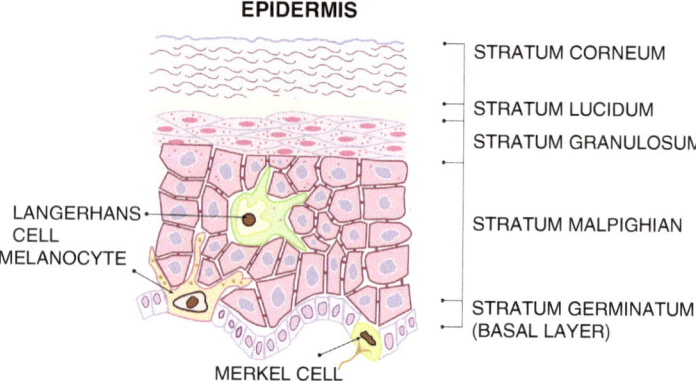

FIGURE 1.1. Epidermal layers: stratum corneum – anucleated cells; stratum lucidum – present only in palms and soles; stratum granulosum – epidermal nuclei start disintegrating; stratum malpighian – thickest and strongest layer; stratum germinatum – the only cells which undergo division. Epidermal cells: keratinocytes – the main cells of the epidermis, present in every layer of the epidermis; melanocytes – dendritic pigment producing cells, seen with a halo around them under ordinary staining, due to the lack of desmosomes. Present amongst the basal cells; langerhans cells – dendritic immunologically competent cells, also seen with a halo around them, due to the absence of desmosomes. Present in the stratum malpighian; merkel cells – present only in hairless skin; related to the sense of touch. These cells can only be seen under an electron microscope. Present amongst the basal cells.

1.1.1.1 Keratinocytes

The main function of keratinocytes is to produce keratin. Keratin forms the internal skeleton of the keratinocytes, and is composed of intermediate filaments. The keratins are a family of 30 proteins each produced by a different gene; different keratins are found in different levels of the epidermis, depending upon the stage of differentiation.

Keratinocytes are arranged in layers. The innermost layer is the basal layer; changes occur in the cells as they move up to produce the tough, impermeable, fibrous protein keratin present in the outermost layer, the stratum corneum. The cells get larger, thinner, and flatter as they move upwards.

Basal Cell Layer (Stratum Germinatum)

These are the innermost cells, present as a single layer over the basement membrane. These are the only cells of the epidermis that divide. The cells are columnar in shape with large, dark-staining nuclei. The basic component of the cytoplasm is the tonofilament – the keratin filament.

The cell cycle time is the time between two successive episodes of mitosis, or the time taken for the individual cells to divide. The normal cell cycle time is 163 h; in psoriasis it is reduced to 37.5 h.

Stratum Malpighian (Stratum Spinosum)

This layer consists of a number of layers (four to ten) of polyhedral cells. The cells have a central oval nucleus; the cytoplasm is packed with tonofilaments. Intercellular bridges called desmosomes connect the cells to one another. The cells also have a number of organelles, which help in the formation of keratin and intercellular adhesion of the stratum corneum.

Stratum Granulosum

The layer is so called because of the granules it contains. These granules (keratohyaline granules) contain proteins that help in the aggregation of the keratin filaments. It also consists of proteins that help to bind the cells of the stratum corneum together. It is three to four layers in thickness; the cells are diamond shaped.

Stratum Lucidum (Only in the Palms and Soles)

This layer lies between the stratum granulosum and stratum corneum; it is only present in the palms and soles, where the skin is very thick. The cells are nucleated, have opaque membranes and dense cytoplasm.

Stratum Corneum

An abrupt transition occurs as the cells move up from the stratum granulosum to the stratum corneum. The viable nucleated cells of the stratum granulosum change to anucleated dead cells of the stratum corneum. The cells of the stratum corneum are large, flat polyhedral, and filled with keratin; they vary in thickness from 15 to 25 layers. The cells are held together by firm lipid-rich cement. The cells overlap each other; this further helps in making this layer more impenetrable.

The upper layers of the stratum corneum are shed from the skin surface in the form of microscopic scales. The same number of cells lost from the surface are replaced by the cells of the basal layer. It takes about 26–42 days for the cells to migrate from the basal layer to the top of the granular layer, and another 13–14 days for the cells to cross the stratum corneum to the surface, from where they are shed. Total transit time is 52–75 days. In psoriasis, it is reduced to 8–10 days.

1.1.1.2 Melanocytes

These are the pigment producing cells of the epidermis; they are derived from the neural crest. They are present in the basal layer. The number varies in different parts of the body; on an average there is one melanocyte to every ten basal cells. Melanocytes are dendritic cells; they transfer melanin through the dendrites to the keratinocytes to protect them from ultraviolet light and to give color to the skin. Melanin granules form a protective cap over the outer part of the keratinocyte in the inner layers of the epidermis. In the stratum corneum, they are uniformly distributed to form a UV-absorbing blanket, which reduces the amount of radiation penetrating the skin. The melanin is present within granules called melanosomes. Melanin is formed from the aminoacid tyrosine with the help of the enzyme tyrosinase.

The number of melanocytes is the same in every individual; it is the size of the melanosomes and the distribution of melanin, which is responsible for the complexion of their skin.

1.1.1.3 Langerhans Cells

These cells are derived from the bone marrow; they are antigen presenting cells and form the first line of immunological defense of the skin. They have a lobulated nucleus and are recognized by their racket-shaped granules (Birbeck granules). These granules can be seen under an electron microscope.

1.1.1.4 Merkel Cells

These cells are also found in the basal cell layer, in close proximity to the hair follicles. They act as transducers of fine touch. Their cytoplasm contains neuropeptide granules, as well as neurofilaments and keratin.

1.1.2 Dermoepidermal Junction

The epidermis is ectodermal and the dermis mesodermal in origin; they are interconnected by the dermoepidermal junction (Fig. 1.2).

The dermoepidermal junction also provides nutrients to the epidermis, which is devoid of blood supply. It comprises:

- Plasma membrane of the basal cells with their hemidesmosomes.

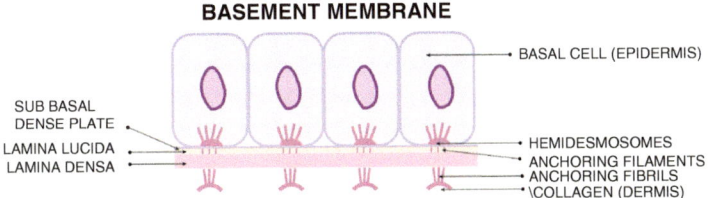

FIGURE I.2. Basement membrane. Constituents of the basement membrane: hemidesmosomes; lamina lucida – composed of structural protein laminin; lamina densa – composed of type IV collagen; anchoring fibrils – composed of type VII collagen.

- Lamina lucida with its anchoring filaments, which connects the hemidesmosomes to the lamina densa.
- Lamina densa consists of type IV collagen fibers.
- Anchoring fibers consist of type VII collagen; these connect the lamina densa to the fibers of the dermis. This completes the connection of the epidermis to the dermis.

1.1.3 Dermis

This is the tough fibrous layer of the skin; it consists of collagen fibers, elastic fibers, ground substance (glucosaminoglycans), fibroblasts, dermal dendrocytes (dendritic cells with a probable immune function), mast cells, histiocytes, blood vessels, nerves, and lymphatics (Fig. 1.3).

The dermis consists of an upper part called the papillary dermis and the lower part, the reticular dermis. There is no sharp demarcation between the two. The fibers in the papillary dermis are thin and they interdigitate with the epidermal rete ridges, while the fibers of the reticular dermis are thick and coarse.

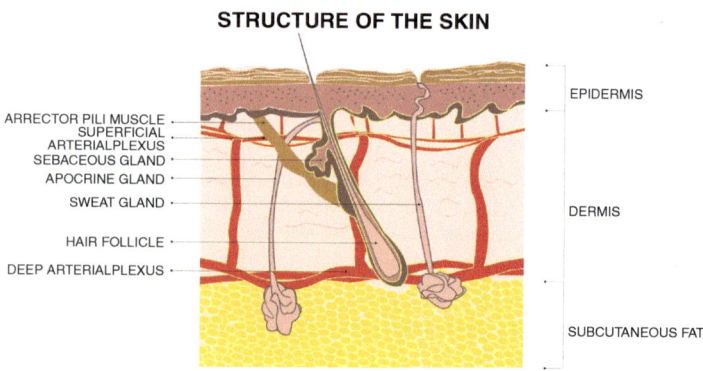

STRUCTURE OF THE SKIN

ARRECTOR PILI MUSCLE
SUPERFICIAL ARTERIALPLEXUS
SEBACEOUS GLAND
APOCRINE GLAND
SWEAT GLAND
HAIR FOLLICLE
DEEP ARTERIALPLEXUS

EPIDERMIS

DERMIS

SUBCUTANEOUS FAT

FIGURE 1.3. Structure of the skin: apocrine glands are found only in the axillae, periareolar region, periumbilical area, and anogenital region. Sebaceous glands and hair follicles are not found in the palms and soles. Arrector pili muscles are not found on the face.

Collagen fibers (collagen fibers 1 and 3) give the tough mechanical support to the skin; they run horizontally in the reticular dermis. Elastic fibers help in the elastic recoil of the skin; damage to these fibers by ultraviolet light in ageing is responsible for the formation of wrinkles. The elastic fibers are loosely arranged in all direction.

Ground substance supports the collagen and elastic tissue; it has a remarkable capacity to hold water, and it helps in the passage of nutrients, hormones, and fluid molecules through the dermis.

Blood vessels of the dermis serve two purposes, to supply the nutrients and to help in maintaining body temperature. The blood vessels of the dermis are arranged in two horizontal plexi that are connected to each other. The superficial plexus is situated at the lower border of the papillary dermis and the deep plexus in the lower part of the reticular dermis. To reduce body temperature, blood is shunted from the deep to the superficial plexus and cooling occurs through the skin. During cold weather, the blood is shunted from the superficial plexus to the deep plexus, thereby conserving heat.

Cutaneous nerves are both myelinated and unmyelinated. The unmyelinated fibers extend to the epidermis up to the granular layer. Myelinated fibers end in specialized end organs in the dermis. These nerve fibers are responsible for cutaneous sensations and prevent us from injury due to heat, cold, pain, pressure, etc. In some diseases in which sensations are absent, the body is prone to injury such as in leprosy.

The smooth muscle of the skin, the arrector pili muscle, helps in the erection of the hair (goose pimples) in cold weather, thereby trapping warm air near the skin, to protect against the cold.

1.1.3.1 Epidermal Appendages

These comprise the hair follicles, sebaceous glands, apocrine glands, eccrine (sweat) glands, and the nails. These are derived from the epidermis during intrauterine life; all of them lie in the dermis except the nails.

Hair Follicles (Pili)

Hair follicles are distributed all over the body surface, except the palms and soles. The hair on the human body is of two types: vellus hair and terminal hair. The vellus hairs are thin, short, and slightly pigmented; they are present all over the body. The terminal hairs are thick, pigmented, and are longer than the vellus hairs, e.g., the hair of the scalp, eyebrows, eyelashes, axillae, and pubis. Some of these are stimulated by androgens, such as the hair of the axillae, pubis, beard, and moustache in men. These appear at puberty (Figs. 1.4 and 1.5).

Each hair follicle consists of a hair shaft and bulb. The upper part of the hair shaft is called the infundibulum. Into the shaft of the hair follicle the ducts of the sebaceous and apocrine gland open; the opening of the apocrine gland is

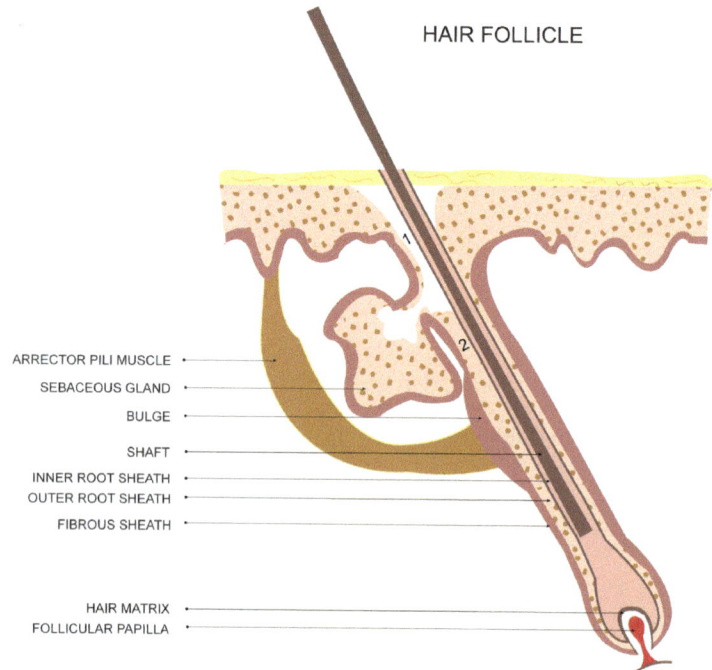

HAIR FOLLICLE

ARRECTOR PILI MUSCLE
SEBACEOUS GLAND
BULGE
SHAFT
INNER ROOT SHEATH
OUTER ROOT SHEATH
FIBROUS SHEATH
HAIR MATRIX
FOLLICULAR PAPILLA

FIGURE 1.4. Structure of the hair follicle: 1 – infundibulum; 2 – isthmus.

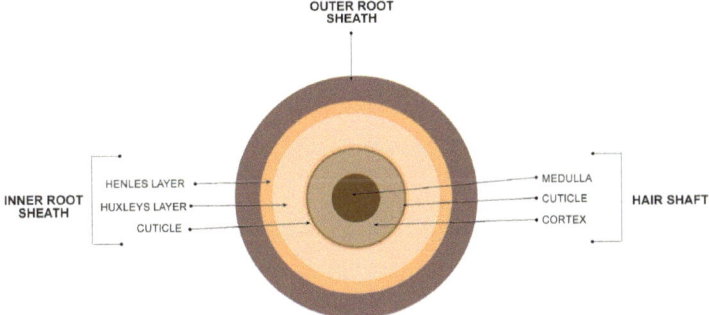

FIGURE 1.5. Cross section of the hair follicle: Lanugo hairs are non-medullated and nonpigmented, present during intrauterine life. Vellus hairs are unmedullated and slightly pigmented, present all over the body, except on the palms and soles. Terminal hairs are medullated and pigmented, present on the scalp, axillae, and pubis.

above that of the sebaceous gland. Below the opening of the sebaceous gland is the attachment of the arrector pili muscle.

The hair bulb consists of cells (matrix) which are responsible for cell division, similar to the basal cells of the epidermis; the cells then differentiate to form the shaft. The shaft is made of hard keratin. The mitotic rate of the hair matrix is greater than that of any other organ in the body. Hair growth is greatly influenced by any stress and disease process that can alter mitotic activity. This explains the hair loss when a patient is treated with cytotoxic drugs.

Hair growth is cyclical with an anagen, catagen, and telogen phase. The cells grow in the anagen phase; catagen is the transitional phase, and telogen, the resting phase. About 80–85% of the hair is in the anagen phase, 1% in the catagen phase, the rest in telogen phase. In the catagen phase growth stops and the hair becomes club-shaped. The hair is shed in the telogen phase to be replaced by new hair from the matrix, similar to the shedding of the stratum corneum. On the scalp on average about 100 hair are shed each day. The anagen phase is the longest (3–7 years) in the scalp; this accounts for the long scalp hair as compared to the terminal hair of other parts of the body. For the eyebrows the anagen phase is only 4 months.

The number of hairs differ in different parts of the body, there are about 600 hair/cm^2 on the face, and the rest of the body has about 60 hair/cm^2. Facial hairs do not have the attachment of the arrector pili muscle; this explains why we do not have goose pimples on the face in cold weather.

The hair plays an important part in the overall appearance of the body; people who have alopecia and those with hirsutism are under great psychological stress. Scalp hair protects the skin from ultraviolet radiation; bald people have a higher incidence of damage due to ultraviolet radiation. Hair could also be helping in the trapping of foreign material from entry in the body, similar to nasal cilia.

Nails

Nails are located at the ends of the fingers and toes; they are made of hard keratin. Each nail is made up of the nail matrix, nail bed, nail plate, and proximal and lateral nail folds. Nail matrix is composed of cells that undergo cell division; the cells then keratinize to form the nail plate. These cells are similar to the matrix cells of the hair and basal cells of the epidermis. The matrix cells lie under the proximal nail fold and form the lunula of the nail. The lunula is the white half-moon seen through the nail plate; it is the distal part of the nail matrix. Most of the nail plate is formed by the nail matrix. Nail plate is hard and translucent, and made of hard keratin (Figs. 1.6 and 1.7).

The nail bed extends from the distal end of the nail matrix to the hyponychium. The nail bed is attached to the nail plate; it produces a minimal amount of keratin. It appears pinkish in color due to the vascularity of the dermis. Proximal and lateral nail folds protect the nail. An extension of the proximal nail fold forms the cuticle of the nail. The cuticle seals the nail matrix from the nail plate and protects it from injury by foreign pathogens and entry of water.

The hyponychium lies under the free edge of the nail plate; stratum corneum produced here forms a cuticle to seal the junction of the distal nail bed and nail plate. The hyponychium

NAIL DORSAL VIEW

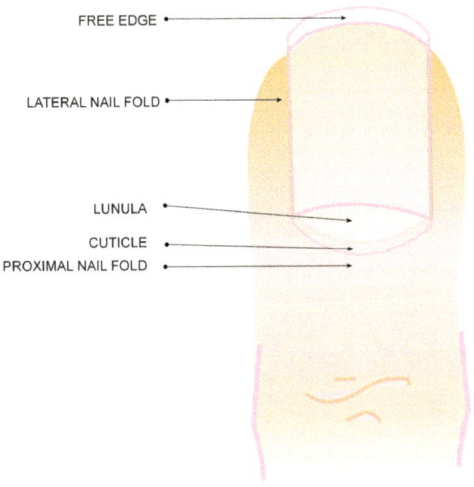

FREE EDGE

LATERAL NAIL FOLD

LUNULA

CUTICLE

PROXIMAL NAIL FOLD

FIGURE 1.6. Structure of the nail (dorsal view).

NAIL SAGITTAL SECTION

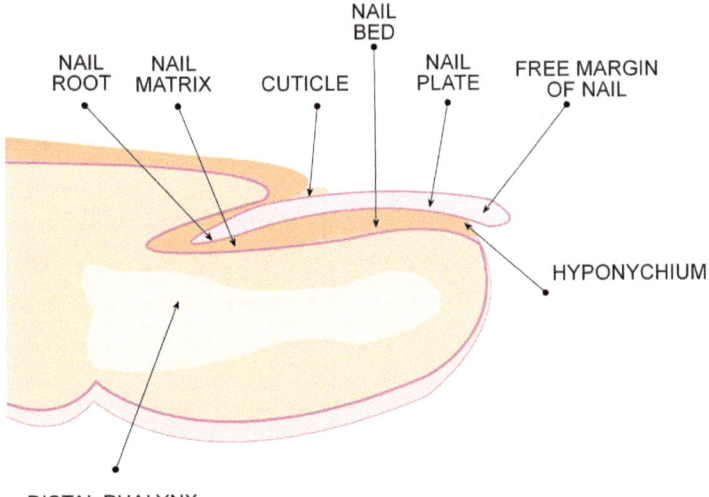

NAIL
BED

NAIL
ROOT

NAIL
MATRIX

CUTICLE

NAIL
PLATE

FREE MARGIN
OF NAIL

HYPONYCHIUM

DISTAL PHALYNX

FIGURE 1.7. Structure of the nail (lateral view).

begins at the distal end of the nail bed and ends at the distal groove.

Nails help in fine movements such as grasping and picking up objects.

Sebaceous Glands

These glands open in the hair follicles which form a part of the pilosebaceous unit; they are therefore found where the hair are present. Sebaceous glands are therefore absent from the palms and soles. They are most prominent on the face, scalp, front of the chest, and back. These glands are androgen-dependent and are stimulated at puberty and they are responsible for the development of acne. The glands secrete sebum; it is greasy due to the presence of lipids and triglycerides. The secretion is fungostatic; this explains why fungal infections of the face and scalp are less frequent in adults.

The secretion of sebum is a halocrine process; cells at the periphery of the gland break down and are completely converted into lipid secretion, as they move to the center of the gland, from where they are secreted through the sebaceous ducts into the hair follicles.

The sebaceous glands are maximum on the face, about $600/cm^2$. Their exact function is unknown, sebum lubricates the skin and prevents it from drying; it is also mildly fungistatic and bactericidal.

Most of the sebaceous glands are formed from the hair follicle, but a few free glands arise from the epithelium. The free sebaceous glands are found in the eyelids (meibomian glands), mucous membranes (Fordyce spots), nipple, perianal region, and gentalia.

Apocrine Glands

These glands are found in certain areas of the body; the axillae, anogenital, periareolar, and periumbilical areas. The ducts of these glands open in the hair follicle above the opening of the sebaceous glands. These glands are also androgen-dependent and become active at puberty. Their secretion is produced by breaking the tip of the secretory cell cytoplasm.

Body odor is due to the secretion of the apocrine glands; although the secretion is odorless when formed, the action of bacteria on the surface of the skin produces the odor.

Sweat Glands

These glands are present all over the surface of the skin; they are maximum on the face, palms, and soles. They help in keeping the skin moist and maintaining the body temperature. During hot weather a large amount of sweat is secreted; this is evaporated on the surface of the skin, thereby reducing the body temperature. During cold weather, the sweat secretion diminishes. Daily secretion of sweat is about 500 mL, but the body can produce up to a maximum of 10 L. Sweat glands also help in the excretion of waste as urea. The sweat glands open independently on the surface of the skin.

The sweat glands are unique in their innervation; they are innervated by the sympathetic nerves, but they secrete acetylcholine instead of adrenaline and are thus cholinergic sympathetic fibers.

The stimuli to produce sweat can be thermal, mental, or gustatory. This explains increased amounts of sweat in times of stress and in some people while eating spicy and hot food.

There are about two to three million sweat glands in the body, ranging in density from 60 to 600/cm^2. Sweat is acidic with a pH of between 4 and 6.8; it has low concentration of sodium and chlorine and high concentration of potassium, lactate, urea, ammonia, and some aminoacids. Only small quantities of toxic substances are excreted in sweat.

Subcutaneous Tissue

This lies below the dermis; it consists of lobules of fat cells and connective tissue septa, which are traversed by nerves and blood vessels. The collagen of the septa is continuous with the collagen of the dermis.

Subcutaneous tissue acts as a heat insulator; it cushions the body against trauma and is a storage of nutritional energy.

1.2 Functions

The functions of the skin are briefly summarized in the following table.

Skin structure	Function
Keratinocytes – stratum corneum	Prevents the skin against external environment. Barrier for shearing forces acting on the skin
	Prevents the absorption of water from outside, and loss of water and electrolytes from the skin
Melanocytes	Protects against the damage by ultraviolet light
Langerhans cells	Acts as the first line of immunological defense for the skin
Collagen tissue	Prevents the body against mechanical forces
Elastic tissue	Provides the elastic recoil to the skin
Ground substance (glucosaminoglycans)	Remarkable capacity to absorb water, gives fullness to the skin Protects the body against compressive forces
Nerves	Provide sensations to and from the skin
Blood vessels	Nutritional and help in maintaining body temperature
Sweat glands	Helps in maintaining body temperature, in keeping the skin moist, and excretion of waste products such as urea
Sebaceous glands	Moisturizes the hair and skin, fungistatic and bacteriostatic
Apocrine glands	Responsible for body odor
Nails	Helps in fine movements such as grasping of objects
Hair	Improves body image, scalp hair protects against ultraviolet damage
Subcutaneous fat	Insulates the body from cold, reserve source of food, and cushions the body from blunt trauma

The skin is the largest organ of the body.

The structure and thickness varies with site.

The mitotic rate of the hair matrix is the highest in the body.

The nerve supply to the sweat glands is sympathetic but the secretion is acetylcholine.

The skin protects the body against the external environment, "it keeps the outside out and the inside in."

The Langerhans cells are the first line of immunological defense in the skin.

Normally about 100 hairs are shed from the scalp everyday.

Sebaceous glands are responsible for acne.

The stratum corneum is the major physical barrier of the skin.

The basal cells of the epidermis are the only dividing keratinocytes.

The number of melanocytes is the same in all individuals.

Chapter 2
Immune System of the Skin

The immune system is divided into two functional components: the innate and the adaptive. In the skin, the stratum corneum is the first line of defense (innate component). The adaptive system comes into play when there is a breach in the innate system. The skin produces specific reaction to each infectious agent and prevents it from attacking the body. These two components comprise the "skin immune system" (SIS).

Two basic types of adaptive immunity occur in the body. In one of these, the body develops circulating antibodies, which are capable of attacking the invading organism. This is called humoral immunity and is brought about by B-lymphocytes, which change to plasma cells to produce the antibodies.

The second type of adaptive immunity is achieved through the formation of large number of activated lymphocytes that are specially designed to destroy foreign agents. This immunity is called cell-mediated immunity. It is brought about by T lymphocytes.

The immune system of the skin can be studied under the following headings:

- Stratum corneum
- Cellular components of the immune system
- Molecular components of the immune system

Z. Zaidi, S. W. Lanigan, *Dermatology in Clinical Practice*,
DOI: 10.1007/978-1-84882-862-9_2,
© Springer-Verlag London Limited 2010

2.1 The Stratum Corneum

This is the tough outer layer of the skin. It consists of 20–25 layers of thin, flattened cells, that overlap each other and consists of completely keratinized cells. Intercellular lipids connect the cells of the stratum corneum with each other. This dry mechanical barrier prevents the loss of fluids from the body and prevents the entry of microorganism and chemicals into the body. It also removes the contaminated organisms and chemicals from the body, through desquamation.

2.2 Cellular Components

These are the Langerhans cells, keratinocytes, T lymphocytes, mast cells, and dermal dendritic cells.

2.2.1 Langerhans Cells

These form the first line of cellular immune system of the skin. They are dendritic cells derived from the bone marrow; they contain cytoplasmic organelles called Birberk granules. These cells play an important role in antigen presentation. These cells can be identified by their surface markers CD1a and S-100 (present also in melanocytes).

2.2.2 Keratinocytes

These cells in addition to their protective role have immunological functions of their own. These cells produce large number of cytokines and produce α-melanocyte stimulating hormone, which is immunosuppressive. The keratinocytes express on their surface immune reactive molecules such as

MHC class 11 antigens, e.g., HLA-DR and intercellular adhesion molecules (ICAM-1).

2.2.3 T Cells

These cells circulate through the normal skin. There are different types of T cells depending upon their function. These are:

- Helper T cells (Th), these cells are CD4 positive. There are two type of T helper cells; Th 1, these promote inflammation, secrete IL-3, interferon, and tumor necrotic factor. Th 2 cells stimulate B cells to produce antibodies, and secrete IL-4, IL-6 and IL-10. B cells are not found in normal skin, only in disease states.
- Cytotoxic T cells (Tc) are CD 8 positive. These cells are recognized by MHC Class 1 molecules on their surface. These cells are capable of destroying allergenic and virally infected cells.
- Suppressor T cells (Ts), these cells regulate other lymphocytes.

2.2.4 Mast Cells

These cells are present in most connective tissues, predominantly around the blood vessels. They release histamine and other vasoactive molecules when stimulated. Mast cells play an important role in urticaria.

2.2.5 Dermal Dendritic Cells

These are poorly characterized cells, present around the small blood vessels of the papillary dermis. They bear MHC Class 11 antigen on their surface. Like Langerhans cells they probably play a role in antigen presentation.

2.3 Molecular Components

2.3.1 Antigens and Haptens

Antigens are molecules with large molecular weight that are recognized by the immune system, producing an immune response, usually in the form of a humoral response. Haptens are chemicals of low molecular weight that cannot provoke an immune response, unless they combine with a protein. They are important sensitizers in allergic contact dermatitis.

2.3.2 Super-Antigens

These molecules, often bacterial toxins, do not require to be recognized by an immune system, they directly signal to different classes of T cells, causing their proliferation and cytokine production, e.g., toxin produced by phage group 2 *Staphylococcus aureus* causes staphylococcal scalded skin syndrome.

2.3.3 Histocompatability Antigens

The tissue type antigens of an individual are found in the major histocompatibility complex (MHC), located in man on the HLA gene cluster on chromosome 6. HLA-A, -B and -C are expressed on all nucleated cells and are referred to as Class 1 antigens. HLA-DR, -DP, -DQ and -DZ antigens are expressed only on some cells, e.g., Langerhans cells. They are poorly expressed on keratinocytes except during disease process. These antigens are vital for tissue recognition, but are also involved in transplant rejection.

2.3.4 Antibodies

A number of antibodies are produced in response to antigens. Antibodies (IgA, IgD, IgE, IgG, and IgM) are produced by the differentiation of B-lymphocytes to plasma cells. The antibodies neutralize or opsonize antigens and activate the complement system. The highly specific mechanism of the immune system serves to recognize the particular antigen whose elimination is then accomplished in a relatively nonspecific way. In addition, the antigen (with T and B memory cells) is held in memory.

- IgG is responsible for the secondary response to most antigens. It can cross the placenta, activate complement (classical pathway), coat the neutrophils and macrophages, and act as an opsonin by cross-bridging the antigen.
- IgM is the largest antibody; it does not cross the placenta, and it is responsible for most of the primary response to antigens.
- IgA is the most common antibody in secretions; it does not bind complement but can activate it by the alternate pathway.
- IgE is bound to the receptors in the mast cells and basophils. Its release causes Type I immediate hypersensitivity reactions such as hay fever and asthma. It is present in very small quantities in the blood.
- IgD has some properties of IgG, and is found exclusively on the surface of the B-lymphocytes.

2.3.5 Cytokines

Some cells such as T lymphocytes, macrophages, Langerhans cells, fibroblasts, endothelial cells, and keratinocytes secrete cytokines, these are small proteins. They regulate the amplitude and duration of an inflammation by acting locally on nearby cells (paracrine), on the cells which produce them (autocrine); seldom do they act away from the site of production.

The term cytokine includes a number of substances such as interleukins, interferons, colony stimulating factor, cytotoxins, and growth factors. Cytokines frequently have overlapping actions, some may act synergistically and some may antagonize each other.

2.3.6 Eicosanoids

These are nonspecific inflammatory mediators, e.g., prosta-glandins, leukotrienes, thromboxanes. These are products of arachidonic acid, present on cell membrane lipid, and they play an important part during inflammation, they serve as both intracellular messengers and extracellular mediators.

2.3.7 Cellular Adhesion Molecules (CAMs)

These are surface glycoproteins that are present on different type of cells; they are involved in cell-cell adhesion and cell-matrix adhesions. CAMs are classified in to four families – selectin, integrin, immunoglobulins superfamily (molecules similar in structure to immunoglobulin), and cadherins.

2.3.8 Complement

The complement is a group of about 20 proteins in the blood, which interact with one another and with the other compo-nents of innate and adaptive immune system. Microorganisms activate the complement system. Complement stimulates the antigen antibody complexes via the alternative or classical pathway. The principal activities of the complement system are directed at protection against infection. It has a wide range of biological effects. One of its components, C_3, seems to play a role in immunological memory.

The complement helps in the following biological effects: histamine release, neutralization of viruses, release of kinins, increased vascular permeability, leukocyte immobilization, promotion of phagocytosis, promotion of fibrinolysis, and promotion of coagulation.

2.4 Hypersensitivity Reactions

2.4.1 Type I (Immediate)

IgE is bound to the surface of the mast cells. On encountering an antigen, the mast cells degranulate, with the release of inflammatory mediators such as histamine, e.g., urticaria and in severe cases anaphylaxis.

2.4.2 Type II (Cytotoxic Reaction)

Antibodies are directed against an antigen present on target cells; they produce cytotoxicity, e.g., IgG antibodies in pemphigus act on the desmoglein on the keratinocye. This results in separation of the keratinocytes, with the production of intraepithelial blister formation.

2.4.3 Type III (Immune Complex Disease)

Immune complexes are formed by the combination of antigen and antibodies in the blood; these are deposited in the walls of small blood vessels, often to those of the skin, e.g., leukocytoclastic vasculitis.

2.4.4 Type IV (Cell-Mediated or Delayed Hypersensitivity Reaction)

Lymphocytes rather than antibodies mediate this reaction. Specially sensitized T cells have secondary contact with the antigen when it is presented on the surface of antigen presenting cells as the Langerhans cells, e.g., allergic contact dermatitis.

Langerhans cells form the first line of defense of cellular immune system.

Skin contains all the elements of the cellular immune system, with the exception of B cells.

All four types of hypersensitivity reactions occur in the skin.

Keratinocytes are immunologically active cells.

The skin, its afferent blood supply, lymphatic drainage, regional lymph nodes, circulating lymphocytes, and resident immune cells form a regulatory immune unit.

Chapter 3
Diagnosis of Skin Disease

Medical students often pay no attention to cutaneous disorders, they think that skin diseases are the simplest to diagnose. Once these young doctors enter clinical practice, they find skin diseases like a maze and difficult to get out!

The examination of skin diseases requires a lot of patience, listening to what the patient has to say, being sympathetic, and trying to gain the patient's confidence so that they tell you their problems openly and without any hesitation. This is especially important in an Eastern culture where the patients do not want to reveal any problem relating to genital disorders.

3.1 Approach to a Skin Patient

This incorporates a history taking, examination of the lesion, investigations where necessary, and then giving the appropriate treatment.

3.1.1 History Taking

History taking is similar to the history taking in other branches of medicine, e.g., history of the present complaints, past illness, family history, systemic illness, etc. Particular emphasis is laid on the drug history. In the first place, we do not want to give the same medicine that the patient has already been receiving; for example, in acne we would not

Z. Zaidi, S. W. Lanigan, *Dermatology in Clinical Practice*,
DOI: 10.1007/978-1-84882-862-9_3,
© Springer-Verlag London Limited 2010

like to repeat tetracycline if it has shown no response so far. Medicines applied on the skin can change the morphology of the lesion, e.g., the use of steroids leads to tinea incognito, which should be kept in mind while dealing with asymmetric rashes. In many cases, drugs are the cause of lesions, e.g., psoriasis may be due to the use of β-blockers for hypertension.

3.1.2 Examination

To examine the skin *adequate light* is required; daylight is the best, otherwise examine the patient with bright overhead fluorescent light. This can be supplemented by a movable incandescent lamp. A *magnifying glass* helps in enlarging subtle skin changes, which can be missed by the naked eye.

In the first visit, it is advisable to examine the whole body, even if the patient insists that the lesion is only on one part of the body. The patients may be unwilling to show lesions on the genitals, or the lesions on the back can be missed if not examined. Many melanomas, of the back have been diagnosed this way. Always *palpate* and examine the lesions; this not only reassures the patient but also helps in the diagnosis. For example, induration is characteristic of squamous cell carcinoma; some dermal nodules if they are deep down can only be felt (primary and secondary lesions are described at the end of chapter).

Examine the *oral mucosa, scalp, and nails*. The examination gives important clues for diagnosis of diseases such as lichen planus, collagen disorders, syphilis, etc.

A Wood's lamp, diascopy, and a dermatoscope when required can assist in diagnosis of skin disease. *Wood's lamp* emits long-wave ultraviolet radiation; it helps in the examination of some fungal infections, tinea versicolor, erythrasma, and vitiligo. In patients with porphyria, the urine shows coral pink fluorescence due to porphyrins when examined with a Wood's lamp. The subtle pigmentations of the epidermis become prominent with Wood's lamp; the dermal pigmentations show no prominence. *Diascopy* helps to differentiate erythema from purpura. Erythemas blanch and purpuras do not. *Dermatoscope* – this is an illuminated handheld magnifying device; it helps in the diagnosis of pigmented lesions especially for the diagnosis of malignant melanoma. The lesion is covered with oil or water, and the site examined with a dermatoscope. The fluid eliminates the surface reflection and makes the horny layer translucent, so that the pigmented structures in the epidermis, superficial dermis, and superficial vascular plexus can be assessed.

Common skin lesions are rashes or growths. Other conditions such as ulcers, disorders of the hair, nail, and mucous membrane may be grouped as the miscellaneous lesions.

The important points to be noted in a *rash* are: whether the rash is acute or chronic, localized or generalized, dermatomal or nondermatomal, symmetrical or asymmetrical, eczematous or noneczematous, permanent or evanescent, scaly or nonscaly. Color of the rash should also be noted, whether it is erythematous, skin-colored, pigmented, purplish, yellowish, or white. The morphology of the rash also provides a clue to diagnosis; note whether the rash is nummular (round), discoid (disc-like), annular (ring-like), oval, irregular, gyrate (wave-like), reticulate (net-like), and arcuate (curved). The type of rash helps in categorizing the skin disease; see whether the rash is composed of macules, papules, vesicles, bullae, and pustules. Note the symptoms; is the rash pruritic or nonpruritic, painful or nonpainful? Lichenification and scratch marks are indicative of pruritic disorders. Finally, look for scarring in a lesion; it is specific of some disorders such as discoid lupus eythematosus. Scarring should be especially noted in hairy areas, as the scar indicates that hair growth will not occur at these sites.

The important points to be noted for a skin *growth* are: the onset, whether slow or rapid; site of growth, whether head and neck, sun-exposed areas, trunk or extremities. Is the lesion single or multiple, if multiple is it localized or generalized? Size and morphology of the growth should be noted, is it papular, plaque-like, or nodular? Is the size <6 mm or >6 mm? Is the growth umbilicated or nonumbilicated? Does it have a punctum or not? Is the surface of the growth smooth, verrucous, scaly, or nonscaly? Color of growth helps in diagnosis; pigmented growths should be examined carefully to exclude melanoma. See whether the pigmentation is uniform, or are there color variations. Large pigmented growths with irregular color variations should be considered suspicious of malignancy. Is the color of the growth pearly, yellowish, erythematous or skin-colored? (Color variations can occur due to different skin photo types; this should be kept in mind.) Is the growth painful or nonpainful? Finally, the consistency of the growth is felt, is the growth soft, firm, indurated, rubbery, malleable, or hard?

For all erythematous rashes, check whether they are due to dilatation of blood vessels or is it due to purpura, by diascopy. Lesions due to dilation of blood vessels blanch; purpuric lesions do not blanch.

Examine for any specific lesions present such as target lesions in erythema multiforme, café au lait spots in neurofibromatosis, burrows in scabies, ash leaf macules in adenoma sebaceum, and comedones in acne.

Palpation is important while examining a patient with acne. A nodule will be missed on visual examination alone and could result in not treating acne according to its appropriate staging.

Note presence or absence of cutaneous sensation. This is important in tropical countries, where leprosy is endemic and in neurological disorders.

A proper history and examination should lead the clinician to come to a provisional diagnosis. A few questions asked after the examination will help the clinician to come to a final diagnosis, e.g., psoriasis may be due to drug intake. In only a few cases will further investigations be required.

3.1.3 Investigations

3.1.3.1 Potassium Hydroxide Mounts for Dermatophytes

The most common investigation is scraping of the skin for examination of scales. For undiagnosed scaly lesions, a fungal infection should be excluded. Scraping is done with a number 15-scalpel blade. Scrape the scales from the edge of a lesion onto a glass slide. Put one to two drops of 10% potassium hydroxide on the scales; cover it with a cover slip. Gently heat the slide to break down the keratin; this makes the examination of the fungal hyphae clearer. Examine the slide under a microscope. First scan under low power; once the hyphae are found then confirm under high power.

For candidiasis the pustule is examined for hyphae and pseudohyphae; pustules are the initial lesions of candida infection. Microscopy is more confirmatory for candidiasis, as the spore can grow on culture, which is not indicative of infection. The spores when converted to hyphae are pathogenic to man.

3.1.3.2 Tzanck Test

This test is useful for viral infections and acantholytic disorders such as pemphigus. The specimen is collected from the base of the blister. The material is placed on a glass slide, dried, and then fixed with methanol. The specimen is then stained with Giemsa or Wright's stain. Multinucleated giant cells are seen in herpes simplex and varicella zoster infections. In pemphigus, acantholytic cells are found. These are rounded cells with large basophilic nucleus and a rim of mildly eosinophilic cytoplasm.

3.1.3.3 Scraping of a Burrow for Scabies

The finding of a scabies mite under a microscope confirms the diagnosis of scabies. Scraping of a burrow will show the mite, its faeces or eggs. The burrows can be made more visible by outlining them with black ink. The scraping is done with a number 15 scalpel blade moistened with oil, so that the contents of the burrow adhere to the blade. The contents are transferred to a glass slide; a drop of oil is added on it and examined under a microscope. The key to a positive result is vigorous scraping.

Scabies mites can also be examined on the skin with a dermatoscope.

3.1.3.4 Skin Biopsy

Skin is the most accessible organ of the body for histological examination. A biopsy can be excisional, incisional, punch, or shave. For most lesions a punch or shave biopsy is taken. Punch biopsies vary in size from 2 to 8 mm; a 4 mm punch is commonly used. The skin is infiltrated with local anesthesia, the punch drilled through the skin with a gentle rotating action. The specimen is then gently lifted and snipped off. The defect can be closed with sutures, or bleeding controlled with pressure packing.

Very superficial lesions can be removed by a shave biopsy such as seborrhoeic keratosis, warts, etc.

For most skin lesions the specimen is taken from a fresh lesion through the center; the exception is bullous disorders, where the specimen is taken from the edge of a fresh lesion. This is needed to identify the exact site of the split in the skin.

The biopsy specimen is placed in formalin for most examinations. For examination under electron microscopic, the specimen is placed in gluteraldehyde. For immunofluorescence, the specimen should be frozen immediately or placed in a special buffered transport medium.

3.1.3.5 Immunofluoresence Tests

This test is used for the diagnosis of bullous disorders such as pemphigus, pemphigoid, dermatitis herpetiformis, and for other autoimmune disorders such as lupus erythematosus. The test can be direct (on skin) or indirect (on the patients serum). The direct test detects the site of antibody antigen reaction in the skin, e.g., in pemphigus this reaction occurs in the epidermis at the intercellular cement of the keratinizing cells, and immunofluorescence will be seen at this site. The indirect test detects the level of antibodies in the sera; this test is of help in the prognosis of pemphigus.

3.1.3.6 Patch Testing

This test is valuable in detecting the allergens in allergic contact dermatitis. Batteries of suspected allergens in diluted standardized forms are placed on the back of the patient, under occlusive dressing for 48 h. The patches are then removed and inspected for any reaction; a final reading can be taken after 96 h if no reaction occurs in 48 h. If the test is positive steps are taken to determine the clinical relevance. The offending substance is then removed from the patient's environment. Unknown chemicals should not be patch-tested.

3.2 Primary and Secondary Lesions of the Skin

While examining the skin one should have a clear picture of the different kinds of skin lesions. These give a clue to the diagnosis and prevent unnecessary investigations. The skin lesions can be primary or secondary.

3.2.1 Primary Lesions

The primary lesions are those, which are not affected by trauma, manipulations such as scratching, scrubbing, etc., or regression over time. They arise on normal skin. The common primary lesions are:

Macule. It is a flat circumscribed discoloration of the skin; it lacks elevation or depression. These may be round, oval, angular, or irregular in shape. These may be due to transient dilatation of the blood vessels (erythema), permanent dilatation of the blood vessels (capillary naevi), escape of blood in the skin (purpura), they may be due to deposition of melanin as in freckles, lentigenes; macules may be hypochromic as in leprosy or achromic as in vitiligo.

Papule. This is an elevated solid lesion less than 5 mm in diameter. The lesions may be round, oval, polygonal, flat, or angular in shape. The color may be red, pink, purple or pigmented. The surface may be smooth, scaly or verrucous, e.g., pruritic purple papules of lichen planus.

Plaque. This is an elevated lesion more than 5 mm in diameter often formed by confluence of papules. It lacks a deep component, e.g., psoriasis, tinea corporis.

Nodule. Nodules are circumscribed solid, palpable, deep, and indurated lesions. They are larger than 1 cm in diameter. When above the skin they are round or dome-shaped, e.g., erythema nodosum. Nodules below the skin should be palpated, e.g., some nodules of acne.

Cyst. This is a cavity containing fluid, which is more than 5 mm in diameter; it may contain pus, blood, sebaceous secretion, mucous, etc.

Vesicle. This is a circumscribed accumulation of fluid that it is less than 5 mm in diameter. The content is usually serous, seropurulent, or hemorrhagic. It often develops on inflamed skin. Vesicles arise in the epidermis and heal without scarring.

Bullae. This is a vesicle larger than 5 mm in diameter; it may be tense or flaccid. Bullae located in the epidermis are flaccid and rupture easily, e.g., pemphigus, those situated in the dermis are tense and remain intact for a longer time, e.g., pemphigoid.

Pustule. This is a localized collection of pus. It may appear as such or develop from a vesicle. They may be isolated or grouped. Large groups form a lake of pus. Pustules may be caused by infection or may be sterile as in pustular psoriasis.

Wheal. This is a firm transient edematous elevation of the skin varying in shape and size, pale pink in color. It is caused by edema of the dermis and capillary dilatation. By coalescence large plateau-like elevations are formed. Wheals are characteristic of urticaria and urticarial reactions.

Tumor. This is a circumscribed swelling larger than 2.5 cm in diameter. Tumors are located within or beneath the dermis or are attached to it by a pedicle, e.g., neuroma, fibroma, lipoma, etc.

3.2.2 Secondary Lesions

Secondary lesions are those that are superimposed on an existing skin lesion. These are:

Scales. These are desquamated horny flakes produced as a result of abnormal keratinization. Under normal condition, the stratum corneum is desquamated but this is scarcely perceptible. Scales are produced due to increased proliferation or increased cohesion of keratinocytes. Scales may be dry and silvery (psoriasis), greasy (seborrheic dermatitis), small (dandruff), scales of discoid lupus erythematosus are studded with a keratinous plug at their bottom; in pityriasis rosea, they form a centripetal collarette. Furfuraceous scales are fine and loose as in pitryriasis versicolor, ichthyotic scales are large and polygonal. Large sheets of desquamated epidermis are seen in toxic epidermal necrosis and staphylococcus scalded skin syndrome.

Crust. This is a dry accumulation of exudate or secretion upon the skin. Crusts may be serous (yellow or honey coloured), purulent (yellowish green), bloody (reddish black) or a mixture of these.

Fissure. This is a small vertical crack of the epidermis, which is usually painful. Fissures are normally found in inflamed, inelastic, thickened skin, such as the palms and soles, over the joints, mucocutaneous junctions, rhagades at the angle of the mouth, and anal fissures.

Excoriation. These linear erosions result from scratching and are often covered with bloody crusts. Erosions are usually found in linear, parallel or punctate patterns.

Erosions. This is a partial loss of the epidermis. It may result from breaking down of a vesicle, bulla, or a pustule. It could be due to trauma or chemicals. Erosions heal without scarring.

Ulcer. This is a full-thickness focal loss of the epidermis and dermis; it heals with scarring. Its location, size, configuration (round, oval, angular, annular, or circinate), borders (flat, undermined, punched out, rolled), base (soft, infiltrated, membranous, washed leather), discharge (serous, seropurulent, bloody), color (bright red, livid), surrounding (edema, erythema, fibrosis, pigmentation), symptoms (burning, painful, painless), and regional lymph node involvement should be noted.

Scar. This is the formation of new connective tissue. Scars may be hypertrophic or atrophic. Scars of certain diseases have a diagnostic value, e.g., scars of lupus erythematosus are shiny thin, telangiectatic, and minutely pitted. Some scars become thick and tough, such as hypertrophic scars and keloids. These hypertrophic scars are thick and elevated with increased growth of fibrous tissue. Atrophic scars are thin and wrinkled, such as syphilitic scars. In some individuals, certain areas of the body are especially prone to scarring such as the anterior chest region and over the deltoids.

Atrophy. This is thinning of the skin, atrophy may be epidermal, dermal, or of the subcutaneous tissue or a combination. Atrophy may occur in the normal process of ageing, healing of disease, or as a side effect of drugs such as steroid therapy.

Sclerosis. This localized or diffuse induration of the dermis and subcutaneous tissue gives the skin a hard rigid feel when palpated. The overlying skin is pale, smooth, and shiny as in scleroderma, but it may be rough and show keratotic plugs as in lichen sclerosis et atrophicus.

3.2.3 Special Lesions

Burrow. These are short, linear dark elevations of the horny layer characteristic of scabies, due to the presence of the mite in the stratum corneum. Long pink burrows forming bizarre patterns are diagnostic of larva migrans.

Comedone. This is a horny plug filling the orifice of the pilosebaceous duct. It may be closed (white head), or open (black head). Comedones are characteristic of acne vulgaris and acneform eruptions.

Telangiectasia. This is a thin red linear lesion caused by the dilatation of the blood vessels. It may be idiopathic or caused by diseases such as collagen disorders (scleroderma), vasculitis, etc.

Target lesion. The target lesion consists of typically three zones. The innermost zone is dark or contains a blister that is surrounded by a second pale zone. The third zone consists of a ring of erythema. These are characteristic of erythema multiforme.

The language of dermatology is unique; it encompasses terms that are rarely used in other specialities. The use of correct dermatological terms is important; we can accurately describe a disease by looking at its morphological characteristics. Papules of lichen planus, for example, are violaceous, polygonal, flat, pruritic with Wickham's striae; these are located on the flexural surface of the wrist and ankles. It is therefore important to know the lesions, their distribution, the symptoms they produce to come to a diagnosis by simple examination of the skin; investigations should be done when necessary.

> *The diagnosis of skin disorders depends upon the skill of the examiner's inspection of the skin – "see and then reason."*
> *A correct diagnosis is the key to correct treatment.*
> *The general questions asked for every rash are: duration of the lesion, any medications used and does it have symptoms.*
> *Rapidly growing growths are often indicative of malignancy.*
> *Drug history is an important aspect of every dermatological examination.*
> *The whole body should be examined on the first appointment.*
> *Good light is essential for examining skin lesions; side lighting helps to detect subtle lesions.*
> *The scalp, oral cavity, and the nails should be examined, especially on the first appointment.*
> *Palpation not only helps in diagnosis, but also reassures the patient that they are not infectious.*
> *Chronic ulcers should be examined histologically to exclude malignancy.*
> *Determine which component of the skin is involved in the skin disease.*

Chapter 4
Bacterial Infections

The skin surface harbors a number of saprophytic flora, which are most numerous in the hairy areas that are rich in sebaceous glands. The resident flora are Staphylococcus epidermidis, Micrococci, diphtheroids, and yeasts. Aerobic diphtheroids are present on the surface and anerobic diphtheroids deep in the follicles. The skin's own defenses (unsaturated fatty acids and sebum) keep the flora in check. These flora help to defend the skin against other outside pathogens by bacterial interference or by the production of antibiotics. Overgrowth of diphtheroids can lead to clinical problems such as acne, pitted keratolysis, and trichomycosis axillaris.

4.1 Impetigo

This is a common infectious superficial pyogenic infection of the skin. The causative organisms are Staphylococci, Streptococci, or a combination of both. Impetigo is common in children; the face is the most common site affected. It can be bullous or nonbullous. The initial lesion in nonbullous impetigo is a vesicle, which rapidly ruptures to form yellowish-brown crusts (Fig. 4.1). In bullous impetigo the bullae rupture less rapidly and they last for 2–3 days. The disease is asymptomatic and heals without scarring (Fig. 4.2). Regional lymphadenopathy is common. Glomerulonephritis, scarlet fever, and erythema multiforme complicate streptococcal impetigo.

Z. Zaidi, S. W. Lanigan, *Dermatology in Clinical Practice*,
DOI: 10.1007/978-1-84882-862-9_4,
© Springer-Verlag London Limited 2010

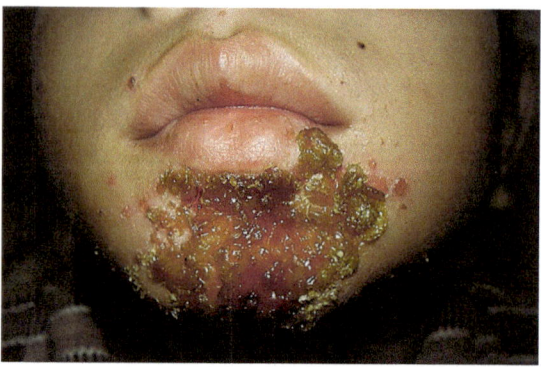

FIGURE 4.1. Impetigo-nonbullous.

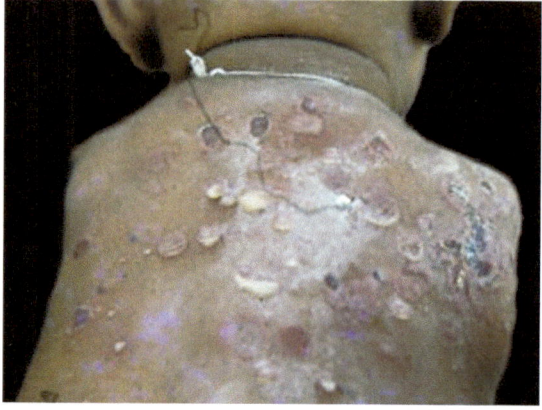

FIGURE 4.2. Impetigo-bullous.

4.1.1 Treatment

Good general hygiene should be maintained, use antibacterial soap, daily change of towels, etc.

Mild and superficial infections are treated with topical antibiotics such as fusidic acid applied three times daily, with an antiseptic such as povodine iodine or potassium permanganate for cleaning the lesions.

If the infection is widespread and severe, then oral antibiotics are required. Most Staphylococci produce pencillinase, so penicillin is not an appropriate antibiotic. The preferred treatment is with oral cephalosporin (cephalexin 250 mg q.i.d. or penicillinase-resistant penicillin such as dicloxacillin 250 mg q.i.d.).

As impetigo is infectious, children should avoid attending school until disease resolution.

If impetigo appears resistant to treatment or is recurrent, then nasal swabs are taken for culture. Nasal mupirocin is useful to eradicate staphylococcal nasal carriage.

Practical points

Staphylococcus aureus can colonize the skin without producing skin infection; this is particularly true in cases of atopic dermatitis. Impetiginization of the skin readily occurs, even if the trauma to the skin is subclinical.

Streptococci do not colonize normal skin. They enter the skin, when it is damaged by trauma, insect bites, scratching, etc.

In developing countries resistance to antibiotics should be considered, especially to erythromycin, penicillin, and tetracycline.

Tilbury Fox (1836–1879)

Tilbury Fox was an able and eminent English dermatologist. He was the first to describe dyshidrosis and impetigo. He also described urticaria pigmentosum, lymphangioma circumscriptum, and epidermolysis bullosa but did not name these conditions.

4.2 Folliculitis/Furunculosis/Carbuncle

Folliculitis is a superficial infection of the orifice of the hair follicle, represented by a pustule (Fig. 4.3). Furuncle or boil is an abscess of the hair follicle infecting the entire length of the follicle, represented as a small inflammatory nodule, soon becoming pustular and necrotic (Fig. 4.4). Carbuncle is a group of continuously infected follicles, these present as a hard red nodule, suppuration develops after sometime; pus is discharged through multiple follicular openings (Fig. 4.5).

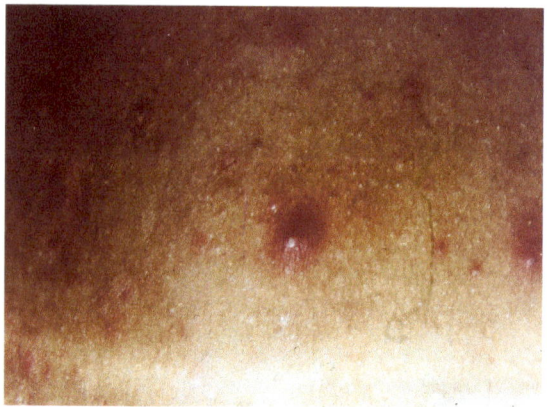

FIGURE 4.3. Folliculitis.

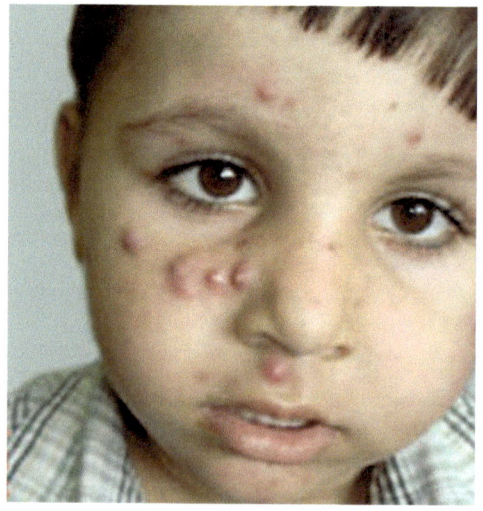

FIGURE 4.4. Furuncles.

Folliculitis is often caused by Staphylococcus aureus, or physical and chemical irritation. The lesions do not coalesce. They are common in the buttocks, thigh, beard area, and the scalp. Clinically the lesion is a pustule with a central hair. It is usually asymptomatic.

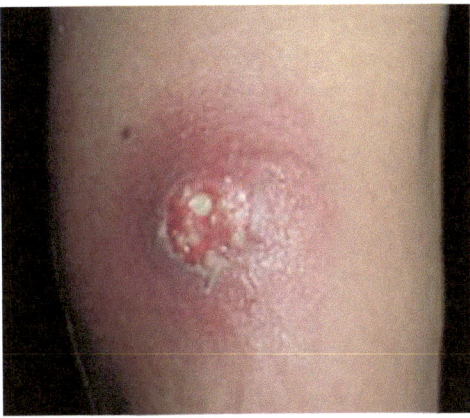

FIGURE 4.5. Carbuncle.

Furuncles are uncommon in children but increase in frequency after puberty. Staphylococcus aureus is the most common organism involved. The organism can be found in the
nares and perineum during quiescent periods. They are often
found in the flexures such as the groin and axillae, due to
maceration by heat and moisture in these areas. Pain is
intense, especially in areas where expansion is limited such as
the external ear. There is no fever and there are no associated
systemic symptoms.

Carbuncles are aggregates of furuncles. The condition is
associated with fever, malaise, and chills. Carbuncles are most
commonly found in the neck, back of the trunk, and thigh.

4.2.1 Treatment

Folliculitis is often self-limiting or responds to topical
antiseptics.

Furunculosis and carbuncles need warm compresses and
oral antibiotics. A furuncle, which does not resolve with antibiotics, needs excision and drainage.

A carbuncle will generally have to be incised and drained.
The abscess is ready for drainage when the skin has thinned
and the underlying mass becomes soft and fluctuant.

4.3 Recurrent Furunculosis

It is best to exclude diabetes, malnutrition, severe anemia, debilitation due to any cause, and immunodeficiency. Often the nose or the perineum may be a source of foci of infection.

4.3.1 Treatment

Treat the predisposing causes when found.

For nasal carriers, application of mupirocin ointment on the anterior nares twice a day for 5 days. Other members of the family who are carriers also need to be treated. Culture secretions from the anterior nares every 3 months, to check for effectiveness of the above treatment.

A combination of 500 mg of cloxacillin every 6 hours and 600 mg rifampicin once a day for 7–10 days may be more effective in eradicating coagulase positive staphylococci from the anterior nares.

A 3-month course of oral clindamycin 150 mg daily is also effective.

4.4 Erysipelas/Cellulitis

Erysipelas is an inflammation of lower dermis and superficial subcutaneous tissue. It is characterized by erythema with a well-defined raised edge, representing the more superficial dermal involvement (Fig. 4.6). Cellulitis is infection of the subcutaneous tissue, it presents as confluent erythema without any raised border (Fig. 4.7). The two conditions often coexist.

The most common pathogens are Streptococci (Streptococcus pyogenes) and Staphylococcus aureus. In young children, Hemophillus influenzae can cause facial cellulitis, this is usually unilateral. In immunosuppressed patients Cryptococcus neoformis is often the cause of infection. Saphenous venectomy in coronary bypass surgery can be a site of cellulitis. In adults the lower legs are often affected, an injury or fungal infection between the toe webs, may serve as a portal of entry for the pathogen. Cellulitis may also be due to a middle ear infection.

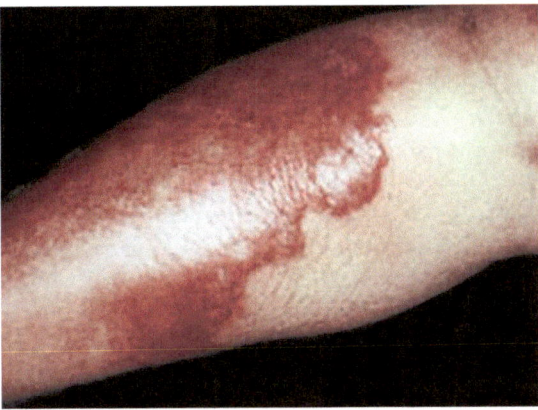

FIGURE 4.6. Erysipelas.

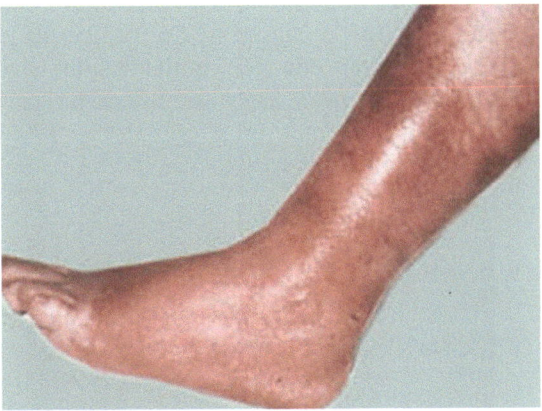

FIGURE 4.7. Cellulitis.

Bacteria may enter the skin from a break in its continuity, or it may be by hematogenous spread. In immunocompetent patients the source is usually external. Proteolytic enzymes produced by the bacteria such as group A streptococci, contribute to the spread of infection. Damage to the local lymphatics during an acute episode can result in residual lymphoedema; this predisposes to recurrent episodes of cellulitis.

4.4.1 Treatment

Oral antibiotics (cephalexin 500 mg, dicloxacillin 500 mg every 6 hours) are required for mild infection; in more severe cases an appropriate antibiotic should be given by the I/M or I/V route.

In recurrent cases long-term penicillin or erythromycin is given. Some patients may require lifelong prophylaxis. Treat any local skin damage including tinea to prevent recurrent episodes.

4.5   Ecthyma

This is a pyogenic infection of the skin, characterized by the formation of crusts, beneath which ulceration occurs. Like impetigo, the infection is caused by Streptococcus pyogenes and Staphylococcus aureus. The initial lesion is a vesicle, which ruptures to form an ulcer; the infection spreads into the dermis, with the formation of crusts (Fig. 4.8). Healing occurs in 2–3 weeks with scarring.

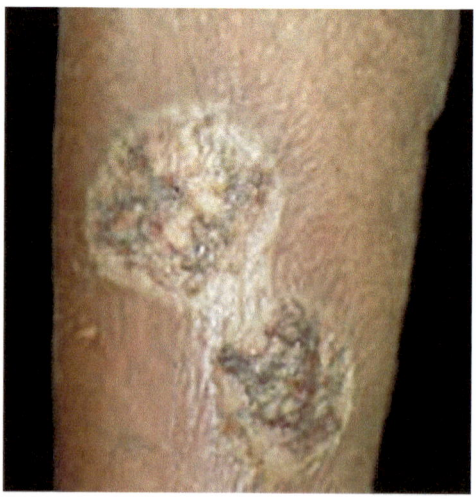

FIGURE 4.8. Ecthyma.

The infection is common in tropical climate; children from disadvantaged backgrounds where hygiene may be poor are usually affected. The lesions are common on the limbs.

4.5.1 Treatment

- The adherent crusts should be removed with a starch poultice.
- Application of topical antiseptic.
- Systemic antibiotic.

4.6 Necrotizing Fasciitis

This is a dangerous, rapidly progressive, and destructive inflammation of the dermis and underlying tissues including the deep fascia. It can be a polymicrobial infection following surgery, especially in a diabetic or imunocompromised patient; or it may be caused by Streptococcal pyogenes leading to Streptococcal gangrene. Necrotizing fasciitis is associated with profound toxemia and multisystem failure.

The condition often arises suddenly after a minor skin trauma. The clue to the presence of this infection is a rapidly spreading cellulitis in a very toxic patient, despite antibiotic therapy. Necrotizing fasciitis is initially manifested as erythema and edema, the lesion progresses to brawny induration and cyanosis. Blister formation and gangrene rapidly follow. The central area of the lesion is anesthetic due to cutaneous nerve damage; the surrounding area is extremely tender and erythematous. The legs are the most common site of infection.

4.6.1 Investigations

Aspiration or incision for culture and sensitivity, exclude clostridial infection with wound smear. Baseline laboratory tests should be performed, and then monitored for leukopenia, hypocalcemia (fat necrosis), and elevated creatinine (muscle necrosis).

4.6.2 Treatment

Necrotizing fasciitis requires immediate treatment with generous surgical debridement. An appropriate antibiotic cover should be started immediately, without waiting for culture and sensitivity results; as the mortality rate is very high. Usually intravenous benzyl penicillin, a quinolone, and clindamycin or metronidazole for gram-negative organisms is started immediately. Even with prompt treatment, mortality rate is high; in some cases amputation of the limb may be required.

4.7 Erythrasma

Erythrasma is a bacterial infection caused by Corynebacterium (C) minutissimum. The most common sites of infection are: in the fourth interdigital toe space, axillae, groins, and submammary folds. The lesions appear as velvety brown scaly plaques (Fig. 4.9). C minutissimum produces porphyrin which fluorescences coral red with a Woods lamp. This helps to differentiate it from fungal infections.

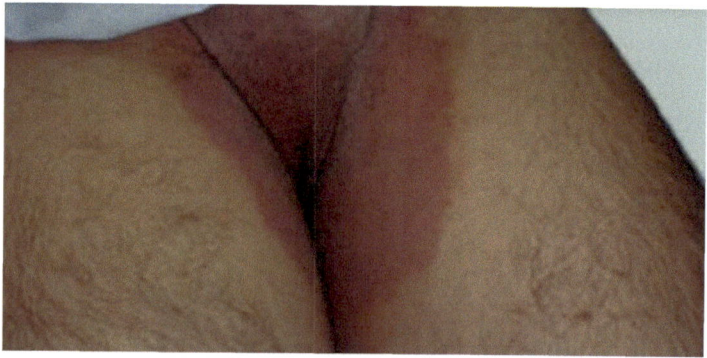

FIGURE 4.9. Erythrasma.

4.7.1 Treatment

Erythrasma often responds to topical imidazole antifungal agents. For more extensive or chronic lesions oral erythromycin 500 mg four times a day for 10 days is required.

4.8 Pitted Keratolysis

This is an eruption on the weight-bearing areas of the sole: the toes, balls of the feet, and the heel. Several bacteria have been implicated to cause pitted keratolysis. The commonest are the aerobic diphtheroids. These bacteria produce an enzyme keratinase, which degrades the keratin and produces pits in the stratum corneum, when the skin is hydrated and the pH rises above neutrality. The condition is associated with hyperhidrosis of the feet.

The disease is characterized by circular or longitudinal punched out, malodorous depressions (Fig. 4.10). Most cases are asymptomatic, but some patients complain of pain if the lesions are large. The eruption is superficial and there is no inflammation of the skin

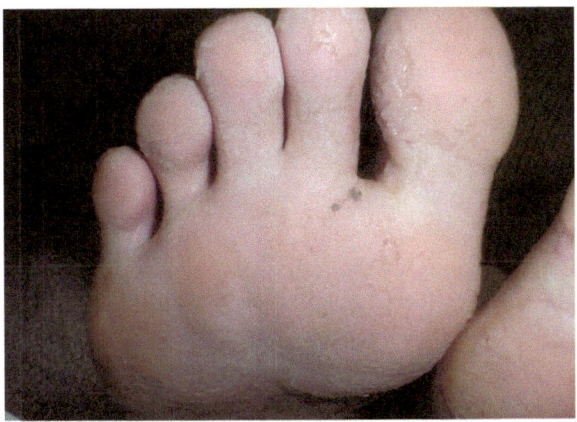

FIGURE 4.10. Pitted keratolysis.

4.8.1 Treatment

Treat the hyperhidrosis with 20% aluminum chloride twice a day, 10% formaldehyde is also a good antiperspirant.

Local therapy with acne medications such as clindamycin, erythrocin, and benzyl peroxide are helpful. Topical antibiotics such as fucidin ointment can also be used.

Oral erythromycin is also effective.

4.9 Trichomycosis Axillaris

This is a common condition and is seen in about one quarter of adult males. It is caused by the aerobic diphtheroids similar to those seen in pitted keratolysis, but the species is different. Yellow, black, or red concretions are present on the hair shaft. These concretions are tightly packed with bacteria. The underlying skin is normal. The axillary sweat may be yellow, red, or black depending upon the color of the concretions. Yellow is the most common and black the least. Clothing becomes stained in the armpit.

4.9.1 Treatment

Clipping the affected hair and application of topical antibiotic ointment is effective.

4.10 Tuberculosis

Tuberculosis is a chronic granulomatous disease that principally affects the lungs, but may affect any tissue or organ of the body. It is present worldwide, with an extremely high prevalence in Asia. Cutaneous tuberculosis can present in a number of ways, the common forms being lupus vulgaris, scrofuloderma, tuberculosis verrucosa cutis, or as tuberculids: in the form of erythema nodosum, erythema induratum.

All cases of cutaneous tuberculosis should have an X-ray of the chest to exclude tuberculosis of the lungs. The cutaneous lesion should be biopsied to confirm the diagnosis.

Lupus vulgaris – presents as a reddish brown plaque with nodules resembling apple jelly. The peripheral extensions are gyrate or discoid in shape; these edges may become scaly and psoriasiform. Irregular scarring is present in chronic lesions. The lesion may ulcerate, produce areas of necrosis, or become deeply infiltrating and present as soft smooth nodules (Fig. 4.11a, b).

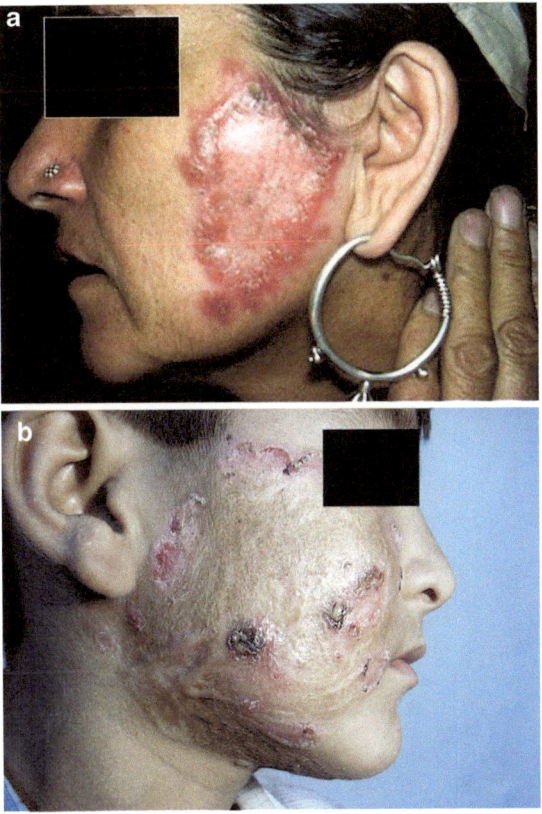

FIGURE 4.11. (**a**, **b**) Lupus vulgaris.

Lupus vulgaris should be differentiated from cutaneous leishmaniasis and discoid lupus erythematosus.

Scrofuloderma – this is an extension of tuberculosis to the skin from the underlying bones, lymph nodes, intestines, epididymis, etc. It commonly affects the sides of the neck, parotid, submandibular region and the axillae. The overlying skin presents as nodules and sinuses. The cervical lymph nodes are commonly affected with discharging sinuses (Fig. 4.12).

Scrofuloderma should be differentiated from hidradenitis suppurativa, actinimycosis, and deep fungal infections.

Tuberculosis verrucosa Cutis (Warty tuberculosis) lesions appear in areas exposed to trauma such as the hands, knees, ankles, soles, and buttocks. It appears as a verrucous plaque with irregular extensions, often with atrophic scars (Fig. 4.13). This should be differentiated from common warts.

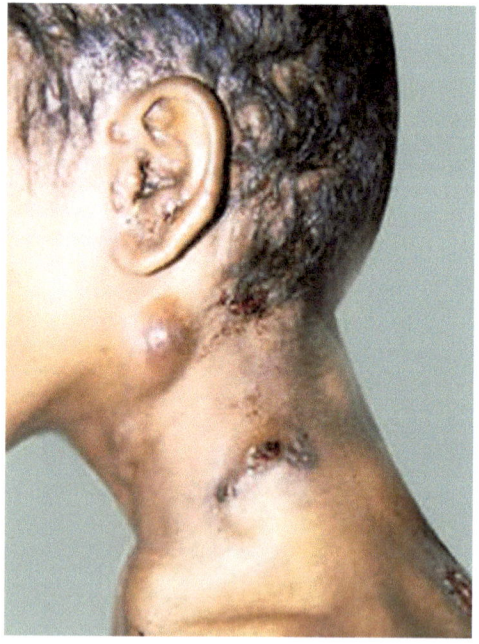

FIGURE 4.12. Scrofuloderma.

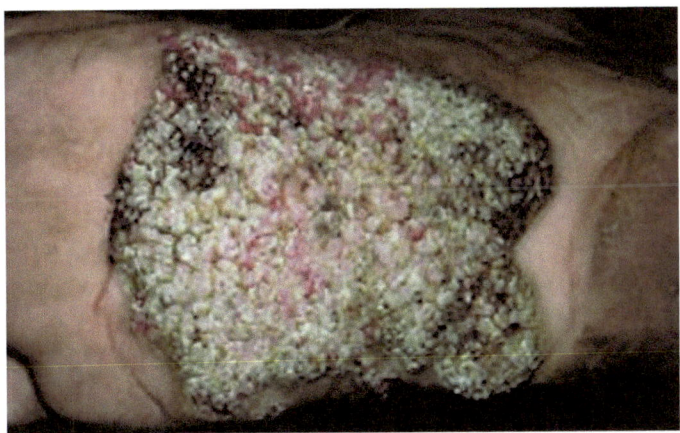

FIGURE 4.13. Tuberculosis verrucosa cutis (Warty tuberclosis).

4.10.1 Treatment

Standard drug regimen consists of two phases: Initial and the continued phase.

Initial phase – consists of three drugs given for 8–12 weeks

- Isoniazid (INH) – 300 mg daily
- Rifampicin – 450 mg < 50 kg, 600 mg > 50 kg
- Pyrazinamide – 1.5 g < 50 kg, 2.0 g > 50–74 kg, 2.5 g > 75 kg
- Or Ethambutol – 15 mg/kg of body weight

All the drugs should be taken on an empty stomach once daily, usually before breakfast; absorption of rifampicin is influenced by food.

Continuous phase – this is continued with INH and Rifampicin for 6 months.

Robert Koch (1834–1910)

Koch received the Nobel Prize for medicine in 1905. He qualified from Gottingen and worked with Virchow in Berlin. In his amateur laboratory, he proved that anthrax was due to a transmitted bacillus. Ten years later in 1882 he discovered the tubercle bacillus and in the next year the cholera vibrio. In 1885, he became the professor of Hygiene in Berlin. He also described the old and new tuberculin. He travelled widely and discovered a number of infectious diseases in India and Africa.

Rokitansky and Virchow described the histopathology of tuberculosis.

4.11 Leprosy (Hansens Disease)

The disease is common in tropical and warm temperate climates all over the world. About two-third cases of leprosy patients are found in Asia. The manifestations of leprosy depend upon the degree of delayed (type IV) hypersensitivity response in the individual to Mycobacterium leprae. Patients with strong cell-mediated immunity develop tuberculoid leprosy, and those with failure of cell-mediated reactivity develop lepromatous leprosy. Borderline status is seen when the immune status is between the two types. Indeterminate leprosy is the form that does not have the features of either polar group – tuberculoid or lepromatous. The disease primarily affects the peripheral nerves, and secondarily affects the skin and other organs. Leprosy still leads to social stigmatization, which is more troublesome than the disease itself.

Lepromatous leprosy – represents a failure of cell-mediated immunity; any organ of the body may be affected, except the central nervous system. The lesions teem with lepra bacilli and it is the most infectious form of leprosy. Infection occurs from the nasal discharge. The first symptoms are stuffiness of the nose, nasal discharge, and epistaxis. Skin lesions occur in the form of macules, papules, nodules, and plaques. The lesions are symmetrical and extensive (Fig. 4.14). Leprosy affects the cooler areas of the body; lesions are not present in the flexures and the scalp, except when the patient is bald. Infiltration is most noticeable in the earlobes. Thinning of the lateral margins of the eyebrow is characteristic. With progression of the disease, typical leonine facies becomes apparent. Nerve involvement occurs late. The involvement of the nerves is bilateral and symmetrical. The nerves commonly involved are the facial, greater auricular, median, radial, posterior tibal and common peroneal. The nerves are thickened and palpable. Glove and stocking anesthesia, gynecomastia, testicular atrophy, ichthyosis, and nerve palsies can develop. Neurotrophic atrophy affecting the phalanges leads to gradual disappearance of the fingers and toes. Involvement of the corneal nerves causes anesthesia, which may later lead to blindness. Involvement of the facial nerve leads to lagophthalmos.

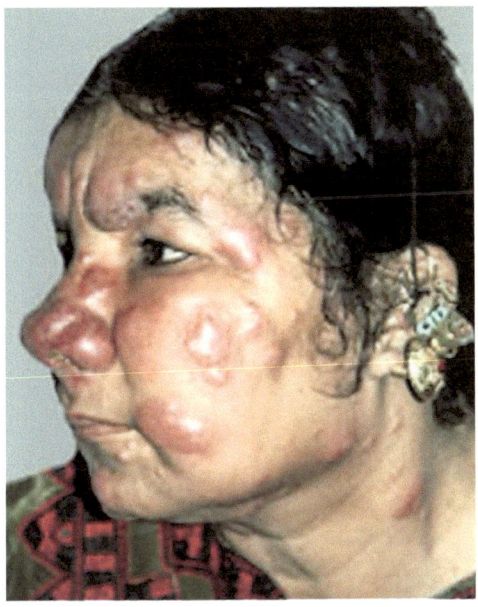

FIGURE 4.14. Lepromatous leprosy.

Tuberculoid leprosy – the cell-mediated immunity is strongly expressed and the infection is localized to one or few lesions, or the disease could be purely neural. The lesions have only a few lepra bacilli. The characteristic lesions are usually single or a few hypopigmented anesthetic, hairless plaques in which sweating is absent; the edge is thickened and clearly demarcated, often with central healing and atrophy (Fig. 4.15). Often an enlarged nerve can be felt at the periphery of the lesion. The lesions on the face are not anesthetic. Enlarged nerves are associated with sensory loss and weakness.

Borderline leprosy – represents the disease between the polar forms, it maybe borderline lepromatous (BL), borderline borderline (BB), or borderline tuberculoid (BT), depending upon the status of impaired cell-mediated immunity. Neurological signs are often present before the skin lesions appear. The nerve enlargement is bilateral and asymmetrical. The cutaneous lesions are multiple; they may be in the form

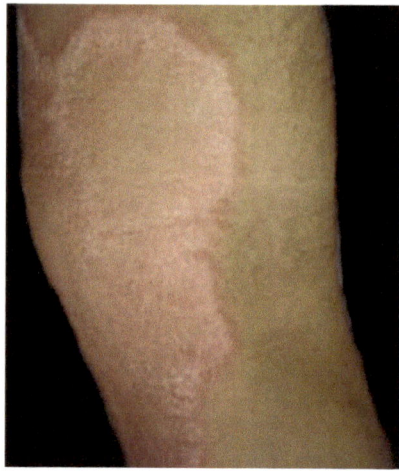

FIGURE 4.15. Tuberculoid leprosy.

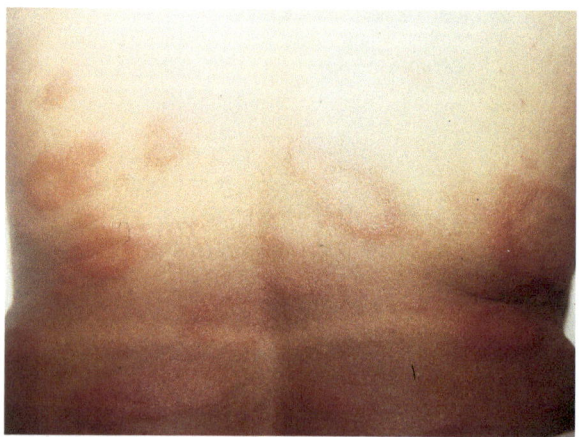

FIGURE 4.16. Boderline leprosy.

of macules, papules, nodules, and plaques. Plaques with a
punched out appearance is characteristic of BB leprosy;
annular and bizarre-shaped lesions are also present (Fig. 4.16).

The lesions are asymmetrical. In BT leprosy the lesions are few and these are drier.

Indeterminate leprosy – this is the early and transitional stage of leprosy; it occurs in those in whom the immunological status has not been determined. It usually presents as hypopigmented or erythematous patch, which is poorly defined. Hair growth and nerve functions are unimpaired.

A pure neural form of leprosy may also present, with asymmetrical enlargement of the peripheral nerves. The disease is diagnosed by a cutaneous nerve biopsy.

4.11.1 Diagnosis

All cases of leprosy should have a skin smear for lepra bacilli and skin biopsy. Scraping from the nasal mucosa and nerve biopsy should be performed when required.

4.11.2 Complications

Neuropathic ulcers, shortening of the fingers and toes from repeated trauma, saddle-shaped nose, and secondary ichthyosis. Testicular atrophy, liver and kidney failure complicate lepromatous leprosy.

4.11.3 Differential Diagnosis

Indeterminate leprosy with hypopigmented patches should be differentiated from pityriaisis alba, tinea versicolor, vitiligo, and postinflammatory hypopigmentation. Lepromatous and borderline leprosy from mycosis fungoides, psoriasis, neurofibromatosis, generalized leishmaniaisis, yaws. Tuberculoid leprosy from tinea corporis, granular annulare, annular erythemas.

The characteristic features of leprosy are:
Early signs of leprosy

- Bilateral edema of the legs and ankles
- Burns that form a blister but do not cause pain
- Development of ENL (erythema nodosum leprosum) in pregnancy
- Numbness and clumsiness of the fingers

  Cardinal signs of leprosy

- Anesthetic skin lesions
- Enlarged peripheral nerves
- Presence of acid fast bacilli in skin or nasal mucous membrane

  Diagnostic tests

- Skin smears for mycobacterium leprae
- Skin biopsy
- Nerve biopsy

4.11.4 Treatment

Leprosy should be treated at specialist centers, with adequate physiotherapy and occupational therapy support. Multidrug therapy is essential because of drug resistance.

4.11.4.1 Treatment of Multibacillary Leprosy (Polar Lepromatous and BL, BB)

The treatment is for 24 months, and a follow-up for 5 years. The drugs used are:

- Self-administered. Dapsone – 100 mg daily, clofazamine – 50 mg daily
- Monthly supervision – Rifampicin 600 mg, clofazamine – 300 mg

4.11.4.2 Treatment of Paucibacillary Leprosy (Polar Tuberculoid, BT)

The treatment is for 6 months, and a follow-up for 2 years.

- Self administered. Dapsone 100 mg
- Monthly supervision – Rifampicin 600 mg

Special care is needed when the two types of *lepra reactions* occur during treatment. The reactions occur due to the sudden change in clinical stability of the disease on treatment. During lepra reactions treatment of leprosy should be continued.

4.11.4.3 Type I (Reversal Reaction)

This is seen in all forms of borderline leprosy, the polar forms are exempt. Lesions become red and angry looking; pain and paralysis may follow neural inflammation. Constitutional symptoms are unusual. Treatment is with salicylates, chloroquine, nonsteroidal and steroidal antiinflammatory agents.

4.11.4.4 Type II (Erythema Nodosum Leprosum ENL)

These reactions are common in lepromatous leprosy; they are caused by an immune complex syndrome of humoral antibody response. Constitutional symptoms are present as fever and malaise. Clinically, new nodules develop, while the preexisting ones remain unchanged. The reactions also include nerve palsies, arthritis, iridocyclitis, proteinuria, and epididimoorchitis. The patients are treated as for type I reactions; thalidomide can also be used.

Newer drugs under evaluation for leprosy treatment are ofloxacillin, perfloxacin, minocycline, and clarithromycin.

Gerhard Armauer Hansen (1841–1912)

Hansen was a Norwegian bacteriologist and leprologist, he discovered the lepra bacillus, Mycobacterium leprae; 14 years before Koch's discovery of the closely related Tubercle bacillus. Fourteenth-century writings refer to chalmoongra oil obtained from the seeds of an Indian tree as a specific cure for leprosy. This oil remained the principle antileprous drug even in the West for decades.

4.12 Pseudomonas Infections

Pseudomonas (P) aeruginosa, a gram-negative rod, is a common human saprophyte; it rarely causes disease in healthy persons. Infection occurs when the body resistance is lowered as in immunosuppression, diabetes mellitus, and general debilitating diseases. P aeruginosa is responsible for a broad spectrum of disease. It causes a wide variety of cutaneous infections, ranging from harmless to life-threatening.

Pseudomonas paronychia is characterized by distal onycholysis and green discoloration of the affected nails. The nail folds are swollen and erythematous. Toe web infection is often superimposed on a fungal infection of the toes; the lesions are macerated, and foul smelling.

Otitis externa often develops secondary to swimming. Pain and swelling occur, erythema is pronounced, there is foul smelling discharge from the ear. In diabetics, the immuno-compromised, or in untreated cases infection can penetrate the floor of the ear canal at the bony cartilaginous junction and spread to the base of the skull and beyond (Malignant otitis externa).

Ecthyma gangrenosum is characterized by hemorrhagic vesicles and blisters, which may be isolated or in groups. The vesicles rupture to form ulcers with a black necrotic center. The most common sites of involvement are the gluteal or perineal regions.

Pseudomonas cellulitis may be localized and secondary to infection of the toe web, ulcers, or wound infection or it may occur during pseudomonas septicemia. The skin is painful and dusky, red in color. The lesion then becomes macerated, eroded, and foul smelling.

Pseudomonas folliculitis occurs after bathing in hot tubs or public baths; the affected users develop folliculitis, and the lesions may become pustular. There is little risk of severe disease; the condition resolves in 2 weeks without treatment.

4.12.1 Diagnosis

Bacterial and fungal cultures should be performed, as pseudomonas can be superimposed with other opportunistic organisms. Wood's light examination reveals a green fluorescence.

4.12.2 Treatment

Dry the area, as pseudomonas infection often follows excessive hydration of the skin. Address any predisposing factors such as diabetes, chronic diseases, and immunosuppression. The infection can often be associated with other pathogens such as Candida, which should be treated concomitantly. Broad spectrum antibiotics such as quinolones (ciprofloxacin) are effective for pseudomonas, but should be guided by the culture results. In ecthyma gangrenosum, two anti-pseudomonas drug therapies are usually recommended for initial treatment.

Antibiotics effective against pseudomonas – piperacillin, ticarcillin, ceftazidime, imipenem, meropenem, tobramycin, gentamycin, ciprofloxacin, and aztreonam.

4.13 Rocky Mountain Spotted Fever (RMSF)

The disease is caused by Rickettsia rickettsii; it is transmitted to humans by the bite of ticks. Children are more commonly affected; most of the cases occur between April and September. The disease is common in the United States and some parts of Europe.

Rickettsia affects the endothelium of blood vessels; as a result hemostasis is affected. The symptoms vary from minor reduction of platelets to severe coagulopathies such as deep venous thrombosis and disseminated intravascular coagulation.

A week after the bite, there is a sudden onset of fever, headache, malaise, myalgia, and vomiting. The rash appears on the fourth day, first on the wrists and ankles; it spreads to the palms and soles, and later becomes generalized. The rash is discrete and macular later becoming petechial. Small areas of gangrene may appear on the fingers, toes, and genitals Involvement of the genitals helps in the diagnosis.

Fever subsides in 2–3 weeks; and the rash fades with residual hyperpigmentation. In about 15% of cases there is no rash, these cases are called Rocky Mountain Spotless Fever.

In some cases dissemination of infection occurs, especially in patients who are not treated in the early stage of the disease. Dissemination of infection leads to increased vascular permeability, pulmonary edema, azotemia, shock, acute tubular necrosis, and meningoencephalitis. Many such patients have a fulminant course and die within a week.

Laboratory diagnosis is rarely helpful as the antibodies are only detected in convalescence. Treatment should be given for any case of suspected disease, in order to prevent the dissemination and complication of disease.

4.13.1 Treatment

Doxycycline is the treatment of choice except for pregnant women. Tetracycline, chloramphenicol, and fluoroquinolone are also effective. Most other antibiotics such as penicillin, cephalosporin, and sulphonamides drugs are ineffective.

> Patients who have received antirickettsial treatment within 5 days of the onset of symptoms are less likely to die than those who received the treatment after 5 days of illness.
>
> Thrombocytopenia and hyponatremia should arouse the possibility of RMSF.

4.14 Lymes Disease (Erythema Chronicum Migrans)

Lymes disease is caused by a spirochaete, Borrelia burgdorferi. It is transmitted to humans by the bite of a tick. It is said to be the most frequent arthropod infestation in the United States.

Like the other spirochetes, the disease manifests itself in stages.

Stage 1. A small papule is formed at the site of the bite; this rapidly expands to form an annular erythema. The size of the annular erythema should be more than 5 cm to qualify for erythema migrans, cases as large as 68 cm have been recorded. The borders of the erythema are macular, not elevated like tinea corporis. The skin lesion is asymptomatic. The sites favored by the mite are the extremities, waistband, and the intertriginous areas. Systemic symptoms such as fever, malaise, arthralgia, and headaches occur.

Less classic features may include alternating rings of erythema and clearing, and a centre which may be hemorrhagic, vesicular, necrotic or ulcerating. The margins may be raised and papular.

Stage 2 (Early disseminated infection). The spirochaete is spread hematogenously to distant sites. The skin is affected in 50% of cases, with annular lesions smaller than the primary infection. The patient is ill with fever, myalgia, arthralgia, and fatigue.

Infection to other organs results in arthritis, meningitis, cranial nerve palsies, carditis, and atrioventricular septal defects. The joints are affected in 60% of cases predominantly as intermittent, asymmetrical arthritis affecting the larger joints; the knee is commonly affected.

Stage 3. Without treatment, the disease enters the third stage. This may manifest as continued arthritis, lasting more than 1 year. Cutaneous lesions manifest as acrodermatitis chronica atrophicans, which manifests as dry atrophic skin (like cigarette paper), over the distal extremities. The lesions initially begin as erythematous plaques, after weeks or months, these become atrophic with loss of subcutaneous fat, and the underlying blood vessels can easily be visualized. Hypopigmentation or hyperpigmentation can be seen in the affected areas. Central nervous system involvement leads to ataxia and encephalomeningitis.

Laboratory investigations are not specific. Serological tests are positive after 2–4 weeks of infection; false negative or false positive results are not uncommon. Serology may remain positive for years after infection; it is then difficult to differentiate the active from the inactive disease.

4.14.1 Treatment

The preferred antibiotic is doxycycline; 100 mg b.i.d. for 10–21 days.

Others are:

- Amoxicillin 500 mg t.i.d. for 10–21 days.
- Cefuroxime 500 mg b.i.d. for 10–21 days.
- Involvement of the CVS or CNS requires parental therapy.
- Ceftrioxone 2 g daily for 10–21 days.

For Lymes arthritis:

- 100 mg doxycycline 100 mg b.i.d. for 30 days
- Amoxicillin 500 mg q.i.d. for 30 days

  Arthritis is the most common manifestation of systemic disease.

  Erythema migrans should be 5 cm in diameter to qualify for Lymes disease.

  Lymes disease is the most frequent arthropod-borne disease in the United States.

4.15 Sexually Transmitted Diseases (Bacterial)

Sexually transmitted diseases (STD) are a diverse group of infections caused by multiple microbial pathogens. There are three ways by which microorganisms can be transmitted during intimate sexual contact. Cutaneous inoculation is the most common route for the five classical STDs (syphilis, gonorrhea, chancroid, lymphogranuloma venereum, and granuloma inguinale), as well as for herpes simplex. Blood-borne infections transferred are HIV, hepatitis B, and cytomegalovirus. Enterically acquired infections are Shigella, Entamoeba, and hepatitis A. Scabies and molluscum contagiosum can be sexually transmitted.

4.15.1 Syphilis

Syphilis is a sexually transmitted disease caused by Trepanoma (T) pallidum. Unlike gonococcus, T pallidum is fragile and dies when removed from the body. It can infect any organ and can have many presentations. Thus the old adage "he who knows syphilis knows medicine." If untreated the disease passes through four stages: primary, secondary, latent and late.

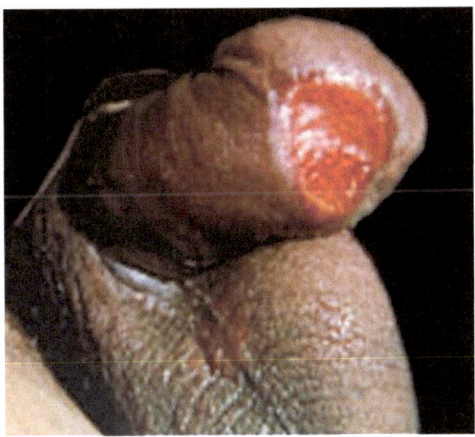

FIGURE 4.17. Syphilis – chancre.

4.15.1.1 Primary Stage

The lesions are usually present on the genitals, they begin as a papule, that undergoes ischemic necrosis and forms a painless indurated punched out ulcer (syphilitic chancre). The base is clean with a scanty yellowish serous discharge. A narrow red border surrounds the ulcer (Fig. 4.17). This is followed by enlargement of the inguinal lymph nodes, first on one side and then the other. The lymph nodes do not suppurate or coalesce, unless secondarily infected. Painless vaginal and anal lesions may go unnoticed unless looked for.

4.15.1.2 Secondary Stage

Begins 6–8 weeks after the appearance of the primary chancre. The manifestations are generalized rashes on the skin and mucous membranes. It is an inflammatory respond to the hematogenously disseminated Trepanoma pallidum. There can be many presentations but the most common is the development of symmetrical coppery red papules and plaques. Occasionally nodules may occur, but vesicles and bullae do not develop, except in newborn babies and those associated with HIV infection. The eruption is generalized, but the lesions on the palms and soles are particularly noteworthy (Figs. 4.18 and 4.19). Pruritus, once thought not to occur in syphilis, may be occasionally noted. Condylomata lata are flat-topped moist papules in the genital areas (Fig. 4.20). Generalized microlymphadenopathy is present; the occipital, preauricular, and trochlear glands are most prominent.

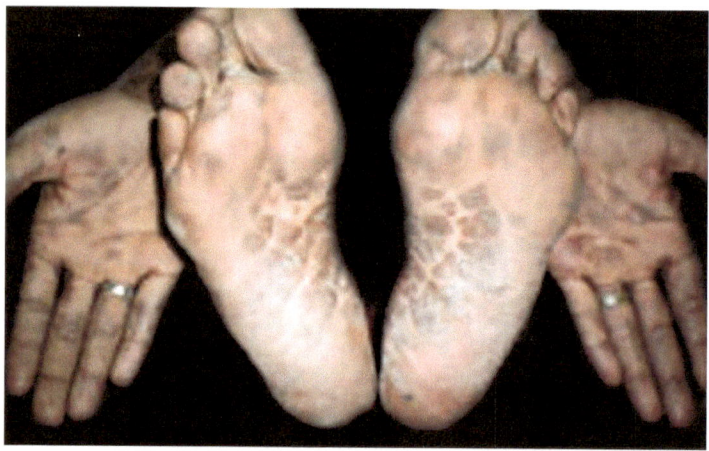

FIGURE 4.18. Syphilis – palmoplantar keratoderma.

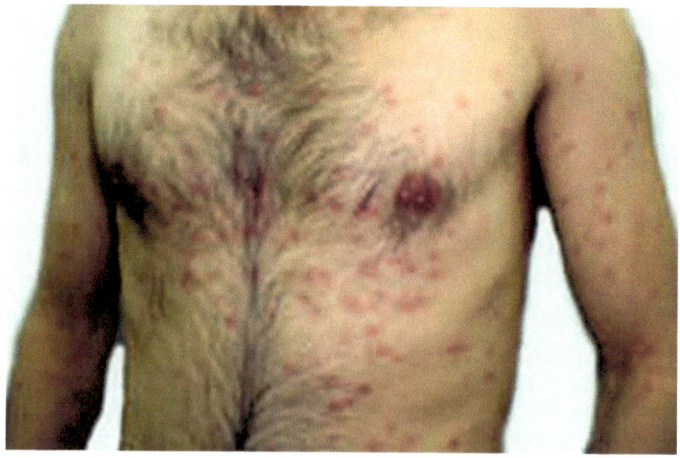

FIGURE 4.19. Syphilis – generalized papular eruption.

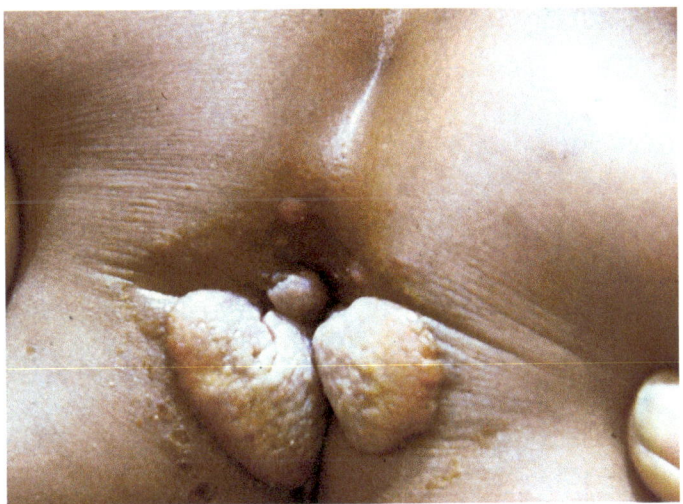

FIGURE 4.20. Condylomata lata.

Systemic symptoms such as fever, malaise, arthralgia, and sore throat are present. Lesions on the oral mucous membrane appear as white plaques known as mucous patches. Spotty alopecia of the scalp is commonly known as the moth eaten alopecia of syphilis.

4.15.1.3 Latent Syphilis

Clear-cut evidence of clinical syphilis is absent; the disease is diagnosed by serological tests.

4.15.1.4 Late or Tertiary Syphilis

This manifests as syphilitic gumma, or as papules and nodules. Cardiovascular, musculo-skeletal and neurological signs are also seen in this stage.

The risk of transmission of infection, are in the primary, secondary, and early latent stages of syphilis. Patients with secondary syphilis are most contagious because of the large number of lesions present.

4.15.1.5 Diagnosis

Primary syphilis. A dark field examination for trepanoma is helpful in differentiating syphilis from other genital ulcers. Alternative to the dark ground microscopy is the direct fluorescent antibody test (DFAT).

Secondary syphilis. A triad of oral ulcers, lymphadenopathy and nonitchy symmetrical skin lesions are almost diagnostic of secondary syphilis. VDRL is positive in all cases of secondary syphilis. RPR (rapid plasma reagin) test is a modified VDRL test. A test specific for syphilis is the fluorescent trepanoma antibody absorption test (FTA-ABS). Serological tests are positive in the latent phase.

Tertiary syphilis. A CSF examination should be done in all cases of tertiary syphilis; this shows an increase in the cell counts and an increase in total proteins. Serological tests are positive in tertiary syphilis.

4.15.1.6 Differential Diagnosis

Syphilitic chancre should be differentiated from the ulcers of herpes simplex, chancroid, anal fissure, and cervical erosion.

Secondary syphilis can mimic a number of diseases such as guttate psoriasis, generalized lichen planus, drug eruptions, pityriasis lichenoides chronica, pityriasis rosea, and urticaria pigmentosa. Always examine the oral cavity, lymph nodes, palms and soles and examine the pattern of hair loss as it aids in diagnosing syphilis. A VDRL test will confirm the diagnosis.

Tertiary syphilis should be differentiated from leishmaniasis, lupus vulgaris, and deep fungal infections; sometimes basal cell carcinoma and squamous cell carcinoma also have to be considered.

4.15.1.7 Treatment of Early Syphilis

This includes primary syphilis, secondary syphilis, and latent syphilis of not more than 2 years duration.

Benzathine penicillin G 2.4 million units in a single session by I/M route (1.2 million units in each buttock).

Alternative Treatment

Procaine penicillin G 600,000 units I/M for 10 days
Patients allergic to penicillin can be treated by erythromycin or tetracycline 500 mg q.i.d. for 15 days.

4.15.1.8 Treatment of Late Syphilis

This includes latent syphilis of more than 2 years duration and late syphilis (late latent, cardiovascular and gumma/nodular cystic skin lesions).
Benzathine penicillin G 2.4 units I/M each week for 3 weeks.

Alternate Treatment

Procaine penicillin G 600,000 units daily for 20 days.
If patients are allergic to penicillin then erythromycin or tetracycline 500 mg are given for 30 days, or doxycycline 100 mg b.i.d. for 30 days.

4.15.1.9 Treatment of Neurosyphilis

Benzathine penicillin G has a low concentration in the CSF, crystalline penicillin G is used in the treatment of neurosyphilis. Crystalline penicillin G 20 million units I/V is given every 4 hours for 15 days.

Alternate Treatment

Procaine penicillin 600,000 units I/M for 15 days, with probenecid 500 mg q.i.d. orally for 15 days.
Cefrtiaxone 2 g I/V daily for 15 days.

4.15.2 Congenital Syphilis

This is seen in undeveloped countries where antenatal care is not well-developed, especially in rural areas. The trepanoma can cross the placenta any time during pregnancy.

4.15.2.1 Early Congenital Syphilis

Signs of congenital syphilis manifest in less than 2 years of age. The signs resemble those of secondary stage of syphilis. Flu-like symptoms and highly infectious nasal discharge are seen in the early stage of the disease. Mucocutaneous lesions include generalized maculopapular rash, deep fissures at the angle of the mouth, desquamative erythema of the palms and soles. Hepatosplenomegaly and lymphadenopathy.

Vesicle, bullae and erosions (pemphigus syphiliticus), osteochondritis, iritis, and alopecia are some of the signs of early congenital syphilis.

4.15.2.2 Late Congenital Syphilis

The signs become evident after 5 years of age. The signs include frontal bossing, saddle nose, high arched palate, Hutchinson's teeth (notched upper central permanent incisors), Mulberry molars (four or more cusps on the first permanent lower molar), Higoumenaki's sign (enlarged sternoclavicular part of the clavicle on one side), rhagades (radiating scars) at the angle of the mouth, nose, eyes and anus, deafness, and iritis.

Hutchinson's triad said to be pathognomonic of congenital syphilis includes Hutchinson's teeth, sensory nerve deafness, and iritis.

4.15.2.3 Treatment

Penicillin G 50,000 units/kg by I/V injection every 8–12 hours, or procaine penicillin 50,000 units/kg by I/M injection for 10–14 days.

> It is often said that syphilis was imported to Europe from Hispaniola (Haiti), by the crews of Christopher Columbus. Syphilitic bone changes have been found in the skeletons of Australians, Africans, and American aborigines.

> An Italian pathologist Giro Lamo Fracastoro gave a complete description of syphilis in 1530, in a poem entitled 'Syphilis Sivi Morbus Gallicus'. In this poem, he describes a mythical shepherd named

Syphilis, who was affected by a sexually transmitted disease as a pun-ishment for blasphemy to the sun god.

Shaudinn and Hoffman in 1905 discovered the causative organism of syphilis: Treponema pallidum. Wasserman, Neisser and Bruck in 1906 detected the lipoidal antibodies in the serum of infected individuals.

Sir Jonathen Hutchinson (1828–1913)

Hutchinson qualified from the medical school at York and then studied under Sir James Paget at St. Bartholomew's Hospital. He later joined the London Hospital and is said to have treated a million cases of syphilis. He was an outstanding clinician of the nineteenth century.

4.15.3 Gonorrhea

Is a disease of adolescence caused by Neisseria gonorrhea; about 40% of the infected patients are symptomless.

In males the disease presents as urethritis causing dysuria and/or urethral discharge (Fig. 4.21). Infection can spread to the prostate, seminal vesicles, and epididymis.

In females the disease is manifested by vaginal discharge, dysuria, and intermenstrual bleeding. Infection can spread to Bartholin glands, uterus, fallopian tubes, and adjacent pelvic structures giving rise to lower abdominal pain.

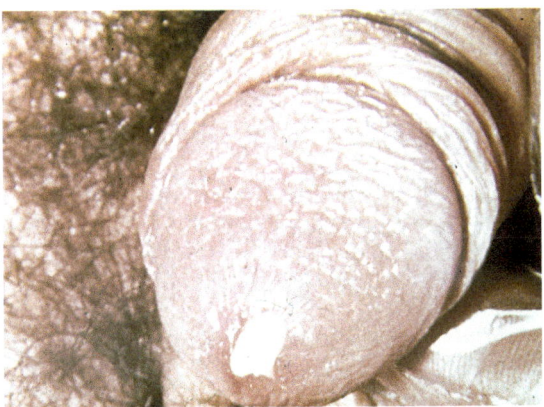

FIGURE 4.21. Gonorrhea.

4.15.3.1 Disseminated Gonorrhea

Neisearia gonorrhae can survive only in blood and on mucosal surface (a moist environment at body temperature) dissemination via the blood stream rapidly occurs. It is more common in females; menses exposes the submucosal vessels and increases the rate of dissemination.

The classical triad of disseminated gonorrhea is arthritis, tenosynovitis, and dermatitis. The cutaneous rash is most prominent on the extensor surface of the extremities. These appear as macules, papules, or vesicles with a red halo, which may develop into pustules or bullae.

Polyarthritis is characteristic; most people have involvement of less than three joints. The wrist and knees are most commonly affected. Joint inflammation is often sterile as the reaction is immunological.

Tenosynovitis is present in two-third of the patients; joints of the hands and fingers are most often affected.

The other disease manifestations include endocarditis, myocarditis, and meningitis.

4.15.3.2 Diagnosis

Acute gonococcal urethritis can be easily diagnosed by examination of the urethral smears; typical intracellular diplococci are diagnostic. Swabs from chronic cases should be cultured.

4.15.3.3 Treatment

Gonococcus is susceptible to a wide range of antibiotics, but there has been an increased resistance to the antibiotics over the last 2 decades. It is best to treat gonorrhea with a single dose of 3 g of amoxicillin with probenicid.

- Spectinomycin 2 g by single I/M injection
- Ceftrioxone 250 mg by single I/M injection

The other drugs used for the treatment of gonorrhea are ciprofloxacillin, cifizine, and erythromycin. It is best to follow the treatment with doxycycline 100 mg for 7 days to treat any concurrent chlamydial infection.

John Hunter (1728–1793)

The Hunter brothers (William and John) were dominant figures in the study of anatomy in England. John Hunter was a brilliant surgeon and experimentalist, who has left a great impression in the history of medical sciences. After becoming an expert anatomist, John studied surgery under Percivall Pott and William Cheseldon.

It was previously thought that gonorrhea and syphilis were caused by a single organism. John inoculated himself with the secretion from a case of gonorrhea. Hunter developed syphilis, as the patient was suffering from both syphilis and gonorrhea. Hunter thought that both the diseases had a common origin. John Hunter died 27 years later of syphilitic heart disease. Philip Record cleared the confusion half a century later.

4.15.4 Chancroid (Soft Chancre)

The disease is caused by Hemophilus ducreyi, a gram-negative rod. The disease is common in males, often acquired from prostitutes. The lesion begins as a painful red papule on the penis; the surrounding skin is inflamed and red. The papule rapidly becomes pustular and ulcerates. The ulcer bleeds easily, is deep with undermined edges, and the base is covered with a yellowish gray exudate. The ulcers are highly infectious and many lesions occur from autoinoculation.

Unilateral or bilateral lymphadenopathy occurs in 50% of cases. The lymph nodes may resolve or suppurate and break down.

A combination of painful genital ulcers and suppurative lymphadnopathy is almost diagnostic of chancroid.

4.15.4.1 Treatment

A single dose of azithrocin 1g orally, ciprofloxacin 500 mg b.i.d. for 3 days or erythrocin 500 mg q.i.d. for 7 days, ceftriaxone 250 mg by a single I/M injection can be used to treat chancroid.

Practical points

The three common ulcers on the genital areas due to sexual contact are syphilis, herpes simplex, and chancroid. All patients with these ulcers should be investigated for HIV infection.

All sexually transmitted diseases must be followed up at regular intervals, to ensure that the infecting organism has been eradicated.

All sexual contacts should be examined and treated if necessary.

Differentiating points between genital ulcers – syphilis, chancroid, and herpes simplex

Characteristics	Syphilis	Chancroid	Genital herpes
Causative organism	Treponema pallidum	Hemophilus ducreyi	Herpes simplex virus
Incubation period	3–4 weeks	2–4 days	3–10 days
Symptoms	Painless	Painful	Painful
Ulcer	Oval or rounded, indurated, narrow rim of erythema, dark, velvety red in color	Shallow inflamed ulcer, soft, yellowish red in color	Grouped vesicles on an erythematous base
Duration	3–6 weeks	Undetermined, usually months	Primary: 2–6 weeks recurrent: 7–10 days
Lymph nodes	Bilateral, firm, mobile, do not break down	Unilateral or bilateral, break down and ulcerate	Bilateral, tender, lymphadenopathy, with primary herpes. No involvement in recurrent herpes
Diagnosis	Treponema in smears, positive direct fluorescent antibody test	Gram staining shows Hemophilus ducreyi	Tzanxk test shows multinucleated cells

Chapter 5
Superficial Fungal Infections

Fungi affect human life in a number of ways. Some fungi help in the production of antibiotics; some are used for brewing and baking, while others destroy crops and produce disease. Fungal infections in humans are common; these are mainly due to two groups of fungi:

Dermatophytes – these are multicellular filaments or hyphae, which reproduce by the formation of spores.

Yeasts – these are unicellular and multiply by budding.

Dermatophytes are fungi that cause superficial fungal infections of the skin. These fungi have the ability to digest keratin. They infect and survive in the dead keratin of skin, hair, and nail. The word tinea (Latin for worm), is used for superficial fungal infections. It is followed by a qualifying term that denotes the location of infection, e.g., tinea faciei for infection of the face, tinea pedis for infection of the feet, etc. Tinea versicolor is the only exception; its name is due to the several shades of color that are present in the disease (the disease is now called Pityriasis versicolor).

The typical lesion produced by dermatophytes is an annular lesion with a scaling border, there is a tendency for the center of the lesion to heal. The characteristic feature of the infection is the active border, which is scaly and slightly elevated. Annular lesions are present on all areas except the palms and the soles. These fungal infections should be differentiated from other annular lesions such as granuloma annulare, the herald patch of pityriasis rosea, annular erythemas, annular impetigo, discoid eczema, psoriasis, etc.

Z. Zaidi, S. W. Lanigan, *Dermatology in Clinical Practice*, DOI: 10.1007/978-1-84882-862-9_5,

Man is infected from other human beings (anthrophilic), animals (zoophilic) or from the soil (geophilic). Zoophilic and geophilic infections are more inflammatory. Dermatophyte infection of the skin is caused by a number of dermatophyes, the most common are: Trichophyton, Microsporum and Epidermophyton species. The clinical reaction depends upon the type of dermatophyte infection. In general, the anthrophilic species produce less inflammation than the zoophilic species. The inflammation is due to the metabolic products of the fungus or to delayed hypersensitivity.

All dermatophytes are keratinophilic; they feed on keratin. Dermatophyte infection does not spread beyond the epidermis, because of the fungistatic properties of transferin and β-globulin.

5.1 Clinical Features

These are given in the following table.

Name	Location	Clinical appearance
Tinea capitis	Scalp	Four patterns: black dot, dry scaly, kerion (boggy swelling) and favus (dry yellow crusts)
Tinea corporis	Body	Typical annular lesion
Tinea cruris	Groin	Sharply delineated symmetrical plaques, central clearing ±, scales not prominent, border elevated and serpiginous
Tinea faciei	Face	Annular, but the pattern is often distorted by various topical applications used by the patient
Tinea barbae	Beard	Superficial resembles T corporis, deep resembles bacterial folliculitis
Tinea pedis	Feet – soles	Interdigital, diffuse dry and scaly or vesiculopustular
Tinea manuum	Hands – palms	Dry and scaly or vesico-pustular
Tinea unguium (onychomycosis)	Nails	Yellow, brittle, and thick, with subungal hyperkeratosis

5.1.1 Tinea Pedis

Is common in adults; it is predisposed by wearing of shoes, swimming, communal washing, and hot weather. The three common varieties are:

Interdigital. Usually found in the web between the fourth and fifth toe; the area is erythematous, soggy, and macerated. Also a diffuse dry, hyperkeratotic, scaling of the soles (moccasin type); the scales are more prominent on the creases of the foot. The more inflammatory type is the vesiculo-bullous variety, in which papules, pustules, and sometimes bullae are found on the sole (Figs. 5.1 and 5.2).

Recurrences can be prevented by wearing of wider shoes and expanding the web spaces with small strands of Lamb's Wool. Powders absorb moisture and should be applied to the feet, not the shoes.

5.1.2 Tinea Manuum

Tinea of the hands, "tinea manuum," is similar to tinea pedis, but the interdigital form is not seen. Tinea pedis can cause pompholyx of the hands. Characteristically a fine scaling

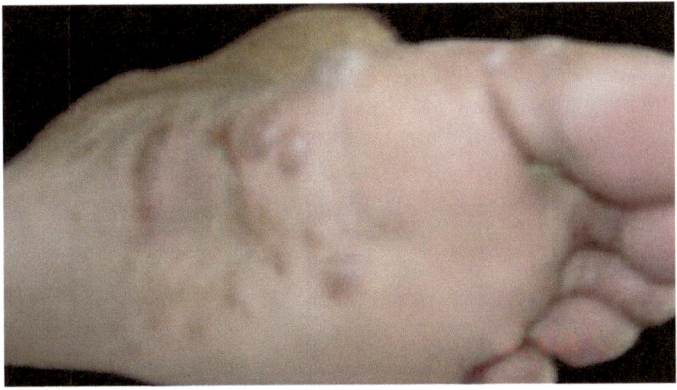

FIGURE 5.1. Tinea pedis. Type – vesiculobullous.

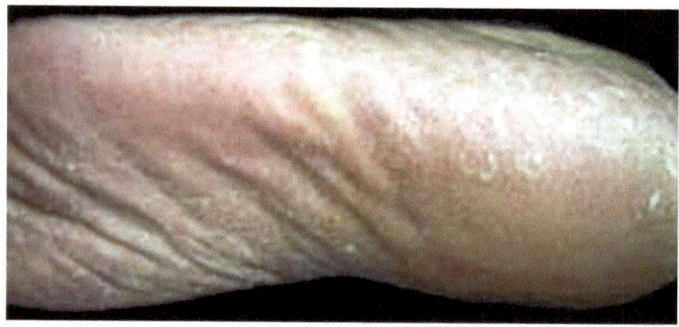

FIGURE 5.2. Tinea pedis. Type – dry and scaly.

occurs in the palmar creases. Always consider tinea in cases of unilateral "hand dermatitis." Always examine the feet when a patient presents with pompholyx.

5.1.3 Tinea Capitis

This is usually a disease of children; a number of morphological forms are seen.

The common variety produces dry, scaly, and bald areas on the scalp; this is due to the fungus acting on the surface of the hair shaft. This type produces the characteristic green fluorescence on Wood's lamp examination. When the fungi invade the hair shaft, they produce the "black dot" variety of hair loss. The affected hair break at the surface of the scalp. Kerion is probably due to a delayed hypersensitivity reaction to fungal elements. Clinically it is characterized by a boggy inflammatory mass discharging pus. Lymphadenopathy is often present. This should be differentiated from bacterial infections such as carbuncle or furuncle. The hair loss may be permanent. In favus, yellowish cup-shaped, foul-smelling crusts called scutula appear around the hair follicles. This can also lead to cicatricial alopecia. Tinea capitis due to favus also shows fluorescence under Wood's light (Figs. 5.3–5.6).

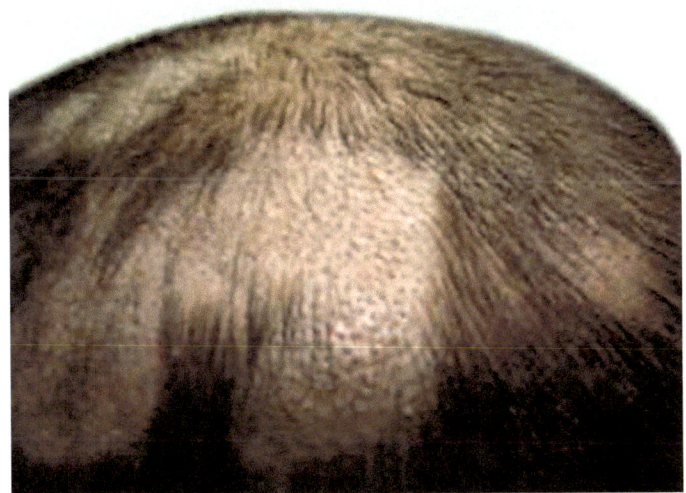

FIGURE 5.3. Tinea capitis. Type black Dot.

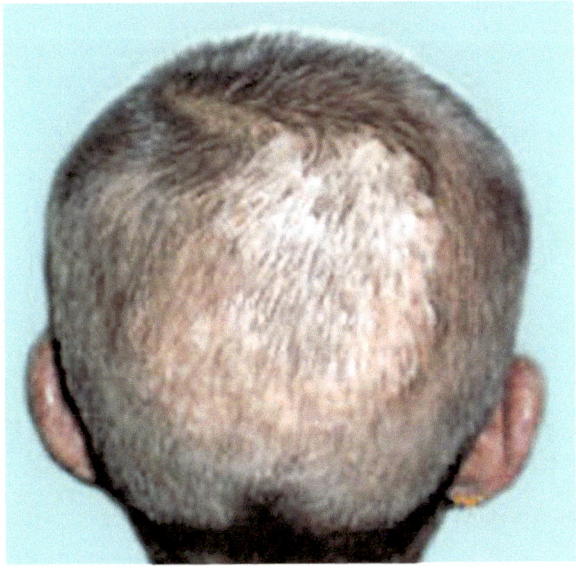

FIGURE 5.4. Tinea capitis. Type dry and scaly.

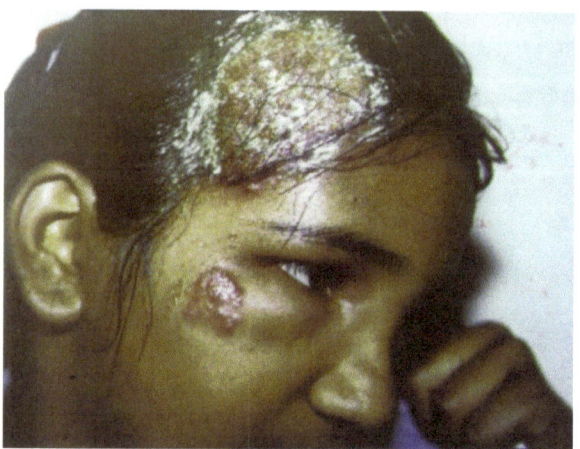

FIGURE 5.5. Tinea capitis. Type kerion.

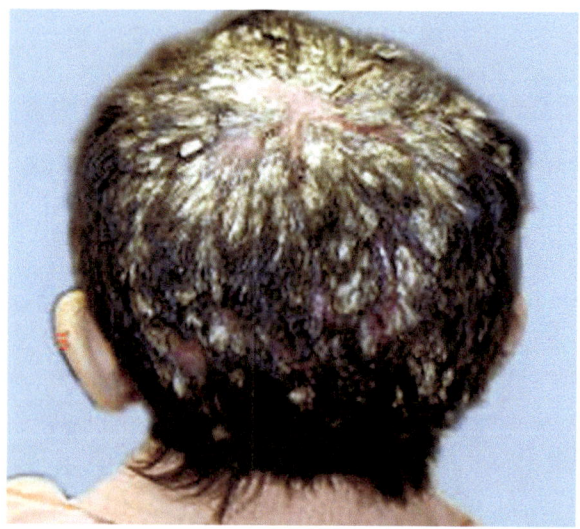

FIGURE 5.6. Tinea capitis. Type favus.

Wood's lamp is useful for screening children in schools where an outbreak of tinea capitis is suspected.

5.1.4 Tinea Corporis

This includes all the superficial fungal infections of the skin, excluding those of the scalp, nails, groins, beard, hands, and feet. It occurs both in children and adults, both sexes are equally affected.

Erythematous, scaly plaques characterize the lesion, which expands slowly with healing in the center, giving the characteristic "ring like" appearance. The erythema and scaling is most pronounced at the periphery of the lesion. Scales should be taken from the periphery of a lesion for microscopic examination for fungal hyphae. The lesions can be single or multiple. A number of lesions can coalesce to involve large areas of the body (Figs. 5.7–5.9).

In some cases, the zoophilic fungi can invade the skin, giving rise to severe pustular reaction, with no central clearing.

5.1.5 Tinea Cruris

Infection of the groin is common in men; a number of cases are due to autoinoculation from tinea of the foot. The lesions are characterized by erythematous well-defined plaque with central clearing. The eruption is sometimes unilateral and asymmetrical. In contrast to candidiasis of the groin, the scrotum is often spared. The lesion extends to involve the thighs and buttocks. Itching is a prominent feature (Fig. 5.10).

5.1.6 Tinea Barbae

This is infection of the beard and moustache area of men. The lesions may be inflammatory like a kerion, or in the less inflammatory cases due to anthrophilic infection, the lesions

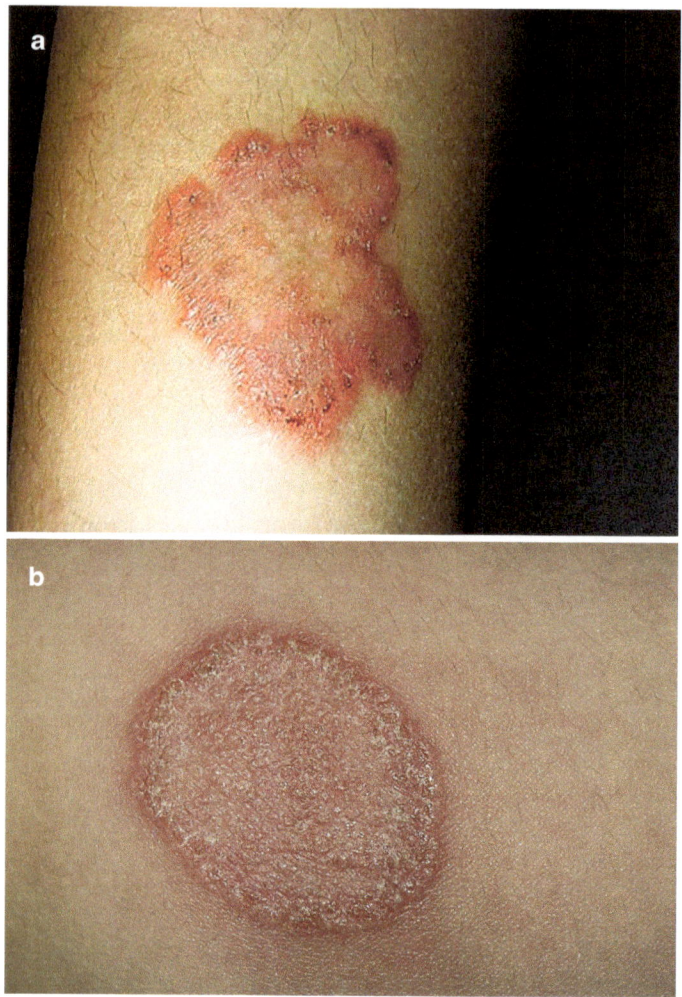

FIGURE 5.7. (**a**, **b**) Tinea corporis.

appear as dry, scaly, erythematous areas of hair loss. Tinea barbae should be differentiated from a bacterial infection, which is painful and there is no hair loss (Fig. 5.11).

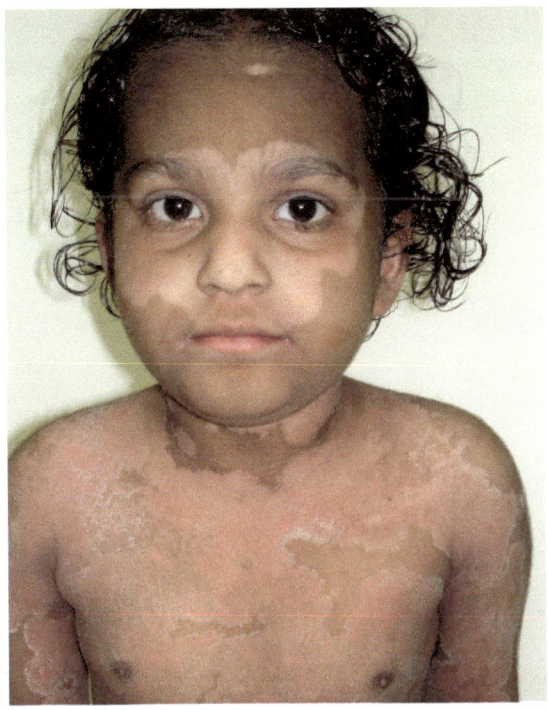

FIGURE 5.8. Tinea corporis – generalized.

5.1.7 Onychomycosis (Tinea of the Nails)

The most type affects the distal end of the nail, which becomes yellow and crumbly. Subungal hyperkeratosis results in separation of the nail from the bed, and thickening of the nail follows. Usually a few nails are infected. There is no paronychia as seen in infections due to Candida (Fig. 5.12).

5.1.8 Tinea Incognito

This is a term used for a tinea infection, which has been altered by the application of topical steroids; which are a

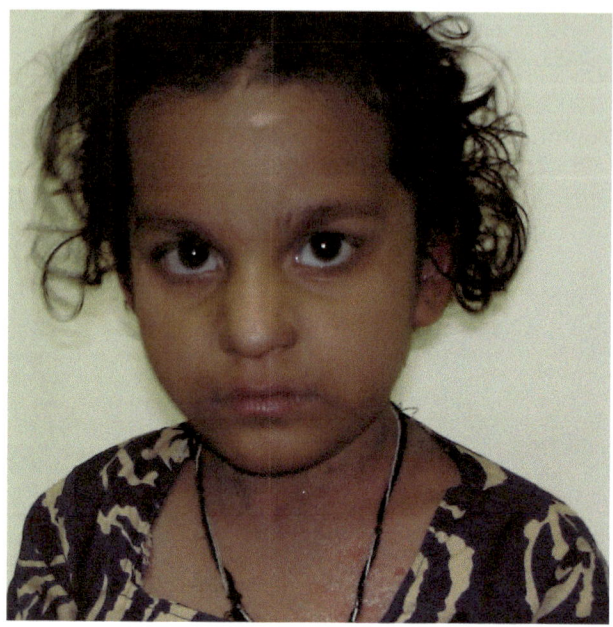

FIGURE 5.9. Same patient after treatment.

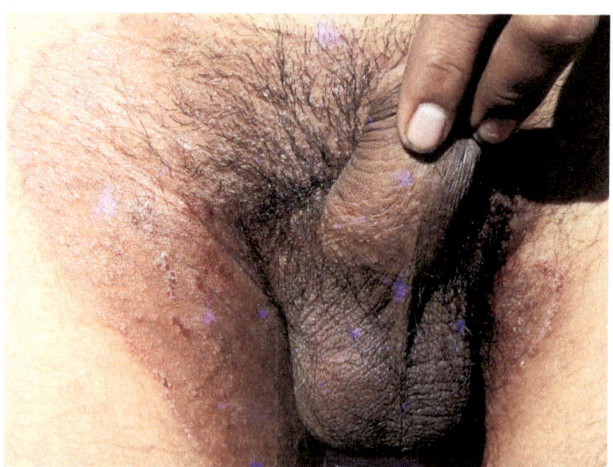

FIGURE 5.10. Tinea cruris.

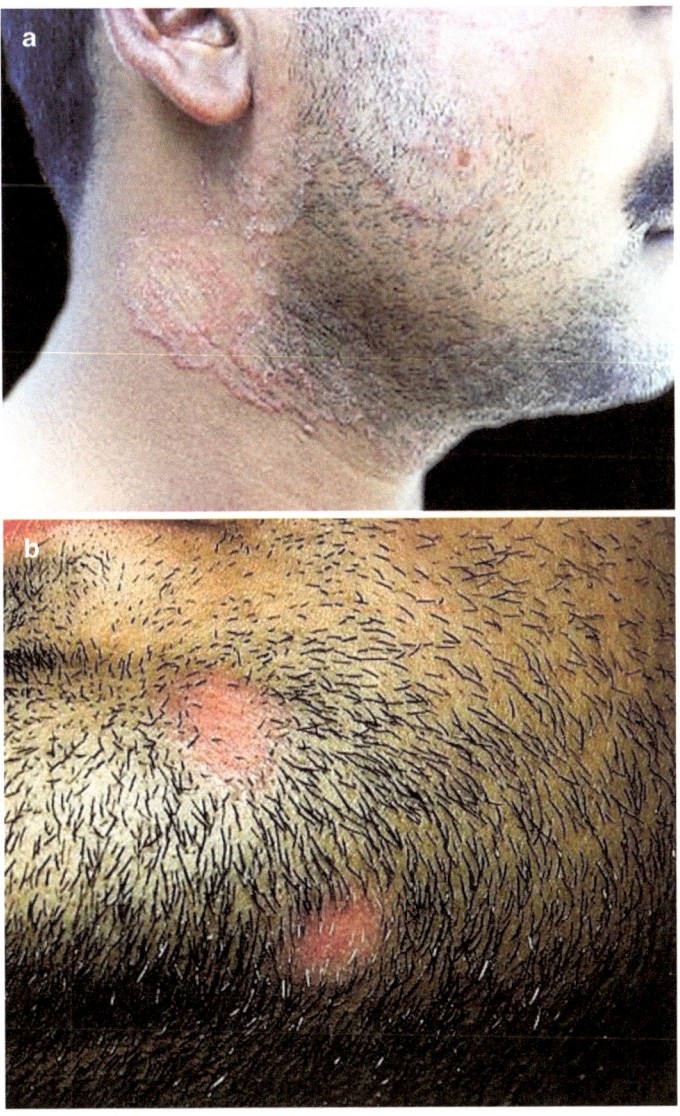

FIGURE 5.11. (**a**, **b**) Tinea barbae.

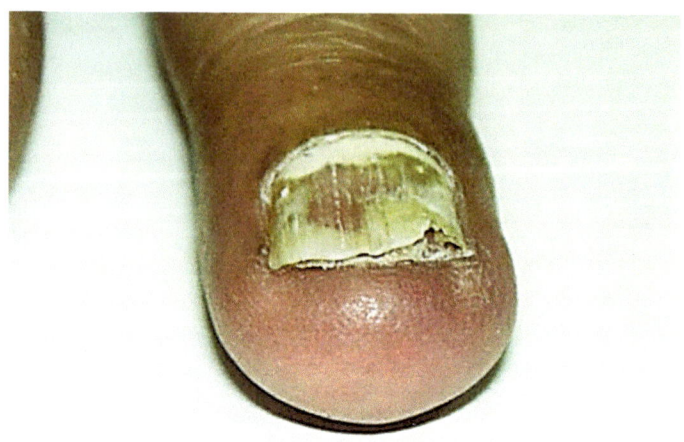

FIGURE 5.12. Onychomycosis.

common household remedy for many cutaneous infections. The typical annular pattern is lost; it may present as diffuse erythema, or diffuse scaling. Scattered pustules may be present, papules and brown pigmentation may also be seen. A well-defined border is absent, and an expanding border may be seen at one end (Fig. 5.13).

5.2 Diagnosis

Microscopic examinations of skin scrapings, nail, or hair are required for diagnosis. The scrapings should be taken from the scaly margins of a skin lesion. The hair should be plucked for the diagnosis of tinea capitis. Positive results from nail scrapings are difficult to get as the active border is at the proximal end of the nail. A dental drill is a useful instrument to take the nail sample.

Culture takes about 3 weeks; the specimen should be sent in a folded black paper in a sealed package to the laboratory. Mycological culture differentiates the different organisms.

Wood's lamp. Examination of the scalp reveals a green fluorescence in mycosporum species and in T schonleini. The

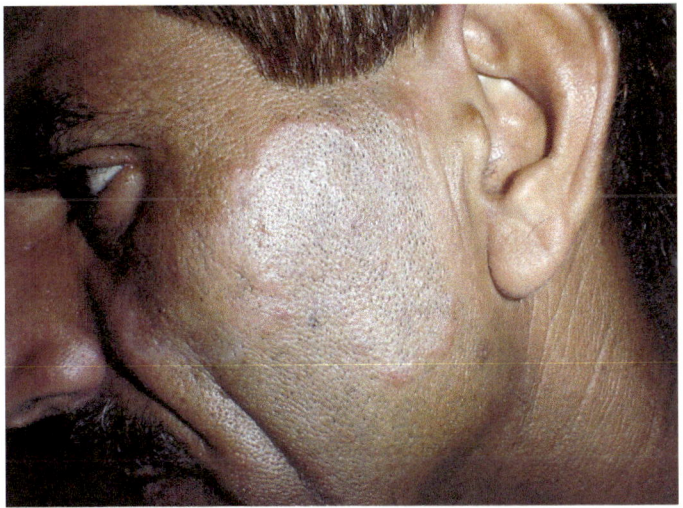

FIGURE 5.13. Tinea incognito.

black dot variety does not fluoresce. Wood's lamp examination is a useful method in screening schoolchildren with tinea capitis.

5.3 Differential Diagnosis

Tinea capitis should be differentiated from alopecia areata, trichotillomania, psoriasis, and seborrheic eczema. Kerion should be differentiated from a boil or carbuncle. These bacterial infections are painful and tender, and will not have hair loss. *Tinea corporis* should be differentiated from granuloma annulare, tuberculoid leprosy, annular psoriasis, discoid eczema, and pityriaisis rosea. *Tinea cruris* should be differentiated from other infections of the flexures such as candida, seborrheic dermatitis, intertrigo, and erythrasma. *Tinea of the palms and soles* should be differentiated from eczema, psoriasis, and lichen planus. *Onychomycosis* should be differentiated from the nail changes of eczema, psoriasis, and chronic paronychia.

5.4 Treatment

Tinea corporis, tinea faciei, and tinea cruris are treated by topical antifungal preparations, while tinea of the scalp, nails, palms, and soles require systemic treatment. The thick stratum corneum in these sites makes the penetration of topical medicines difficult.

Topical antifungal therapy includes preparations such as imidazoles, ketoconazoles, allylamine, Whitfield's ointment, Castellani's paint, undecenoic acid, and tolnaftate. Amorolfine is used as a liquor for the nails. The patient is advised to use the antifungal preparations until the infection disappears and then to apply them for further 1–2 weeks to prevent recurrence.

Systemic therapy for tinea infections include: griseofulvin, ketoconazole, itraconazole, fluconazole, and the allylamines. *Griseofulvin* was the first antifungal drug discovered. It is fungistatic, toxicity is rare, it does not have any residual action, so the relapse rates are high, and it is cheap. Griseofulvin acts only against dermatophytes. The *azoles* include ketoconazole, itraconazole, and fluconazole; they are all fungistatic drugs, and they act on both dermatophytes and yeasts. Liver toxicity limits the use of ketoconazole. The action of itraconazole on cytochrome P 450 is much less than ketoconazole, and it has a residual action on the skin after the drug has been stopped. The drug is widely used to treat fungal infections, both superficial and deep. The action of fluconazole is similar to itraconazole. It can be given on a weekly basis, which makes patient compliance good, but it is teratogenic and should be avoided in pregnancy and lactation. *Allylamines* are newer antifungal drugs; these are fungicidal, they act mainly against dermatophytes, they have a wide margin of safety, and allylamines do not inhibit cytochrome P 450 enzymes. They also have a residual action on the skin after the treatment is stopped.

Tinea pedis can be very refractory to treatment, especially if the patient has nail involvement. Preventive measures are important such as keeping the foot dry, wearing cotton socks, and use of lightweight ventilated footwear. For interdigital tinea pedis, potassium permanganate solution is used if there is bacterial infection of the toe cleft, and if the inflammation is pronounced then an oral antibiotic is needed in addition.

Terbinafine gives excellent long-term remissions in a dose of 125 mg b.i.d. for 4–6 weeks. Itraconazole is also effective in a dose of 100 mg daily for 1 month. Griseofulvin does not act on interdigital tinea pedis; for the moccasin type it is given in a dose of 500 mg b.i.d. for 2–3 months.

For suppression, the patient should use an antifungal powder topically for a long period to prevent recurrence.

Tinea corporis – topical preparation of imidazoles are often used; these should be applied twice a day for 2–3 weeks. Oral treatment is used in chronic or very extensive lesions.

Tinea capitis – terbinafine 250 mg daily for 4 weeks in adults and 62.5 mg daily for 4 weeks in children above 2 years of age. Griseofulvin 20 mg/kg of body weight, for 6–8 weeks. Itraconazole is currently not licensed for treatment of children.

Onychomycosis – terbinafine 250 mg daily for 6 weeks for fingernails, and 250 mg daily for 12 weeks for toe nail infection. Itraconazole 400 mg daily for 1 week every month for 3 months. Griseofulvin 750–1,000 mg daily for 4–6 months for fingernails and for 12–18 months for toe nails. Griseofulvin produces a slow response and the relapse rates are high.

Topical treatment with amorolfine liquor used once weekly may help in obtaining a quicker response in the nail infection.

Sometimes nail avulsion is required, this will reduce the treatment period.

Fingernails respond to treatment better than toenails due to the faster nail growth of fingernails.

> *The most common types of tinea are Tinea pedis and onychomycosis of the nails.*
> *A characteristic feature of the infection is its active border.*
> *Tinea capitis is common in children; adults are protected by their sebaceous secretion, which is fungistatic.*
> *Asymmetrical infections, e.g., of two feet and one hand, or two hands and one foot are typical of tinea.*
> *Synonyms for superficial fungal infections are: dermatophytosis, tinea, and ringworm.*

Common groin rashes are tinea, candidiasis, and intertrigo.
The three genera of dermatophytes are Trichophyton, Microsporum, and Epidermophyton.
Athelete's foot is a superficial fungal infection.
Tinea of the hands and feet should be differentiated from contact dermatitis and psoriasis.
Think of dermatophyte infection if a patient's eczema is not responding to steroids.

5.5 Pityriasis Versicolor (Furfuracae)

This is a superficial fungal infection, caused by Malassezia furfur; there are several species of this lipophilic yeast. The disease results in scaly patches of different color; these may be erythematous, hypopigmented, or hyperpigmented. The scaly patches later coalesce. The hypopigmentation is produced by carboxylic acid produced by the fungus, which inhibits the production of melanin by melanocytes.

The disease is common in young adults; sweat and moisture are important factors for converting the yeast into the active hyphae, which is responsible for the infection. The lesions are commonly present on the upper part of the chest, back, and upper arm. The face and lower arms can also be infected in tropical countries. The patients complain of a patchy change in skin color with mild irritation. The primary lesion is a sharply demarcated macule with slight erythema, and fine branny scales (Fig. 5.14).

The involved skin gives a pale yellow fluorescence with Wood's lamp. Scrapings show a mixture of short hyphae and spores (spaghetti and meat ball appearance).

5.5.1 Differential Diagnosis

Pityriasis versicolor should be differentiated from pityriasis rosea and seborrheic dermatitis.

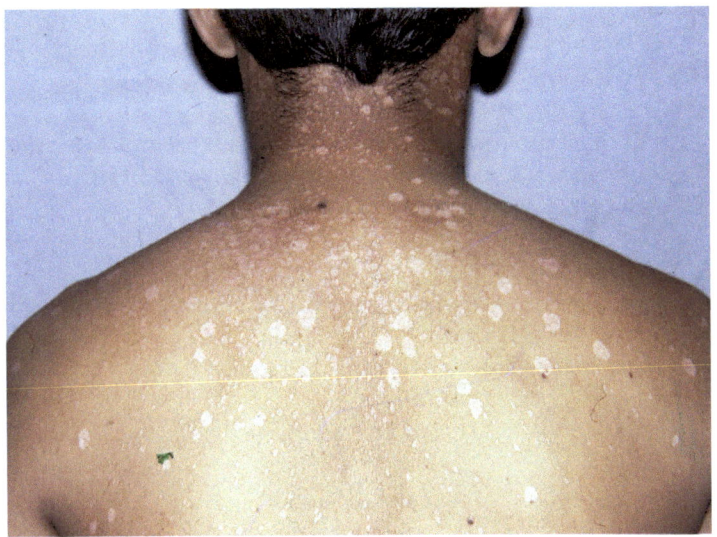

FIGURE 5.14. Pityriasis versicolor.

5.5.2 Treatment

Topical azole antifungal ointments applied twice a day for 2–4 weeks. Terbinafine spray is also effective.

Selenium sulphide shampoo applied to the affected areas for about 10 min before washing for three nights in a row is helpful in a number of cases. The shampoo can also be applied weekly for 3 weeks. The shampoo can be left on the skin at night, and washed off the following morning. Repeat once a week for 4 weeks. The treatment must be repeated every 3 months to prevent recurrences. Ketoconazole shampoo is also effective; it does not have the characteristic odor of the former but is more expensive.

Shampoos cover a large area of the body; at low cost and are easy to apply.

Ketoconazole tablet 400 mg single dose is effective for cases which do not respond to topical treatment. Repeat the treatment every 3 months for 1 year to prevent recurrences.

Itraconazole 200 mg qd for 7 days, for therapy. For prophylaxis 200 b.i.d., once a day, every month for 6 months.
Fluconazole 300–400 mg once. Repeat after 2 weeks.

The hypopigmented areas will repigment much later, after therapeutic cure. The patient should be informed of this prior to treatment.

Terbinafine and griseofulvin are not effective orally in Malassezia furfur.

The fungus is a normal commensal of the skin, so recurrences are frequent.

Treatment is not only directed to eradicate the infection, but also for prophylaxis.

Advise patients to avoid excess exposure to heat and moisture.

5.6 Pityrosporum Folliculitis (Malassezia Folliculitis)

This folliculitis is caused by the same organism that causes Pityriasis versicolor. The areas affected are rich in sebaceous glands, which provide the lipid environment required by the yeast.

The lesions appear as papules and pustules, the lesions are itchy. The itching differentiates it from acne. The eruption is common on the upper chest, back, and upper arms, similar to acne, but it does not have comedones, the pathognomonic character of acne. The face may be affected; on the face the sites are the mandible region, chin, and sides of the face. In acne, the central part of the face is more involved (Fig. 5.15).

5.6.1 Treatment

Same as for Pityriasis versicolor. Topical imidazole creams and antifungal shampoos. Systemic treatment is given if lesions are extensive or not responding to topical therapy.

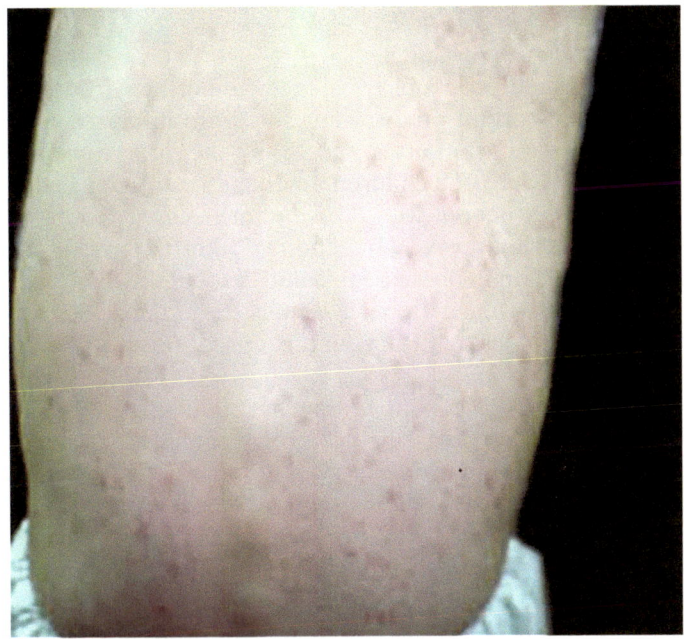

FIGURE 5.15. Pityrosporum folliculitis.

5.7 Candidiasis

Candida albicans is a yeast that colonizes in the skin, mouth, GIT, and the vagina. Infection occurs when the yeast is transformed to hyphae and pseudohyphae. Conditions that favor this transformation are warmth, moisture, diabetes, immunosuppression, antibiotic therapy, pregnancy, and steroid treatment.

When the skin is infected, the organism enters the epidermis and activates the alternate complement pathway, resulting in inflammation that is characteristically bright red in color. Chemotactic factors attract neutrophils, resulting in pustule formation. Cell-mediated immunity is important in host defense.

5.7.1 Clinical Features

Candida can affect people of all ages; a moist environment is the most important predisposing factor. In infants, the most common manifestation is thrush in the oral cavity, and perineum in diapered children. In adults, interdigital candidiasis occurs in people who do wet work such as cooks, bartenders, and housewives. Infection of intertriginous areas is seen more often in obese people and diabetics. Vulvovaginitis is common in women. In old age, moisture at the angles of the mouth due to poorly fitting dentures predisposes to candidal infection.

The most characteristic finding in candidiasis is bright red erythema of the skin, surrounded by satellite papules and pustules. Pustules may not be seen in some patients, but their residua are seen as erythematous scaly macules.

Oral Candida (thrush) – is seen as white patches on an inflamed mucosa. This white curd-like pseudomembrane can be removed easily. The membrane consists of desquamated epithelial cells, fibrin, leucocytes, and fungal mycelium, attached to the inflamed epithelium.

Angular stomatitis (perleche) – best considered as an intertrigo; Candida and other pathogens are involved. Deficiency of vitamin B also play a part.

Candidal intertrigo – any skin fold can be affected. The lesions have a moist, glazed, and macerated appearance, characterized by erythema and pustules at the periphery of the lesion; these often rupture to form erosions (Fig. 5.16).

Interdigital candidiasis – affects the web spaces of the fingers or toes. There is marked maceration of the skin; a thick white horny layer is prominent. The web of the finger is often predisposed to infection with gram-negative bacteria: blastomycetes (Fig. 5.17).

Napkin dermatitis – seen commonly in the buttocks and genitalia of infant; where the skin is moist. The lesion is erythematous with irregular borders, satellite lesions are characteristic.

Candidal paronychia – usually several fingers are affected, the nail fold is swollen, and the cuticle is lost. There is nail

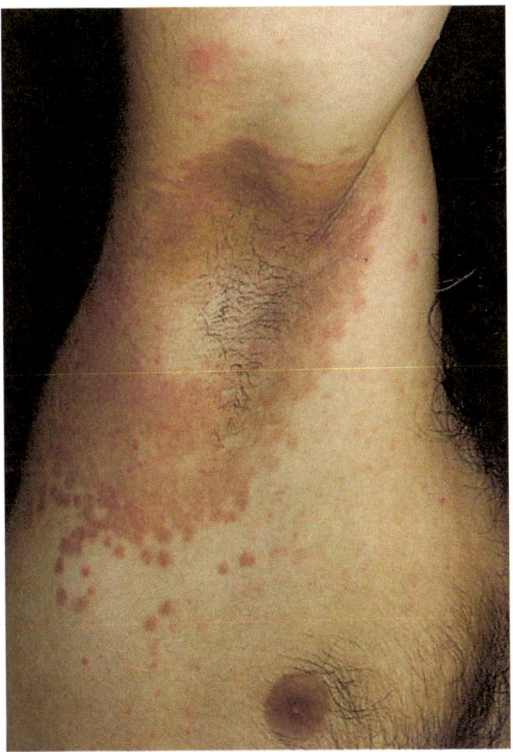

FIGURE 5.16. Candida.

dystrophy, some discoloration, and onycholysis around the lateral fold may occur.

Chronic mucocutaneous candidiasis – this is a rare form of candidiasis, sometimes seen in infancy due to an immune deficiency. The disease is persistent, and comprises infection of the skin, nails, and mucous membranes without dissemination of the infection. Genetic, endocrine, and immunological causes for the infection should be excluded.

Systemic candidiasis – this is seen in severe systemic illness, leucopenia, and immunosuppression. The lesions appear as firm red nodules; these contain yeast and pseudohyphae on microscopic examination.

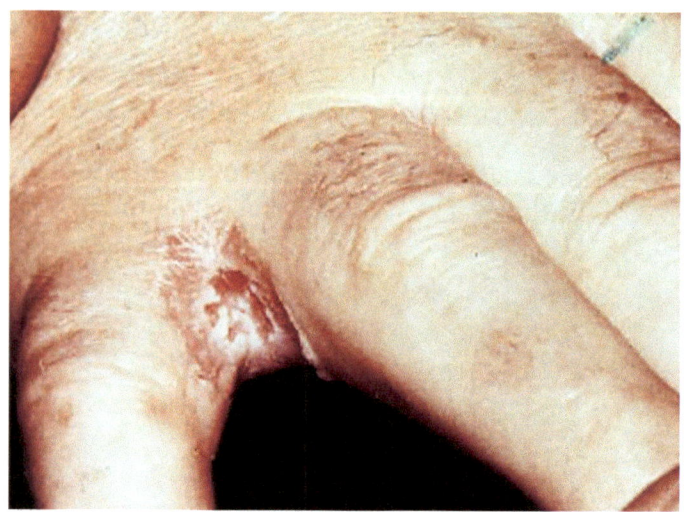

FIGURE 5.17. Interdigital candidiasis.

5.7.2 Investigations

Microscopic examination of material from the pustules will demonstrate hyphae and pseudohyphae in potassium hydroxide preparations. Spores alone are not diagnostic, as Candida can colonize the skin without causing infection.

Swabs from suspected areas should be sent for culture.

Urine should be examined for sugar.

A detailed immunological workup is required in chronic mucocutaneous candidiasis.

5.7.3 Treatment

Remove all predisposing factors, diapers should be changed frequently, keep the hands dry, treat any predisposing cause such as diabetes, obesity, etc.

Oral Candida – suspension of nystatin, amphotericin, or miconazole gel is applied several times a day for 10–14 days.

Unresponsive cases require one dose of fluconazole 150 mg, or itraconazole 100 mg, or ketoconazole 200–400 mg daily for 14 days.

Intertrigo – imidazole, azole, or polyene preparations are used topically three to four times a day for 14 days. In extensive or chronic cases, ketoconazole 400 mg daily, itraconazole 100 mg daily for 14 days. Fluconazole 150 mg once is another choice.

An absorbent powder should be used once the rash disappears.

Vaginal candidiasis – itraconazole 200 mg bd for 1 day, or fluconazole 150 mg once.

Paronychia and onychomycosis – require prolonged treatment with frequent applications of polyene or imidazole preparation; lotions are preferable to creams. The hand should be kept dry. Treat any associated irritant or contact dermatitis. Pulse imidazole therapy; 200 mg bd for 7 days every month for 3 months is the treatment of choice.

For prophylaxis:

- Fluconazole 150 mg once a month.
- Itraconazole 200 mg b.i.d. once a month.
- Ketoconazole ½ of 200 mg tablet, once a month for 6 months.

> *Creams should be applied sparingly in moist areas, as excessive application will contribute to the maceration.*
> *Widespread candidiasis is treated systemically.*

5.8 Subcutaneous Fungal Infections

5.8.1 Madura Foot (Mycetoma)

This is a localized infection of the skin; the infection slowly extends to the subcutaneous tissue and the bone, and it is common in tropical countries. Mycetoma occurs in people who walk barefooted. The disease is caused by various species of fungi (eumycetoma), actinomycetes (actinomycet-oma), and other bacteria. Aggregates of the causative organisms (grains) form within the abscess.

Mycetoma begins as a painless subcutaneous swelling in the foot; usually the insteps or the interdigital spaces are first affected. The lesion then enlarges to form a nontender rubbery mass. The lesion matures by tumefaction, with the formation of nodules and sinuses. The disease gradually extends to the underlying bones; this leads to gross swelling of the foot. The sinuses reveal grains or microcolonies of the causative organism. The grains may be black, yellow, or red. The black color is indicative of fungal infection, yellow of actinomycetes, and red due to streptomyces (Fig. 5.18).

The disease is locally invasive, involving the muscles, bones, and tendons. Blood dissemination does not occur. Lymph nodes are not affected. The clinical triad of tumefaction, sinuses, and grains are suggestive of mycetoma. Longstanding cases should have an X-ray of the foot to exclude bone involvement.

Madura foot should be differentiated from Price's disease. Podomycosis (Price's disease) resembles madura foot; it is due to penetration of sand in people walking barefoot. The disease is an allergic reaction to the salicylates in the soil. In addition to the enlarged foot; the regional lymph nodes are also enlarged.

5.8.1.1 Treatment

Treatment is difficult; patients often come for treatment when the disease is far advanced. Fungal mycetoma responds poorly to antifungal therapy; ketoconazole, griseofulvin, itraconazole, and fluconazole are worth attempting. Mycetoma caused by actinomycetes responds to chemotherapeutic agents. Dapsone, streptomycin, and sulphamethoxazole-trimethoprim are effective. Alternately, rifampicin can be used.

Localized lesions should be excised, without causing any residual disability.

5.8.2 *Sporotrichosis*

This subcutaneous fungal infection is caused by Sporothrix schenckii. The earliest manifestation of the disease is a small nodule at the site of inoculation. In the course of a few weeks, new nodules develop along the lymphatics. The nodules may remain hard, or soften and ulcerate. A chronic localized form is present in about one-third of cases.

5.8.2.1 Treatment

Itraconazole 100–200 mg daily for 3–6 months. Fluconazole 400 mg daily for 3–6 months.

Saturated solution of iodine is also effective, starting with a dose of 5 drops three times a day in milk, increasing the dose gradually up to 30–40 drops at each dose. Treatment should be continued for 4 weeks after the clinical cure.

Amphotericin B is also effective.

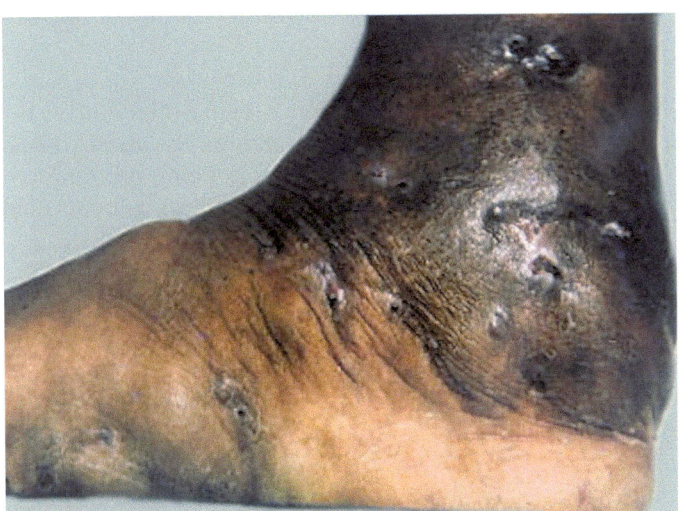

FIGURE 5.18. Madura foot.

5.9 Deep Fungal Infections

Deep fungal infections involve the skin secondarily. When the skin lesions occur in systemic mycosis, the prognosis is poor. In most cases the primary infection is in the lung, the cutaneous spread is manifested by granulomas, which present as papules, nodules, sinuses, and abscesses.

5.9.1 Cryptococcosis

The yeast is found in soil, particularly that which is contaminated by pigeon excreta. The portal of entry is usually inhalation via the lungs; central nervous system manifestations are predominant as meningitis. In the disseminated form the skin is involved; the lesions are most frequent in the head and neck. A variety of skin lesions is present, as tumor-like growths, molluscum contagiosum, sinuses, plaques, ulcers, and cellulitis.

5.9.2 Histoplasmosis

The disease begins as an acute pulmonary infection; at times erythema nodosum may be the presenting lesion. Histoplasma is unique amongst pathogenic fungi in being predominantly intracellular, found within the cells of the reticuloendothelial tissue in the form of budding yeasts.

5.9.3 Blastomycosis

The disease first affects the lungs, with pulmonary changes resembling tuberculosis. The disease is confined to the rural areas of the USA. Disseminated lesions to the skin are rare, these occur as wart-like, hyperkeratotic nodules, which spread peripherally with a verrucose edge, with a tendency to clear and scar centrally.

5.9.4 Coccidioidomycosis

The disease is present in the arid zones of the USA. The lungs are affected through inhalation. Human infection can be caused by very little exposure to the organism, so that through foreign travel cases of coccidioidomycosis are reported in many parts of the world. The skin lesions present as abscesses that remain localized for several years. Some lesions are similar to those of mycosis fungoides, in the form of plaques and nodules.

5.9.5 Treatment of Deep Mycosis

Most of the deep mycosis are treated by itraconazole or amphotericin B. The duration of treatment is long; usually 6–8 months.

Some characteristics of deep fungal infections:

They have a chronic course.

Systemic symptoms are usually mild or absent. When the lesion disseminates from the primary focus constitutional symptoms become severe.

Each disease has its own geographic distribution.

The diagnosis is often made by finding the causative fungus in the lesion, exudate, or sputum and in the histological examination of the tissue.

Chapter 6
Viral Infections

Viruses are the most prevalent of all organisms, yet they are not found on human skin, like bacteria and yeasts, because they multiply in living cells. Viruses cannot be seen on ordinary light microscopy; an electron microscope is needed for examination. Viruses have a central core of nucleic acid either DNA or RNA, a protein coat that surrounds the central core, and an outermost lipid envelope. Viral infections are diagnosed by cell culture, examination under an electron microscope, and detection of antiviral antibodies by immunoflourescence studies.

6.1 Herpes Simplex

Herpes virus are large DNA viruses, they multiply in the nucleus and produce typical intranuclear inclusions. A typical feature of all herpes virus is that after clinical recovery the virus persists in the patient as a latent infection. Under certain conditions, the virus becomes reactivated, to produce an acute infective episode with cellular damage.

Herpes simplex (HS) is one of the commonest infections worldwide. There are two strains of herpes simplex virus, type 1 and 2. Type 1 causes oral and type 2 genital infections. HS has two phases of reactivity; primary infection caused by direct inoculation of the virus; the virus then becomes established in the nerve ganglion. The secondary phase is characterized by the transfer of the virus, from the ganglion via the nerves to cause recurrent disease at the same site. Recurrent

Z. Zaidi, S. W. Lanigan, *Dermatology in Clinical Practice*,   101
DOI: 10.1007/978-1-84882-862-9_6,

attacks may be triggered by sunlight, infection, systemic upset, stress, etc. Genital recurrences are six times more frequent than the oral recurrences.

Type 1 infection is common in children, and type 2 in adults causing genital infection.

The lesions of primary HS are more numerous than secondary eruptions, and consist of scattered vesicles and indurated papules. Bullae may also occur. Prodromal symptoms of itching and burning are severe. Primary infections are frequently accompanied by fever, malaise, headache, and regional adenopathy. In secondary HS the lesions classically occur as grouped vesicles on an erythematous base. The vesicles soon become pustules, which rupture and form a crust. The prodrome occurs within 24 h of the rash and is much milder than that of primary HS.

Infections due to herpes virus 1 are seen on the face, most commonly around the lips and those due to herpes virus 2 occur on the genitals (Figs. 6.1–6.2). Direct inoculation of the virus into the fingertip results in *"herpetic whitlow."* This may be secondary to herpes virus 1 or 2. *Eczema herpeticum* is a generalized cutaneous infection of herpes virus in patients with atopic dermatitis; it may also occur in immunosuppressed patients from any cause. It is accompanied by a severe toxic reaction and can be fatal. The eruptions are most common on areas of active atopic dermatitis or recently healed lesions of the disease. Normal appearing skin becomes

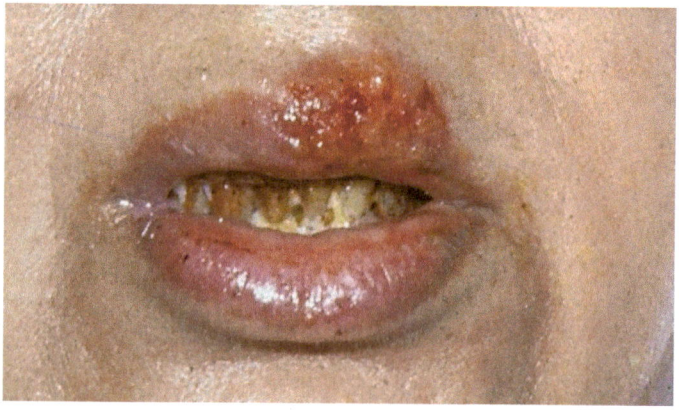

FIGURE 6.1. Herpes simplex.

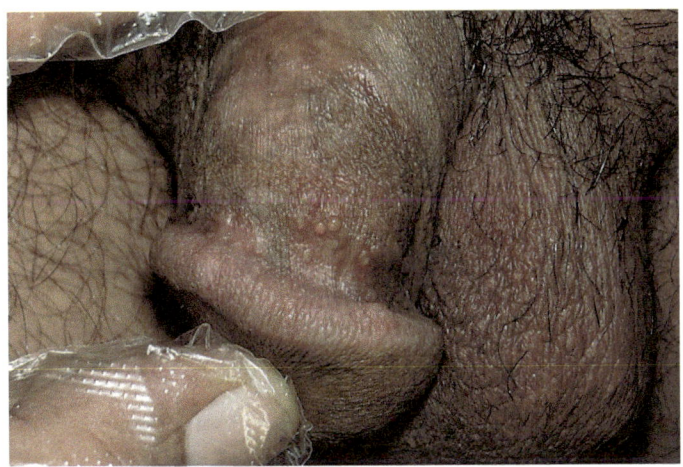

FIGURE 6.2. Herpes genitalis.

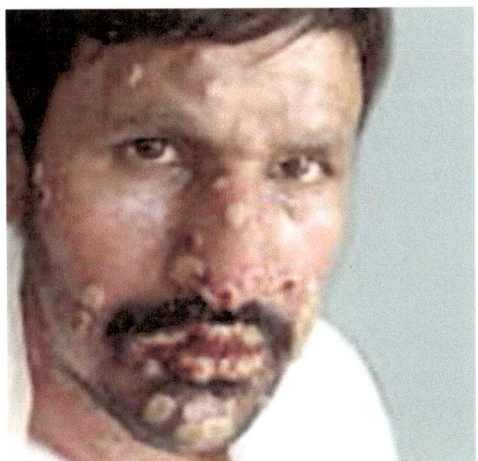

FIGURE 6.3. Eczema herpeticum.

involved ultimately. The numerous vesicles become pustular and umbilicate markedly. Secondary staphylococcal infection often follows (Fig. 6.3). This is a medical emergency; early treatment with parental antivirals is life saving. Recurrent disease is milder and usually without constitutional symptoms.

Primary herpes simplex infection can also occur in newborns, from HS infection of the mother through vaginal secretions. The infection is devastating in infants. It should be diagnosed, and treated promptly.

6.1.1 Complications

Disseminated herpes simplex can occur in newborns and immunosuppressed patients. Eczema herpeticum can occur in atopic patients, and cancer of the cervix in patients with herpes simplex type 11 viruses. Herpes simplex is the most common cause of recurrent erythema multiforme.

6.1.2 Differential Diagnosis

Herpes simplex though easy to diagnose, should be differentiated from impetigo, discoid eczema, and fixed drug eruption.

6.1.3 Diagnosis

Usually no investigations are required for the diagnosis of herpes simplex. The infection can be confirmed with Tzanck's test, which shows the presence of multinucleated giant cells.

6.1.4 Treatment

Mild uncomplicated cases require only symptomatic treatment with calamine lotion. Secondary bacterial infection can be reduced by topical fuscidic acid, mupirocin, or bacitracin. For more severe cases, topical acyclovir cream applied five or six times a day can cut down the severity of the infection if applied early in the disease. For widespread and systemic involvement cases, oral antiviral drugs may be used as follows:

- Acyclovir 200 mg given five times a day, for 5–7 days, or 5 mg/kg of body weight given I/V, 8 hourly for 5–7 days
- Suppression acyclovir 200–400 mg b.i.d. for 4–6 months
- Famciclovir – 250 mg t.i.d for 7 days

- Suppression famciclovir 250 mg b.i.d. for 4–6 months
- Valaciclovir – 500 mg b.i.d. for 7–10 days
- Suppression valaciclovir 500 mg – (less than ten episodes a year) b.i.d. for 4–6 months. 1,000 mg – (more than ten episodes a year) b.i.d. for 4–6 months

> *A history of repeat vesicular eruption on the same site should arouse the suspicion of herpes simplex.*
> *Fixed drug eruptions also occur at the same site, but the morphology is different.*
> *Pregnant women with active herpetic vaginal lesions should be delivered by Caesarian section.*

6.2 Herpes Zoster (Shingles)

This is an infection of the varicella zoster virus along a nerve trunk. It is caused by the reactivation of the varicella zoster virus, in persons who have had varicella in childhood. This may be along a cranial or spinal nerve, depending upon the ganglia where the varicella virus is present in a dormant state.

Most cases of herpes zoster occur in people older than 50 years of age. Initial symptom is pain, which can be very severe; this is followed by the eruption of grouped vesicles on an erythematous base, along a nerve trunk. This eruption is characteristic of herpes zoster, it stops at the midline. The initial pain is so severe that it may be mistaken for appendicitis, myocardial infarction, or pleurisy. The infection is most common in the thoracic region. This is probably because varicella infection is most concentrated on the trunk (Fig. 6.4).

Disseminated and hemorrhagic herpes zoster should raise the suspicion of underlying malignancy or immunosuppression.

6.2.1 Complications

Ophthalmic zoster may lead to eye complications. Postherpetic neuralgia is one of the most common complications of herpes

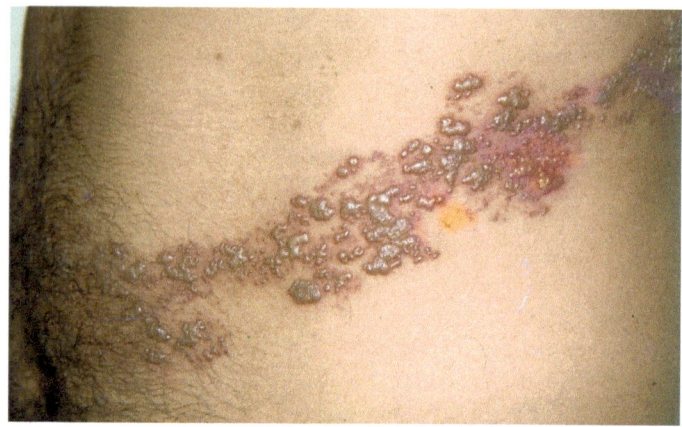

FIGURE 6.4. Herpes zoster.

zoster; the incidence of postherpetic neuralgia increases with age. Scarring can follow secondary infection.

Rarely, the infection can lead to motor complications such as bladder or rectal incontinence and paralysis of the diaphragm and ocular muscles.

6.2.2 Differential Diagnosis

Before the eruption of the rash, the pain in the dermatome is so severe that it may be mistaken for a myocardial infarct or appendicitis.

6.2.3 Diagnosis

The clinical signs are so diagnostic of herpes zoster that no tests are required for its diagnosis. Tzanck test, biopsy, and culture are required in unusual cases.

6.2.4 Treatment

Mild attacks of herpes zoster require only symptomatic treatment, but in the elderly and immunocompromized patients, systemic treatment is required. Oral acyclovir 800 mg is given five times a day for 7–10 days, or I/V acyclovir 10 mg/kg of body weight 8 hourly for 7–10 days.

The other antiviral drugs, which may be used, are valaciclovir 1 g t.i.d for 7 days, famciclovir 500 mg t.i.d for 7 days. In the elderly, the dose can be increased to 750 mg.

In cases of herpes zoster oticus, steroid therapy is also indicated to avoid the inflammatory swelling on the facial nerve. Prednisone 60 mg daily for 2 weeks and then taper the dose in the third week.

Management of postherpetic neuralgia (PHN). This is the most frustrating complication of herpes zoster in elderly patients. The aim of treatment in the elderly should be to prevent this complication from occurring. Analgesics should be initiated immediately; if less potent analgesics are ineffective then stronger agents should be prescribed until pain is relieved.

Antiviral therapy should be initiated within 72 h of the rash.

Treatment with amytriptiline 25 mg daily, soon after development of the rash, and continued for 3 months, may help prevent sensitization of the CNS. The dose is increased in continuous pain with paresthesias.

Some people advocate the addition of steroids with acyclovir to reduce the incidence of postherpetic neuralgia.

For stabbing pain, carbamazipine is of value. Initially 100 mg one to two times a day, increase gradually accordingly to response.

Application of topical aspirin (two tablets dissolved in 15–30 mL of chloroform) or capsaicin 0.025% cream may relieve pain in some patients.

> *If the tip of the nose is involved, then think of eye infection due to involvement of the nasociliary branch of the ophthalmic nerve.*
>
> *Blisters in the ear canal can be associated with facial palsy, and hearing loss is indicative of Ramsay Hunt syndrome.*
>
> *Herpes zoster in infancy indicates intrauterine exposure of the fetus to varicella infection.*
>
> *Treat herpes zoster in the elderly vigilantly, to prevent or decrease the incidence of postherpetic neuralgia.*
>
> *Herpes zoster patients can transmit the virus to another person, who has not been previously infected with chickenpox.*

6.3 Varicella (Chickenpox)

Chickenpox is an infectious disease caused by the varicella zoster virus; it is common in children. Transmission occurs via airborne droplets or vesicular fluid. The patients are infectious from 2 days before the onset of eruption until all the lesions have crusted. The disease is characterized by the development of a polymorphous eruption of macules, papules, and vesicles more prominent on the trunk than the extremities. Constitutional symptoms are proportional to the lesions. Varicella is the primary infection and zoster is the reactivation of the residual latent infection.

After an incubation period of 2–3 weeks, there is fever, malaise, anorexia, and sore throat. The eruption begins on the trunk and then spreads all over the body. The mucous membranes of the mouth and conjunctiva are also involved. The lesions begin as macules; develop into papules and vesicles and pustules when infected. Secondary infection is common in tropical countries because of heat and moisture, and in children living in unhygienic conditions. Crusting of the lesions precedes the healing. The patient is infectious until the appearance of crusts (Fig. 6.5).

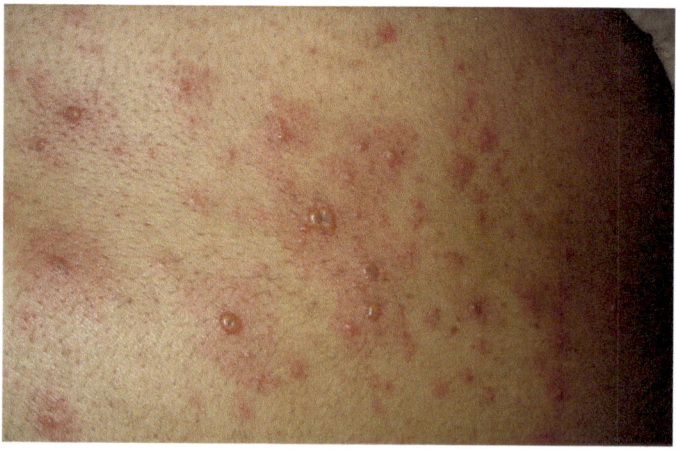

FIGURE 6.5. Chickenpox.

Dissemination of the virus can result in pneumonia, encephalitis, nephritis, and hepatitis. Systemic symptoms and complications are common in adults.

6.3.1 Diagnosis

The lesions of varicella are diagnostic. The condition can be confirmed by Tzanks test, culture, and biopsy but these are generally not required.

6.3.2 Differential Diagnosis

The disease is easy to diagnose. Small pox, which used to be in the differential diagnosis, has now been eradicated from most parts of the world; the infection was monomorphic and centrifugal. Varicella infection should also be differentiated from pityriasis lichenoides acuta and ricketsiall pox.

6.3.3 Treatment

Mild cases of varicella require only symptomatic treatment.

Antiviral therapy is indicated in adults, and immunocompromized patients. Oral acyclovir 800 mg given five times a day for 7–10 days, or I/V injection of acyclovir 10 mg/kg of body weight is given 8 hourly for 7–10 days.

Oral antiviral therapy is also required in children who are receiving long-term salicylate therapy to avoid the complication of Reyes syndrome (acute encephalopathy with fatty degeneration of the liver).

Pregnant women should receive high doses of acyclovir 1 8 mg/kg every 8 h.

Varicella vaccine is given to children at 12–18 months of age in a single dose. Above the age of 13, two doses are given at 4–8 weeks interval.

> Salicylates used during varicella may increase the risk of Reyes syndrome.

Varicella during the first trimester of pregnancy results in congenital varicella syndrome of the newborn.

Varicella vaccine should not be given to patients with immune deficiency or blood dyscrasias.

6.4 Warts

A wart is an overgrowth of differentiated squamous epithelium, caused by human papilloma viruses; these are small DNA viruses. More than 70 subtypes of the virus are known; these can be differentiated by DNA hybridization. Some may be oncogenic, e.g., type 16 and 18; these viruses are found in the genital areas, type 5 and 8 can also lead to squamous cell carcinoma. Human papilloma virus has still not been cultured in vitro. The main histological feature is vacuolation of cells in and below the granular layer; the infected cells are called koiliocytes. Warts interrupt the normal skin lines, and are studded with black puncta. These represent the thrombosed capillaries

Warts are most common in children, and young adults. Genital warts are seen in adults. Warts commonly appear at the sites of trauma. Hands and fingers (periungal warts) are the common sites affected.

Warts are flesh-colored or reddish brown; they can be verrucous (*common warts*), plane, or filiform. These appear as symptomless growths, but those on the soles, palm, and periungul regions may be painful due to pressure on the underlying nerves. *Plantar warts* occur at the site of maximum pressure on the foot, i.e., the head of the metatarsal bones, thick painful callus forms in response to the pressure. Plantar warts tend to grow inwards, due to the pressure of the foot; these appear as sharply demarcated round lesions, with a rough keratotic surface, surrounded by a smooth collar of thickened horn. The surface when pared shows small bleeding points. Multiple plantar warts can coalesce in a mosaic configuration (mosaic warts), or remain discrete. Sometimes, multiple small warts surround a large central wart. *Filiform warts* are elongated growths with a horny cap, most commonly seen on the face and neck. *Plane warts* are small, flat, skin-colored or pigmented growths, often multiple, and found on the face or hands. They have no black dots within them. *Anogenital warts (condylomata acuminata)* are transmitted by sexual contact. They are soft, elongated, filiform, pedunculated, or sessile. Syphilitic condylomata lata are flatter and smoother (Figs. 6.6–6.10).

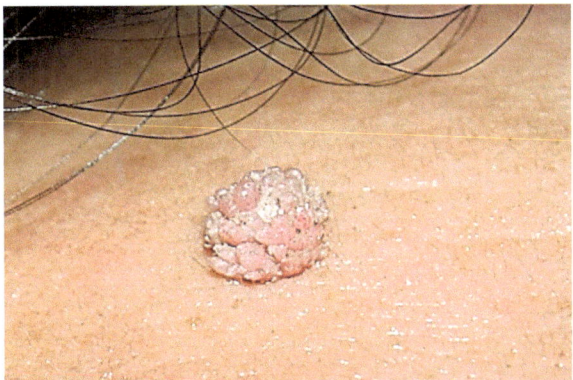

FIGURE 6.6. Verruca vulgaris.

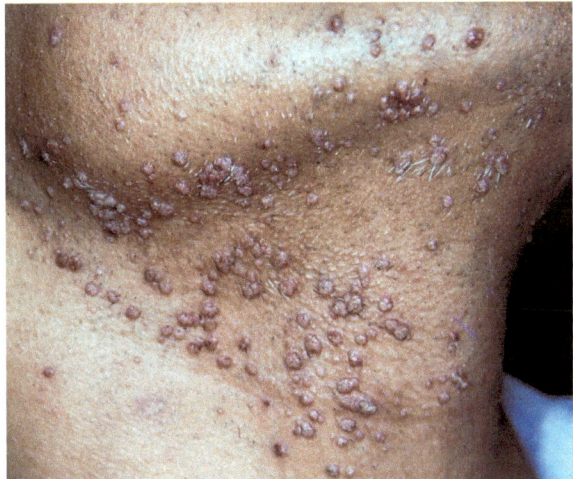

Figure 6.7. Plane warts.

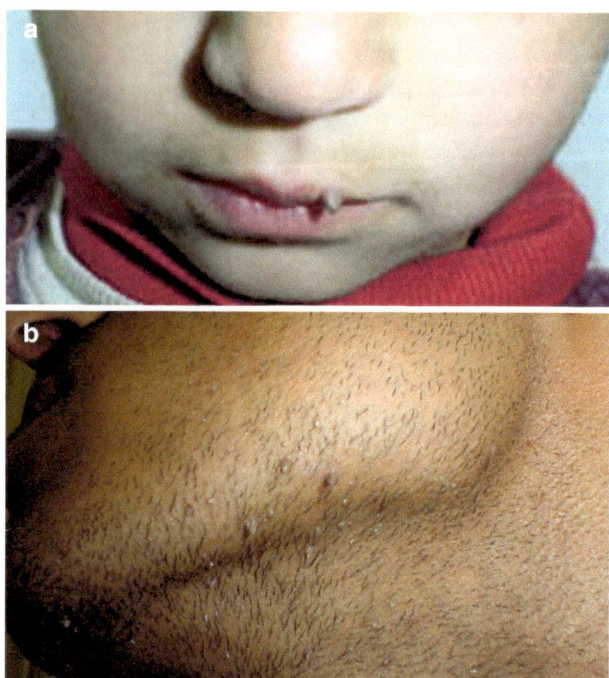

FIGURE 6.8. (**a**, **b**) Filiform wart.

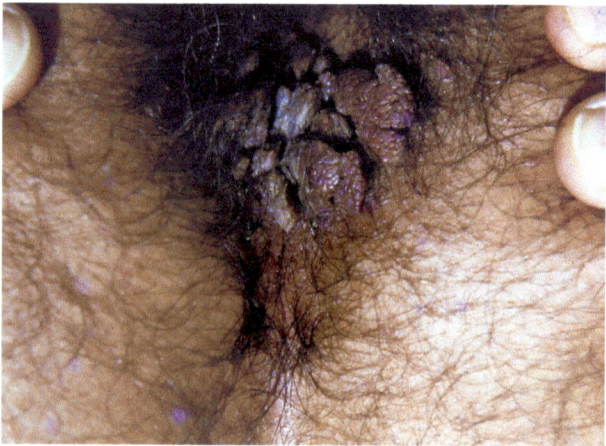

FIGURE 6.9. Condylomata acuminata.

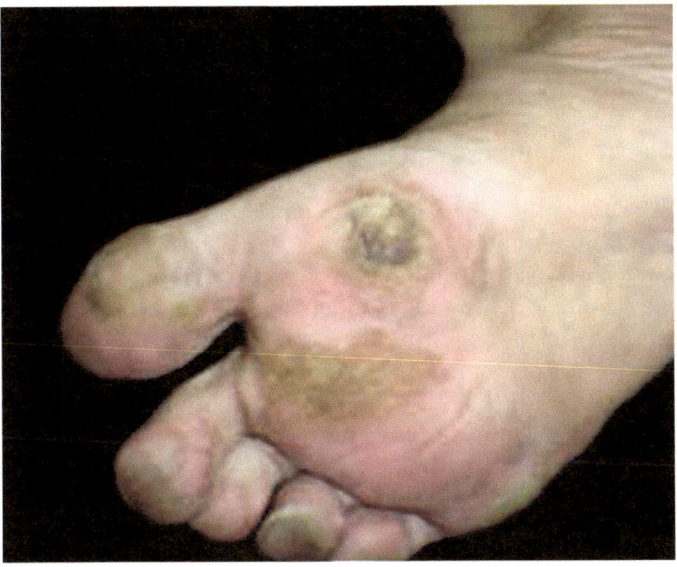

FIGURE 6.10. Mosaic warts.

6.4.1 Differential Diagnosis

Plane warts on the face should be differentiated from intradermal naevi, sebaceous hyperplasia, and molluscum contagiosum; common warts from lichen scrofulosorum and tuberculosis verrucosa cutis; filiform warts from skin tags; plantar warts from corns; and genital warts from condylomata lata of syphilis.

The thrombosed capillaries seen on the surface of a wart can help in the diagnosis warts; gentle paring will reveal the bleeding spots. The skin markings are present on a wart and are absent from corns. Condylomata acuminata have a verrucous surface and are skin-colored or slightly pigmented; condylomata lata have a smooth surface and are pinkish in color, and other signs of syphilis should be looked for.

6.4.2 Treatment

There are a number of ways by which warts, can be treated. The treatment depends upon the age of the patient, site of the wart, number of warts, previous treatments, etc. The most common is the use of keratolytic agents, the concentration of which depends upon the site of the wart and the age of the patient.

6.4.2.1 Common Warts/Plantar Warts/Periungal Warts

A preparation of 10–30% of salicylic acid, possibly with the addition of lactic acid (duofilm-16.7% salicylic acid and 16.7% lactic acid), is the treatment of choice for plantar warts. Daily application, for up to 3 months with weekly paring will clear the wart in the majority of cases. Adhesive skin plaster containing 40% of salicylic acid is also a suitable preparation.

Cryosurgery is also a suitable outpatient procedure repeated at 2–3 week interval. Liquid nitrogen is applied to the lesion until a rim of iced tissue about 2 mm in width develops in the normal skin surrounding the wart. The main disadvantage of freezing is pain; oral aspirin and potent topical steroids may help to reduce the pain. Scarring is unlikely with freezing if it is applied for less than 30 seconds.

Chemical cautry, with monochloracetic acid and trichloracetic acid, though irritant can be used in resistant cases.

Electrocautry is used in resistant cases; the disadvantage is scarring and persistent pain.

> *Use of aggressive cryosurgery over the volar and lateral aspects of the proximal phalanges has caused neuropathy; damage to the matrix may also occur, resulting in permanent nail damage. The nail may have to be removed if the wart is large and embedded in the nail.*

6.4.2.2 Filiform Warts

These are the easiest warts to treat. They can be removed by a curette, liquid nitrogen, or by light electrocautery.

6.4.2.3 Flat Warts

These warts are very resistant to therapy. They are present on the face and hands where aggressive methods cannot be used for treatment because of scarring. Tretinoin is useful; its efficacy probably results from its irritant effect. Very light touch with electrocautery or freezing of individual lesions, with liquid nitrogen can be attempted. For difficult cases imiquimod cream every other day, or 5-fluorouracil once or twice a day for 3–5 weeks may be tried.

6.4.2.4 Genital Warts

Podophylin is used for anogenital warts. A 25% solution in tincture benzoin is applied to the genital wart; the surrounding skin is protected with white soft paraffin. The solution is washed off after 4–6 hours. Application is repeated weekly until the wart clears. Podophylin is ineffective in other areas due to the lack of penetration.

6.4.2.5 For Resistant Plantar Warts

- Gluteraldehyde in 20% solution with aqueous ethanol in a gel base is used for plantar warts; it colours the skin brown and is therefore not used in other areas.
- 2–3% formalin (about 37% of formaldehyde in water) is helpful in plantar warts, but difficult to apply to the affected skin. The affected area has to be soaked in the solution for 15–20 minutes, using white soft paraffin as a barrier for the surrounding normal skin.

6.4.2.6 Recalcitrant Warts

- Cidofovir a purine nucleotide applied topically as a 1% gel or I/L 2.5 mg/mL is effective in plantar, anogenital, and laryngeal warts.
- Aldara cream 5% (imiquimod) is an immunomodulator with antiviral and anticancer properties. It is applied three times a week, for 16 weeks. Apply at bedtime and then wash off in the morning. Imiquimod cream is an immune response modifier that induces keratinocytes to produce cytokines, leading to wart regression. It may help build cell-mediated immunity. It works best on genital warts.

- Difficult warts can also be removed with lasers, surgical excision, contact sensitization, or photodynamic therapy.
- Contact sensitization by squaric acid dibutylester, poison ivy resin, and other allergens will induce allergic contact dermatitis. The wart is destroyed by delayed hypersensitivity reaction that occurs at the site of application of the allergen.

6.4.2.7 Extensive Warts

- These can be treated by oral etretinate.
- An application of 0.5% of fluorouracil with 10% salicyclic acid and 5% dimethylsulfoxide DMSO applied three times a day for 5 days can be used for widespread warts. Five percent fluorouracil applied daily for a month is also effective for the treatment of warts.

  > *The treatment of warts should not result in scarring. Scars can be painful for years.*
  > *It should be explained to the patient on their first visit, that warts require several weeks of treatment.*
  > *It is very important to debride the hyperkeratotic tissue over the wart, so that the medication can penetrate.*
  > *Viral genomes lie deep in the epidermis; this explains their chronicity and treatment failure of many warts.*

6.5 Molluscum Contagiosum

Molluscum contagiosum is caused by a poxvirus; it infects the epithelial cells, creating large intracytoplasmic inclusion bodies (molluscum bodies). The infected cells are large and round and disperse easily on slight pressure. The infected cells cause the disruption of the cell bonds between the cells. This lack of adhesion causes the central core of the lesion to be soft. The center of the papule ultimately disintegrates, forming a crater and releasing the molluscum bodies.

The disease is common in children; the face and trunk are the commonest sites involved. Lesions may be few or many (Fig. 6.11). Pubic and genital areas are affected in adults (Fig. 6.12). The individual lesions appear as firm, pearly papules, with a waxy surface. With time, the center becomes soft

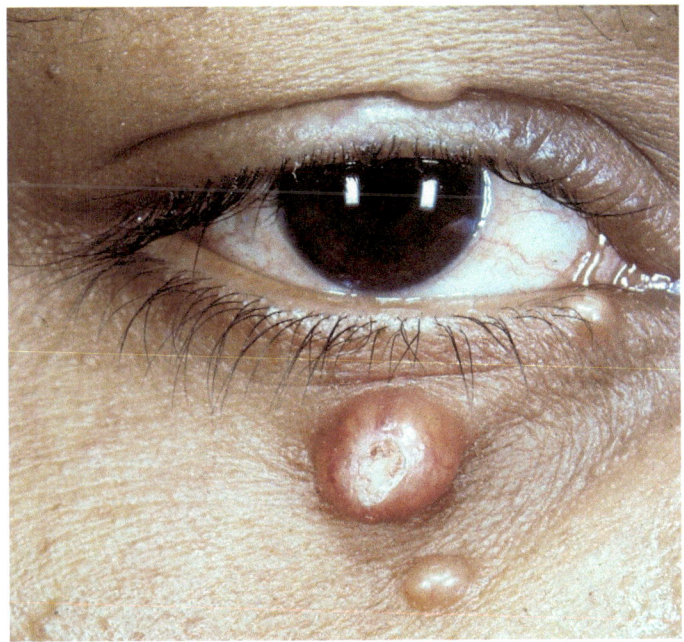

FIGURE 6.11. Giant molluscum contagiosum.

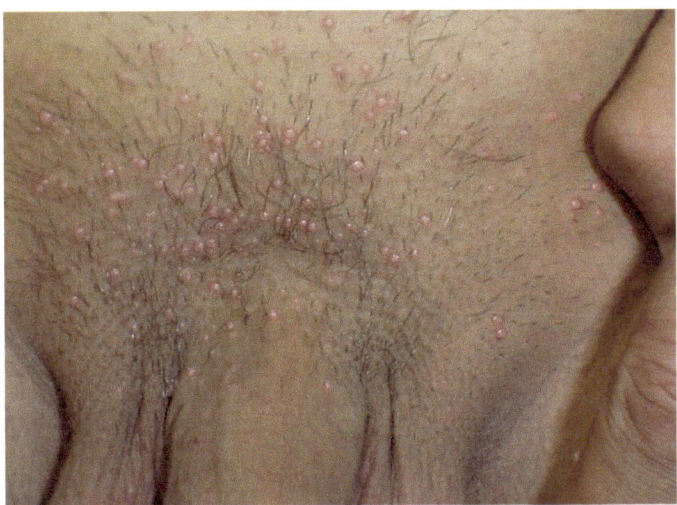

FIGURE 6.12. Molluscum contagiosum-genital.

and umbilicated. Lesions occur singly or in groups. Infection spreads by touch, autoinoculation, scratching, and shaving. Erythema at the periphery of the lesion may be due to scratching or it may be a hypersensitivity reaction. Conjunctivitis and keratitis may complicate lesions near the eyelid.

The diagnosis can be confirmed by examination of the molluscum bodies in a heated potassium hydroxide preparation.

6.5.1 Differential Diagnosis

Molluscum contagiosum should be differentiated from intradermal naevus, early stages of basal cell carcinoma, and sebaceous hyperplasia. An inflamed molluscum can be mistaken for a boil, and a giant molluscum for keratoacanthoma.

6.5.2 Treatment

It depends upon the age of the patient, and the number of lesions present. Cryosurgery is effective in adults applied at 3–4 week intervals. Individual lesions can be manually expressed with forceps, shaved, or by curettage.

Young children will not comply with these physical procedures; it is advisable to apply a local anesthetic before treatment although compliance is not guaranteed. A 5–10% ointment of salicylic acid can be applied to the molluscum daily, and then ask the mother to gently squeeze them when mature. A wart paint can also be applied to lesions that are away from the eyes, once or twice a week. Imiquimod cream or chlortetracycline cream can also be used in children, to produce inflammation, which then helps in the clearance of the molluscum.

Cantharidin is a safe and effective therapy. A small drop of 0.5–0.7% cantharidin solution is applied over the molluscum. Lesions blister and heal without scarring. It is applied with a cotton-tipped applicator (about 20 lesions treated per visit). After 4–6 h the area is washed with soap and water, or earlier if burning appears. The treatment can be repeated after 2–4 weeks (it should not be applied on the face).

An alternative method is to apply a combination of 1% cantharidin, 30% salicylic acid, 5% podophylin and cover the area with a tape for 1 day. The resulting blister is treated with polysporin until the reaction subsides.

A combination of salicylic acid plaster with povidine iodine has been reported to be effective.

Chemical cautery with liquid phenol diluted to 10–20% solution is also helpful

6.5.2.1 Resistant Cases

- Cidofovir 1–3% cream/gel can be applied once or twice daily.
- Oral cimetidine 40 mg/kg/day for 2 months may help in the clearance of the lesion in some cases.
- 5% aldara cream is applied once at night and washed off in the morning, or a 1% cream can be applied three times a day for 5 days.
- 25–50% trichloracetic acid peels.

The disease is infectious; the patient should avoid the use of public pools, baths, and shared towels.

6.6 Hand Foot and Mouth Disease

This is a disease caused by an enterovirus, it mainly affects young children. The disease begins with a low-grade fever, sore mouth, and abdominal pain, followed by a rash in 2–3 days. The rash affects the mouth, palms and soles. It is characterized by the formation of a vesicle surrounded by an erythematous halo. The lesion clears within 2–7 days.

Treatment if required is symptomatic.

6.7 Erythema Infectiosum (Fifth Disease)

The disease affects young children; small outbreaks can occur. An erythema, which looks like a child slapped on the cheeks, appears. This is quickly followed by reticulate erythema on the shoulders. The child feels well and the rash clears in a few days. In some cases, there may be arthralgia. No treatment is required.

6.8 HIV Infection (AIDS)

The infection is predominantly concentrated in developing countries but rapidly spreading in the third world. AIDS is caused by human immunodeficiency virus (HIV). The virus selectively attacks CD4 T lymphocytes, and these cells decrease in number. Symptoms of AIDS appear when the counts fall to 200/mm^3. The disease is manifest by increased susceptibility to infections, and some rare malignancies.

HIV is a retrovirus. Viruses in this group are characterized by lifelong persistence in their host. After seroconversion, there is a long asymptomatic phase before the appearance of clinical symptoms. Retroviruses replicate via a DNA intermediary made by the viral reverse transcriptase enzymes. During viral replication structural proteins are produced. Antibodies against these proteins are used for the diagnosis of HIV infection.

HIV infection is widespread. It is the result of both the direct effect of HIV infection and that associated with immune dysfunction. After an incubation period of 2–4 weeks, the primary illness presents with flu-like symptoms. The illness lasts for about 3 weeks. The patient is then asymptomatic for a variable length of time. However, the virus continues to replicate and the patient is infectious. A phase of generalized lymphadenopathy follows; there are no other signs and symptoms of the disease. The patient may be asymptomatic for 10–15 years. As the infection progresses the CD4 levels fall, the viral load rises, and the patient develops an array of signs and symptoms. AIDS can affect any system of the body.

Infection is transmitted through blood, semen, placenta, and milk. Sexual contact is the most common method of transmission. In children it is through the placenta and breast-feeding from an infected mother. In others, it is through blood transfusions and using infected needles as seen in drug addicts.

The skin is a common site for HIV-related pathology, as the functions of both Langerhans cells and dendritic cells are targeted. Cell-mediated immunity is reduced or absent. Cutaneous manifestations are more widespread, have an unusual character, a more prolonged course, and are more resistant to therapy. Infection with unusual organisms and neoplasms also occur.

The most common cutaneous malignancy is Kaposi's sarcoma; AID-related lymphomas are also common. Kaposi's sarcoma appears as purple or hyperpigmented patches, papules, nodules, or tumors in any part of the body. Common sites affected are the tip of the nose and hard palate. Kaposi's sarcoma may be the presenting sign of HIV disease.

The skin infections correlate with the degree of impaired immunity. It can be bacterial (folliculitis, cellulitis, furuncles, carbuncles), viral (herpes zoster, herpes simplex, warts, molluscum contagiosum), fungal (candidiasis, histoplasmosis, cryptococcosis, sporotrichosis) and parasitic (scabies); these infections are widespread and unusual in morphology. Bacillary angiomatosis and oral hairy leukoplakia are commonly seen in AIDS patients, though seldom seen otherwise. Eosinophilic folliculitis and pruritic papular eruptions are very itchy and can cause great distress to the patient. Drug eruptions are common in AIDS, especially with sulphonamides. Skin is a common site for opportunistic infections.

Various inflammatory disorders may present de novo, or are exacerbated by AIDS. These include seborrheic dermatitis, atopic dermatitis, psoriasis, and vasculitis. Malnutrition and acquired ichthyosis are common.

Internal infections such as encephalitis, pneumonia, diarrhoea, and nephritis are the major cause of death. Infections are severe and disseminated.

6.8.1 Diagnosis

The ELISA test, Western Block Technique, and polymerase chain reaction diagnose HIV infection.

Once the patient is diagnosed with HIV infection CD4 T cell counts should be done after every 3–6 months. On this basis, the infection is categorized in to three types:

Category 1 – CD4 T lymphocytes greater than 500/mm^3

Category 2 – CD 4 T lymphocytes between 200 and 499/mm^3

Category 3 – CD4 T lymphocytes less than 200/mm^3

6.8.2 Treatment

A combination of clinical assessment, viral load, and CD4 counts will influence the treatment of AIDS patients. A specialist in the field, who can monitor the patient and treat accordingly, should carry out the treatment. The four basic principles for the treatment of AIDS are:

- Antiretroviral therapy
- Restoration of immune response
- General management
- Treatment of opportunistic infection

The best combination of antiviral therapy is a combination of two nucleoside reverse transcriptase inhibitors plus a protease inhibitor or a non-nucleoside reverse transcriptase inhibitor, commonly known as HAART (highly active anti retroviral therapy). The commonly used reverse transcriptase inhibitors (RTI) are zidovudine, didanosine, zalcitabine, starvudine, and lamivudine. The protease inhibitors (PI) are saquinavir, indinavir, and ritonavir. The drugs should be carefully monitored; they can cause bone marrow depression with anemia and leucopenia.

6.8.3 Post Exposure Prophylaxis

The use of zidovudine following exposure to needlestick injury or other parental exposure with HIV, has shown to decrease the viral load in HIV infection. A combination of zidovudine and lamivudine, with or without PI is the treatment of choice in the UK.

6.8.4 Prevention

As the disease is spread via sexual contact, the best principle is to avoid contact with infected secretions, mucosal surface, and broken skin of infected persons. The prevention of sex with infected patients includes promoting monogamous relationship, reduction in the number of sexual partners, and avoidance of high-risk partners such as drug abusers and prostitutes. Use of latex condoms is important. No satisfactory vaccine has been found against AIDS; prevention of infection is therefore of paramount importance.

The best way to prevent the spread of AIDS is to encourage safe sex behavior promoting monogamous relationships and the use of condoms.

Regular screening for AIDS in endemic areas helps to identify and treat the infection in its early stages.

Chapter 7
Parasitic Infestations and Diseases Caused by Arthropods

The major groups of animal parasites that affect man are the protozoa, the unicellular organisms, and metazoa, the multicellular organisms. Only diseases of interest to the dermatologists will be discussed in this chapter.

7.1 Scabies

The disease is prevalent in underdeveloped countries, where overcrowding is common. The lesions of scabies are primary and secondary. The primary lesions are those that are due to the mite at the site of infestation, and secondary lesions are those that develop due to hypersensitivity to the mite. The lesions may be superimposed by secondary infection. Scabies is one of the most pruritic skin conditions, itching is marked at night. Family members are often affected, due to unhygienic conditions and overcrowding in poor communities, with cross-infection occurring readily.

Scabies is caused by Sarcoptes scabie (itching mite). After copulation the male dies, the female burrows under the skin, usually at night advancing about 2–3 mm daily, laying about two to three eggs daily for 4–5 weeks, and then dies. The eggs hatch into larvae, which migrate from the burrow and develop into adults. The life cycle from an egg to adult takes about 15 days.

The primary lesion of scabies is the burrow; it may be linear or curved with a vesicle at one end, representing the site of the mite. These are commonly present on the wrist, and side and web spaces of the fingers (Fig. 7.1).

Z. Zaidi, S. W. Lanigan, *Dermatology in Clinical Practice*, 125
DOI: 10.1007/978-1-84882-862-9_7,
© Springer-Verlag London Limited 2010

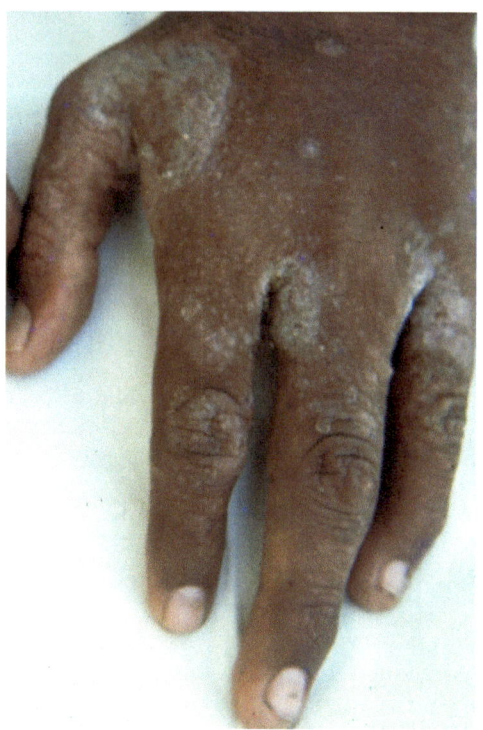

FIGURE 7.1. Scabies – note the interdigital involvement.

After 3–4 weeks hypersensitivity develops, characterized by itchy papules or nodules. The lesions are generalized, and seen particularly in the axillae, periareolar, periumbilical, abdomen, and buttock areas. The presence of papules on male genitalia is highly suspicious of scabies in endemic areas. Scratching spreads the mite to other areas of the body (Fig. 7.2).

The head and neck are not infected in adults, but the lesions may be found in these areas in children, as the mite prefers sites that have a low concentration of sebum. In children, vesicles and bullae may also be present. In patients who are immunodeficient or those with CNS disorders where sensations are impaired, *Norwegian scabies* develops, characterized by excessive crusting with a large number of mites and the patient is highly contagious.

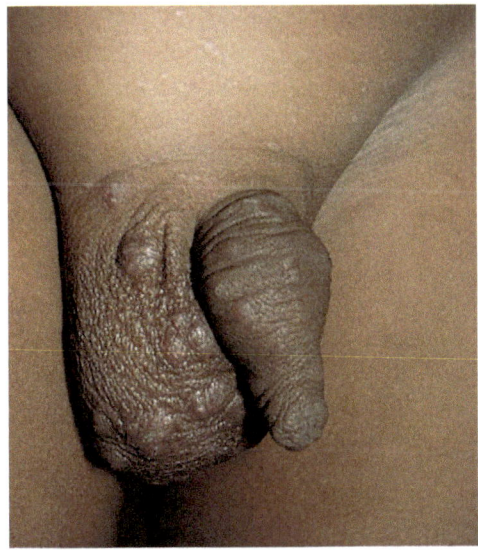

FIGURE 7.2. Nodular scabies – lesions on the genitals are highly suspicious of scabies in endemic areas.

Secondary infection is common due to scratching, with impetigo, folliculitis, and also eczema. Glomerulonephritis may complicate lesions infected by β Hemolytic streptococci. Persistent itchy nodules may remain on the genitalia or axillae for some months after adequate treatment especially in children.

The three characteristic features of scabies are:

- Nocturnal pruritus
- Characteristic distribution of the eruption
- Family members affected

7.1.1 Diagnosis

The diagnosis of scabies is confirmed by scrapings of a burrow, and the finding of the mite, its egg or scybala (feces) under a microscope. A dermatoscope is also helpful in the diagnosis of scabies. Mites may also fluorescence under a Wood's lamp.

7.1.2 Differential Diagnosis

Scabies should be differentiated from other pruritic disorders such as lichen planus, dermatitis herpetiformis, and atopic dermatitis.

7.1.3 Treatment

For the treatment of scabies, the following points should be noted:

All skin below the neck should be treated. Particular attention should be paid to the web of the fingers and toes, and under the nails. All close contacts should be treated at the same time, even if they are symptomless. Reapply the scabicidal to the hands if they are washed during treatment. The scabicidal is kept in contact with the skin for 12–24 h, depending upon the drug used.

Take a bath after the treatment is over. Change to clean clothes and bedsheets after the bath. The patients should be told that the pruritus would persist for 2–4 weeks after the successful treatment of scabies.

The idea of treatment is to kill all stages of the life cycle of the scabies mite (eggs, larvae, nymphs and adults) at the same time. The treatment should be repeated after 7 days, to kill any remaining mites and eggs.

The antiscabies preparations are: 10% sulphur ointment (2 consecutive day application) 25% benzyl benzoate lotion (2 consecutive day treatment), 5% permethrin cream (overnight application), 0.5% malathion lotion (applied for 24 h), 25% monosulphiram diluted in two to three parts of water and applied for 2–3 consecutive days, Gamma benzene hexachloride lotion (applied for 12–24 h; it is a central nervous system stimulant that causes seizures and death of the mite and should not be used for children) and Crotamiton once a day for 5 days (a weak scabicide).

For infants and children these scabicides should be diluted. Because of adverse neurotoxicity, gamma benzene hexachloride is no longer used in the UK.

Any residual itching can be treated with calamine lotion or crotamiton cream applied twice a day. Alcohol should not be ingested after the application of monosulphiram.

Post scabetic nodules can be treated by intralesional steroid injections, persistent cases can be excised.

Oral treatment with ivermectin and cotrimoxazole has been tried, but is not popular due to side effects, especially in adults. Ivermectin is given in a single dose of 200 µg/kg orally, or two tablets of ivermectin 12 mg given orally as a single dose and repeated after 8 days.

7.1.4 Norwegian Scabies

This is so called because it was first discovered in leprosy patients in Norway. Due to the lack of sensations, the disease manifested as excessive crusting (crusted scabies). Crusted scabies also occurs in patients with neurological and mental disorders, senile dementia, and immunosuppression. A lack of immunity and indifference to pruritus are suggested as reasons for Norwegian scabies (Fig. 7.3).

In patients with crusted scabies, there is asymptomatic crusting of the hands and feet, thick subungal keratosis, and dystrophy of the nails. Sometimes the crusting may spread to the trunk and extremities. Generalized lymphadenopathy is present in some cases, eosinophilia is common. These patients often need excessive and prolonged treatment.

7.1.4.1 Treatment

A keratolytic agent is applied before the scabicide to remove the crusts. The scabicide may require two to three applications on consecutive days, to ensure that enough penetrates the skin to kill the mites. It is better to treat Norwegian scabies in an isolated room; empty the soft furnishings and all the furniture of the room. The room should then be cleaned thoroughly, the wall and floors washed with 1% lindane.

Oral ivermectin may be used in difficult cases.

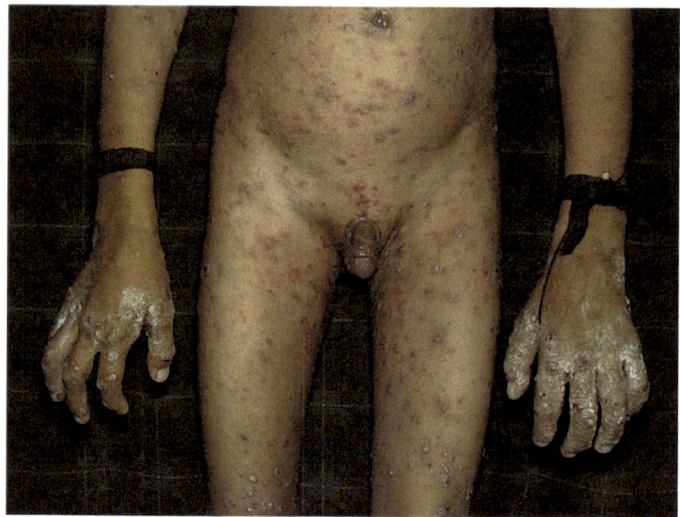

FIGURE 7.3. Scabies – note the crusted lesions on the hands with generalized hypersensitivity reaction.

7.1.5 Animal Scabies

In animal scabies, man is infected from pet animals, the dog being the commonest. The rash is similar to that of human scabies, but the burrows are absent as man is not the definite host. The disease is confirmed by brushing the animal's fur onto a sheet, and then sending the brushings for microscopic examination.

7.1.5.1 Treatment

The pet animal should be treated with 1% gamma benzene hexachloride (lindane) lotion or monosulfiram (tetmasol) soap. Carpets and soft furnishings should be vacuumed, the floor washed with 1% lindane emulsion.

The patient is treated with crotamiton cream until the itching subsides.

7.1.6 Other Mites

Humans can be infected by a number of mites such as the house dust mite, which is responsible for some allergic disorders such as asthma, and allergic rhinitis, and there is an increasing evidence for its role in atopic dermatitis. The Demodex mite inhabits the sebaceous glands of the nose, forehead, chin, and scalp. It may cause folliculitis; its role in rosacea is debated. Chiggers or the scrub mite transmits scrub typhus. Harvest mite is found on low vegetations; an acquired hypersensitivity reaction may occur due to mite's saliva.

> *Treatment failure in scabies is usually due to the scabicide not being applied to the whole body, or failure to treat the entire family and contacts.*
> *All family members and close contacts should be treated.*
> *Papules and nodules on the male genitals are characteristic of scabies.*
> *The disease is confirmed by finding the female mite in the burrow.*
> *A good scabicide is that which acts on all the stages in the life cycle of the mite at the same time.*
> *Look for mites in the burrows and not in the itchy papules.*

7.2 Pediculosis

Pediculosis is caused by infestation with lice. It can infect the scalp (pediculosis capitis), the body (pediculosis corporis), or the pubic area (pediculosis pubis). The body louse is the largest; it is found in people with poor hygiene such as vagabonds. Pediculosis pubis is transmitted sexually; about 30% of patients have at least one other sexually transmitted disease. Crab louse causing pediculosis pubis is the smallest in size.

7.2.1 Pediculosis Capitis

The louse attaches itself to the hair by strong crab like claws. It sucks the blood of the host; feeding about five times each day. The female lice lay about seven to ten eggs per day; the eggs are firmly cemented to the hair. The eggs hatch in about 8 days and the adult lice develop in about 10 days. The infection causes itching, most prominent behind the ears and nape of the neck, which leads to secondary infection. In case of recurrent folliculitis of the scalp with enlargement of the cervical lymph nodes, exclude peduculosis capitis (Fig. 7.4).

Infection is transmitted to others by sharing combs, brushes, and beddings. The lice are active and can travel quickly; this explains why the infection can be so easily transmitted. The adult lice can survive outside the host for 3 days and the nit for 10 days.

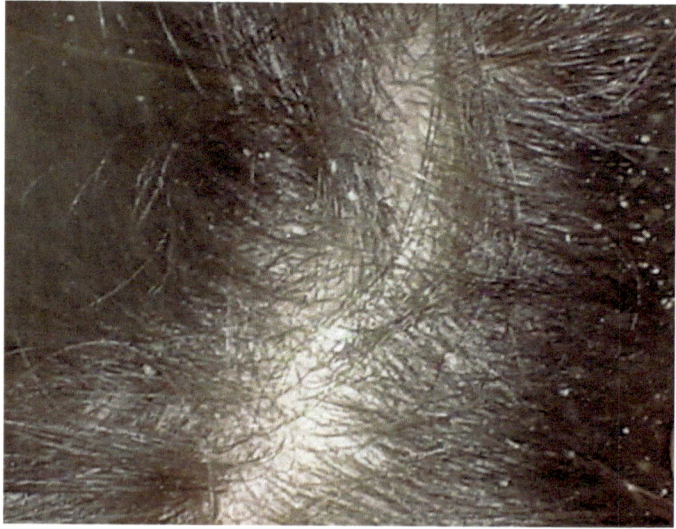

FIGURE 7.4. Pediculosis capitis.

7.2.2 Peduculosis Corporis

The body louse lives in the seams of clothing, found in people who seldom take a bath or change their clothes. The eggs are cemented to the clothing; the adults attack the body only to feed. The infestation is manifested by the scratch marks, most prominent in the interscapular region, posterior aspect of the axillae, hips, and thigh. Long-standing cases show patches of pigmentation, pyoderma, eczematization, and lichenification.

7.2.3 Pediculosis Pubis

This is sexually transmitted; it can also be transmitted through contaminated toilet seats and beddings. In hairy persons, the infestation may spread to the upper thigh, abdomen, axillae, chest, and beard. Adults may spread pubic lice to the eyelashes of children. (Scalp hair is too dense for its habituation) (Fig. 7.5).

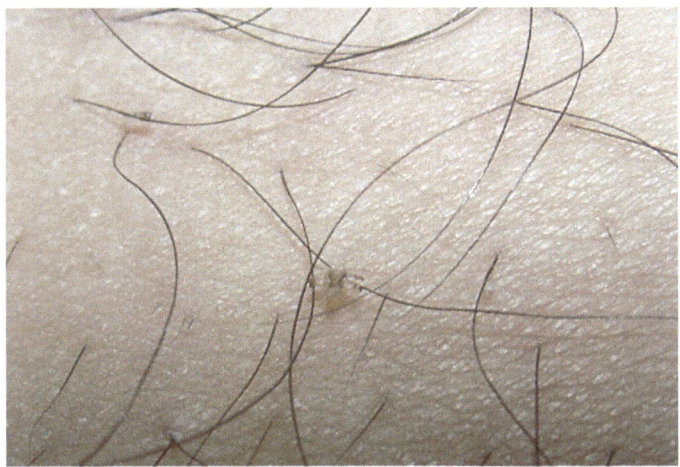

FIGURE 7.5. Pediculosis pubis – pubic lice prefers hair with low density.

Pruritus is the main symptom. In some cases bluish or gray macules are found on the abdomen and pubic area, these are called "maculae ceruleae." The exact pathogenesis for these is not known; it may be due to a toxin injected by the louse, or altered blood pigment.

7.2.4 Diagnosis

This is easy; the symptoms of the disease and the presence of the lice and nits on the scalp and hair are diagnostic. Nits found near the scalp indicate recently hatched eggs; those away from the scalp may not indicate active infestation. Live nits fluorescence, and can easily be detected by a Wood's Lamp; this is useful for detection of lice infestation in school-children. Nits that contain a louse are fluorescence white, while empty nits are fluorescence gray.

7.2.5 Differential Diagnosis

Pediculosis capitis should be differentiated from folliculitis, impetigo, and seborrheic dermatitis of the scalp.

Pediculosis corporis should be differentiated from scabies, eczema, and lymphomas.

Pediculosis pubis should be differentiated from eczema of the pubic area.

7.2.6 Treatment

All members of the family should be treated; their combs and hairbrushes should not be shared. An effective drug should act against both the lice and ova. A hair dryer should not be used to dry the hair after the use of medication for lice as heat degrades the insecticide.

Treatment should be repeated after 7–10 days, as most insecticides used for pediculosis are not completely ovicidal. After shampooing the hair, it should be combed with a fine comb. The fine comb should be used for 1–2 weeks after the application of the insecticide. Lotions are preferable to shampoos, as shampoos are more prone to the development of resistance against the insecticide; they are also too diluted to be effective. A short contact of 10 min does not kill the ova.

Most of the drugs used for pediculosis are the same as those for scabies.

- Permethrin in the form of 1% cream paralyses the nerves that allow the lice to breathe. Lice can close their respiratory passage for 30 min when immersed in water. Therefore, all insecticides should be applied on dry hair. Permethrin is not 100% ovicidal, so a second application is needed after 1 week. Permethrin remains active for 2 weeks after application and can be detected in the hair for 14 days.
- Pyrethrin is also available as a cream, gel, and shampoo. It is not ovicidal and has no residual action.
- Malathion lotion. This is ovicidal and pediculocidal. It binds to the hair and has residual action. Not used for infants and children.
- Gamma benzene hexachloride (lindane), as 1% shampoo, should not be used for children.
- Benzyl benzoate lotion. This is cheap, though slightly irritating to the scalp; it can be used for delousing large families of low income.
- Carbaryl as a 1% solution is also used for pediculosis. The lotion is rubbed well into the scalp at night and washed off the next morning.

Nits can also be removed with 5% acetic acid or white vinegar left for a few hours on the scalp.

For mass delousing 2–5% DDT emulsion or 10%, DDT powder is applied to the scalp overnight and then washed in the morning. Oral treatment with cotrimoxazole has been reported to be effective for the treatment of head lice. The louse ingests the antibiotic which interferes with the synthesis of vitamin B, without which the lice cannot survive. Oral ivermectin is also effective, it causes paralysis and death of the lice, but these medications do not affect the nits, a second treatment is therefore required after 10 days.

A head louse repellent, containing 2% piperonal may be used in patients who are repeatedly infected, and for prevention in other cases. Its value is uncertain.

Pediculosis corporis. It is the clothing and not the patient that requires treatment. High temperature laundering, of the clothes is effective. Lice and the nits are killed by high temperature. Once this has been achieved 5% permethrin cream or 1% lindane lotion may be used on the patient's skin.

Pediculosis pubis. Insecticides used for pediculosis capitis are also used for pediculosis pubis. In view of the possibility of involvement of the body and axillary hair, it is preferable to treat the whole of the trunk and limbs. All sexual contacts should also be treated. The treatment should be repeated after 1 week.

For the eyelashes, a thick layer of petrolatum applied twice a day will suffocate the lice and kill it.

> *Do not apply the drug on broken skin and infected skin, and protect the eyes while applying the scabicide and pediculocide.*
> *Exclude pediculosis of the scalp in patients with recurrent impetigo and eczema of the scalp.*
> *Pediculosis corporis is also the vector for epidemic typhus, trench fever, and relapsing fever.*

7.3 Leishmaniasis

This is a group of diseases caused by several species of the parasite of genus Leishmania; different species cause infection of the skin, mucous membrane, and viscera. Each species has a particular geographical distribution, they are morphologically identical, but can be differentiated by isoenzyme pattern, DNA analysis, and monoclonal antibodies. Leishmaniasis may be cutaneous, mucocutaneous, or visceral. Leishmaniasis can also be conveniently divided into Old World and New World forms.

Cutaneous leishmaniasis (Old world leishmaniasis) – this may occur as a nodule, which resembles a furuncle, developing from a bluish-red papule, at the site of a sandfly bite. This may break down to form an ulcer with raised edges (L major). The other form appears as a slowly extending plaque with a shallow ulcer appearing in the center (L tropica). Chronic leishmaniasis (L recidivans) is the result of a host reaction, in which the cellular immunity fails to sterilize the lesion. Brownish-red papules appear, close to the site of an old lesion. The papules may coalesce to form a plaque closely resembling lupus vulgaris (Figs. 7.6–7.8).

Mucocutaneous leishmaniasis (American Leishmaniasis) – the causative organism is L braziliensis.

In New World leishmaniasis the lesions are frequently multiple, exuberant, nodular, and more destructive. Lymphatic

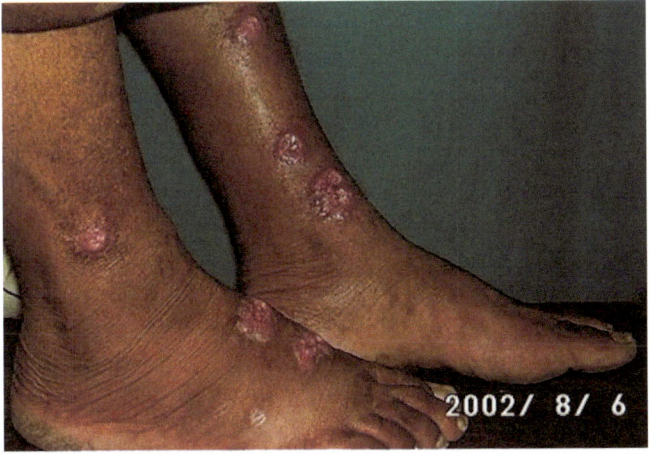

FIGURE 7.6. Leishmaniasis.

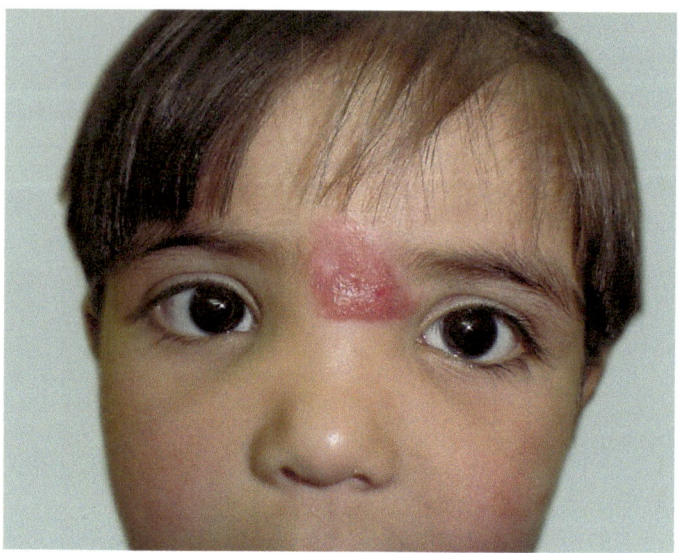

FIGURE 7.7. Leishmaniasis.

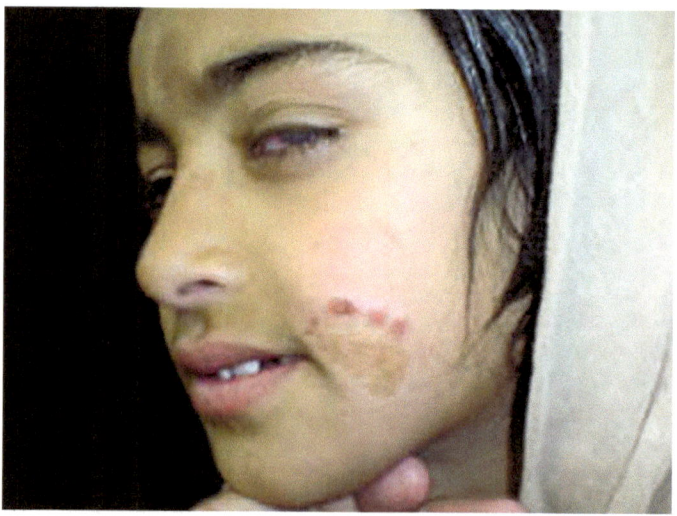

FIGURE 7.8. Leishmaniasis recidivans.

obstruction is relatively common. Another distinguishing feature is the prominent tendency for mucocutaneous lesions to develop. The mouth and oropharynx may be involved. The disease is slowly progressive and can lead to severe tissue destruction.

The parasite first affects the skin and then the mucous membrane of the upper respiratory tract. The anterior part of the nasal septum is first affected, leading to considerable ulceration and destruction

Visceral leishmaniasis – also known as kala-azar, because of the dark macular pigmentation of the skin, that occurs during early infection. The disease affects the reticuloendothelial system of the body. Young people are more commonly affected; there is fever, cough, and diarrhea. The skin is dry, rough, and often pigmented. Post-kala-azar dermal leishmaniasis develops 1–3 years after the disappearance of the disease. The lesions on the skin may be hypopigmented, erythematous, or nodular.

7.3.1 Treatment

Pentavalent antimonials form the basis of treatment. Pentostam (sodium stiboglugonate) or glucantine (meglumine antimonite) are commonly used. It is given in a dose of 20 mg/kg of body weight by I/M injection for 20 days. The dose can be repeated after 10 days if the response is incomplete. Antimonials should be given with care; bradycardia, dysrrhythmia, and circulatory collapse may occur, during treatment. Close monitoring of the pulse and heart sounds should be performed while giving the injection, and for half an hour afterwards. If any side effect occurs, an injection of diazepam should be given immediately.

I/L pentavalent antimonials, curettage, or cryosurgery can also be used in early lesions.

Oral zinc sulphate 5 mg/kg/day for 4 weeks, has shown promising results in a recent Indian trial.

The other drugs used for the treatment of leishmaniasis are dapsone, rifampicin, levamisole, and ketoconazole. Upto four courses of Amphotericin B or pentamidine in a dose of 3 mg/kg of body weight for 10 days may be given in resistant cases.

Treatment is less successful for cutaneous leishmaniasis than for visceral leishmaniasis as antimonials are poorly concentrated in the skin.

Larva migrans is found throughout the hot and humid tropics. The larva penetrates the skin but remains unchanged, as man is not the natural host. The disease is caused by the larva of some nematodes such as Ancylostoma brazeliensis or Ancylostoma canis, which are parasitic to cats and dogs.

The feet, buttocks, and trunk are most frequently affected. Papules appear at the site of inoculation preceded by slight local itching. Pruritus is severe especially at night. Migration occurs in about 4 days after inoculation and progresses at the rate of 2 cm daily. Cord-like superficial burrows develop; these linear lesions may be interrupted by papules, which mark the site of resting larvae. The larvae usually die in 2–8 weeks with resolution of the eruption (Fig. 7.9).

Secondary infection and lichenification may obscure the clinical picture. Larva migrans may be accompanied by Loeffler's syndrome (eosinophilia and pulmonary infiltrate) particularly in severe infection. Similar eruptions can be caused by larva of flies such as Gastrophilus, the horse botfly and cattle warble fly (Hypoderma bovis) and other nematodes.

7.4.1 Treatment

The treatment of choice is topical application of 10% thiobendazole. Two tablets of 0.5 g of thiobendazole are mixed in 10 g of petrolatum and applied twice daily. Ninety-five percent of cases clear within a week. Oral thiobendazole is too toxic to use.

Albendazole tablets, 400 mg daily by mouth for 3 days is safe and often effective.

7.5 Myiasis

Myiasis is an infestation of any part of the body by the larva of diptera. The eggs are laid in neglected ulcers, in which maggots are later found. In ancient times, maggots were used to treat necrotic tissue; this method of treating necrotic tissue is in vogue again.

Lesions may present as:

- Myiasis of a wound, in which eggs and larvae (maggots) are present. This is common in neglected ulcers and wounds in rural tropics. Abscess, lymphangitis, cellulitis, and tetanus may develop.
- Furunculoid lesions.
- Subcutaneous tunnels such as larva migrans.

The nasal, ocular, auricular cavities, and internal organs can be affected by the migration of the larva.

7.5.1 Treatment

- Survival of the mature larva depends upon the availability of oxygen; if the opening on the surface of the wound is blocked the larvae will die. This can be achieved by applying a tape or petroleum jelly on the surface of the wound.

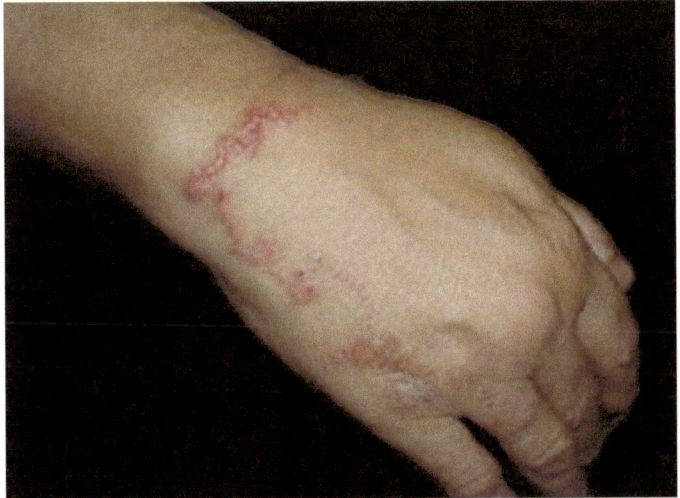

FIGURE 7.9. Larva migrans.

- Wound myiasis is treated by surgical removal of the maggots and douching of the wound for 30 min with 15% chloroform, dissolved in light vegetable oil.
- Treatment of furuncular myiasis is by injections of local anesthetics into the skin, which anesthetize both the skin and the larva. Then incising the lesion or pushing the larva out with pressure from beneath.
- The larva can be suffocated by topical application of thiobendazole. Albendazole can also be used.

7.6 Filariasis

This is a helminthic infection; the infection is caused by Wuchereria bancrofti and Brugia malayi. The disease is widespread in parts of Africa, Asia, North, and South America and in the South Pacific islands.

The larval stage is inoculated in human beings by the bite of a mosquito. The larva develops into adult worms that live in lymphatics. After mating, the female worm produces millions of microfilariae. The microfilariae circulate in large numbers at night in the peripheral blood. These are taken up by the mosquito and develop into infected larva. The onset of the disease in man is characterized by recurrent attacks of acute lymphangitis. The acute inflammation lasts for a few days, but may recur several times a year. The location of the lymphatic damage determines the site and type of clinical manifestation of the disease, e.g., elephantiasis of the lower limbs follows obstruction to the inguinal lymph nodes. Epididymo-orchitis and hydrocele may be associated findings; the scrotum may reach an enormous size. Elephantiasis occurs in association with repeated skin sepsis (Fig. 7.10).

7.6.1 Investigation

In the early stages the disease should be differentiated from thrombophlebitis and infection; a high eosinophil blood

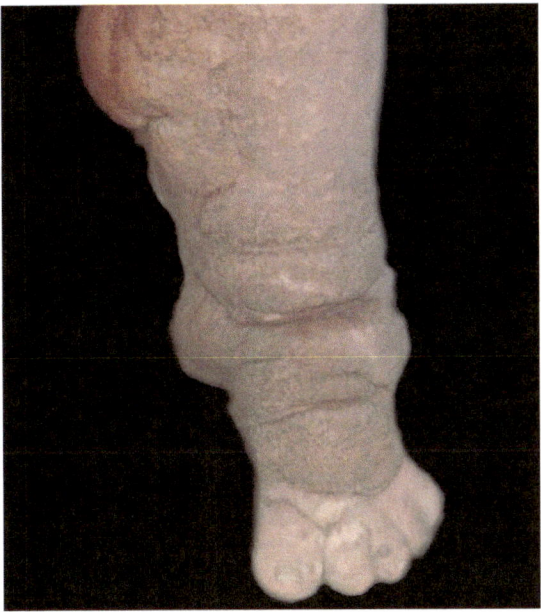

FIGURE 7.10. Elephantiaisis.

count is characteristic of helmintic infection. Microfilariae are seen in the peripheral blood at night, samples of blood should be drawn between 12 pm and 2 am at night. Microfilariae are also found in the peripheral blood after a single dose of diethyl carbamazine.

7.6.2 Treatment

Diethylcarbamazine kills the adult worm and microfilariae in the peripheral blood. The dose should be given as follows:

Fifty milligram od on the first day, 50 mg tds on the second day, 100 mg tds on the third day, and then 2 mg/kg of body weight from the fourth day for 3 weeks. This is to prevent the host reaction to dying microfilariae. It may be necessary to repeat the dose after a few months, if microfilariae appear in the blood. Follow-up is necessary.

Ivermectin 12 mg as a single dose, to be repeated after 2 weeks, improves the cure rate.

Treatment of elephantiasis given on page ....

7.6.3 Prevention

In endemic areas an annual single dose of diethylcarbamazine 100 mg for adults and 50 mg for children have reduced but not eliminated the infection. This is combined with mosquito control measures.

7.7 Onchocerciasis (River Blindness)

This is a filarial disease caused by the bite of a buffalo fly. It is found mostly along fast-moving streams. The disease is found in the tropical regions of America and Africa. These are the largest insects borne filaria; some may be as large as 70 cm in length. The microfilarae reside in the connective tissue and lymphatics of the skin and eye.

The incubation period is about 1 year. The skin is infected first and then the eye. An erysipelas-like eruption, or itchy papules develop at the site of the bite. The lesions later become lichenified with pigmentation and scarring. The skin then loses its elasticity, becomes dry, depigmented, and scaly. Mature worms and microfilaria are sometimes found in the subcutaneous tissue; these later become fibrotic and calcified. These painless lumps are called onchocermata.

Ocular involvement is serious; with conjunctivitis, keratitis, and choroiditis, eventually leading to blindness. The disease is also called River Blindness, as the buffalo fly breeds close to rivers.

7.7.1 Treatment

Ivermectin is the treatment of choice. It is given as a single dose of 100–200 µg/kg. It is nontoxic and does not trigger severe reactions as seen with diethylcarbamazine.

It may be necessary to repeat the dose after a few months if the disease reappears.

7.7.2 Prevention

Mass population treatment with ivermectin.
Onchocerciasis is a common cause of blindness in Africa.
This is also a filarial infestation, caused by the bite of a chrysops fly. The disease is found in the hot, humid climate of equatorial Africa. It is an infection of the subcutaneous tissue, eye, and the viscera. The larva of Loa Loa enters the skin following the bite of the fly; they then enter the viscera and lungs via the bloodstream. The adult worm makes frequent journeys through the skin. In the skin, swelling of the subcutaneous tissue develops; these are known as calabar swellings. Hyperpigmentation occurs when the swellings subside.

Infection of the eye and joints can be incapacitating. When the conjunctiva is infected, the worm can actually be seen crossing the eye. General urticaria and edema of the limbs can occur. The finding of microfilaria in the blood is diagnostic.

7.8.1 Treatment

Diethylcarbamazine is the treatment of choice; the dose schedule should be similar to that of filariasis. Topical antipruritics and oral histamine are helpful.

7.9 Insect Bites

When insects bite, they produce a local reaction at the site of the bite. This may be followed by an anaphylactic reaction, or there may be a delayed hypersensitivity response that occurs 2–3 weeks after the bite. The reaction is due to the injection of foreign proteins or chemicals into the skin by the insect. The degree of host reaction depends upon the degree of immunity present in the patient. Some people do not elicit any reaction, as they are not allergic to the bite. All household members respond in a different way to the bite of the same insect, unless the insect is a carrier of infection such as malaria by a mosquito.

Insects bite out of anger – sting bite; this usually results in immediate pain, or insects bite when they are hungry – hunger bite. Insects that sting include honeybees, wasps, and fire ants. Insects that bite for hunger include mosquitoes, fleas, bedbugs, and lice. Spiders, ticks, and chiggers are other insects that attack human skin.

- The sting bite produces immediate pain and an urticarial reaction at the site of the bite. Of the stinging insects, only the honeybee leaves its stinger behind; this appears as a sharp barb projecting from the skin. In susceptible individuals, a sting bite may lead to anaphylaxis.
- Fire ants produce multiple hives, which later progress to papules, vesicles, and pustules.
- The bite of a spider produces local necrosis and ulceration.
- Fleabites usually occur in groups or clusters. They are capable of jumping approximately to about 2 ft; the lesions are most common on the lower legs and ankles.
- Chiggers favor the leg and areas with tight fitting clothing; they produce papules, vesicles, and occasionally bullae.
- The female tick attaches itself to the skin by sticking in its proboscis, and then sucks the blood of the host from the superficial blood vessels. It remains attached to the skin until it is engorged and then falls off. This usually takes about 12 days. In a few hours at the site of puncture, an urticarial wheal is produced. During this period, the patient may have fever, abdominal pain, and vomiting (tick bite pyrexia). The bite of a hard tick is painless, while that of a soft tick is painful. A pruritic urticarial swelling develops with a central necrosis. Tick paralysis may follow a hard tick bite.
- The bedbug bite is painless; the saliva contains a protein that gives rise to a hypersensitive reaction around the punctum. Papular urticaria and extensive erythemas have been reported. Bedbug bites are found in the covered areas of the body.

Most of the insect bites have a central punctum, by which they are detected, and the patients give a history of the bite. Insect bites can become secondarily infected and eczematized by scratching.

7.9.1 Prophylaxis

Biting insects are attracted by body odor. These insects can be repelled by:

- DEET (*N*, *N*-diethyl-3-methylbenzamide). This is the most effective insect repellent. When DEET-based repellents are applied in combination with permethrin-treated clothing, protection against insect bites is nearly 100%.
- DEET is especially active against mosquitoes, gnats, chiggers, and ticks. It does not repel stinging bites. DEET blocks the ability of theses insects to track the victim's body odor. In hot humid weather the repellent should be applied after every 2 h, in dry weather it can be repeated every 6 h.
- Oil of citronella. This is found in products like candles, lotions, sprays, and towelettes.
- Antihistamines. Prophylactic administration of nonsedating antihistamine is effective for protection against immediate and delayed hypersensitivity reactions.
- Permethrin. This is effective as a clothing spray, against mosquitoes and ticks.
- Thiamine (vitamin B1). A few reports have indicated that 75–150 mg of thiamine hydrochloride taken orally during summer months protect against insect bites. It may be worth trying in children who are bitten often.

7.9.2 Treatment

Cool, wet compresses; calamine lotion; topical steroids; and oral antihistamines are helpful for insect bites.

7.10 Papular Urticaria

Papular urticaria is a common chronic pruritic papular eruption caused by an allergic skin reaction to insect bites. It is
common in children belonging to families of low socioeconomic status; adults develop the disease when they move to a
new environment and are exposed to bites by different
arthropods. In urban areas, the common causes are fleas and
bedbugs. In rural areas mosquitoes, mites, fleas, and chiggers
are the common causative agents.

7.10.1 Clinical Features

The lesions pass through two stages; an urticarial wheal that
fades in 1–2 days and is replaced by a firm papule. A vesicle
often develops at the apex of the papule that becomes excoriated by scratching; each attack may last for 2–10 days. The
lesions occur in crops usually at night, the lesions are discrete
papules a few millimeters in diameter, but they may occur in
groups. Pruritus is severe; scratching causes lichenification
and secondary infection.

The distribution of the eruption may provide a clue to the
causative arthropod. Involvement of the exposed parts suggests a flying insect, infection on the ankles and legs are
frequently caused by fleas, and lesions on the trunk are often
caused by bedbugs. A change in the environment leads to
recovery; residual hyperpigmentation is common. Host sensitivity is probably important since only one member of the
family is usually affected. The disease may gradually disappear due to desensitization following repeated exposure to
the bites. The course of the disease is chronic; the eruption
prevails in warm and rainy weather, and relapses may occur
every summer. New lesions may activate the old ones.

7.10.2 Treatment

The treatment should begin with elimination of the insects;
insecticidal powders such as pyrethrin are effective in

treating furniture and bedding. Bedbugs lie inactive in crevices in furniture during the day and emerge at night.

If the source cannot be isolated, insect repellents may be helpful. Oral antihistamines may reduce itching; antipruritic lotions may be applied topically. Corticosteroids may also be applied in severe cases.

> *Insect bites are usually linear or occur in groups, they have a punctum.*
>
> *Insect bites present as itchy wheals, papules, vesicles, or bullae.*
>
> *The cutaneous reaction is due to a pharmacological, irritant, or allergic response to the introduced foreign material caused by the bite of the insect.*

Chapter 8
Eczema

Eczema is a common inflammatory skin disease. It is an epidermal reaction to specific injurious agents; these agents may be internal or external, acting singularly or in combination. Eczema is a reaction pattern characterized histologically by spongiosis, with varying degrees of acanthosis and superficial perivascular lymphohistiocytic infiltration. Most eczemas share certain general features, and each different type of eczema will have some distinguishing markers of their own. Eczema can be broadly classified as acute, subacute, and chronic, or exogenous and endogenous. Eczemas are easy to diagnose but difficult to define!

8.1 Classification

8.1.1 Clinical

- Acute eczema – this is characterized by erythema, papules, vesicles, oozing, and crusting.
- Subacute eczema – as the eczema becomes chronic, edema diminishes; clinically it is represented by erythema, scaling, and crusting.
- Chronic eczema – presents with thickening of the skin, skin markings become prominent (lichenification); pigmentation and fissuring of the skin occur.

Z. Zaidi, S. W. Lanigan, *Dermatology in Clinical Practice*,
DOI: 10.1007/978-1-84882-862-9_8,
© Springer-Verlag London Limited 2010

Clinically an eczematous disease may start at any stage and evolve into another.

8.1.2 Source of Injurious Agent

- Exogenous – contact dermatitis, photosensitive eczema, infective eczema
- Endogenous – atopic dermatitis, seborrheic dermatitis, nummular eczema, hypostatic eczema, pompholyx, pityriasis alba, asteatotic eczema, lichen simplex chronicus

8.2 Clinical Features

8.2.1 Acute Eczema

Acute eczema is recognized by oozing, weeping, crusting, vesicles, or bullae in severe cases (Fig. 8.1). Another diagnostic feature of eczema is that it has ill-defined borders. Histologically it is characterized by spongiosis (intercellular

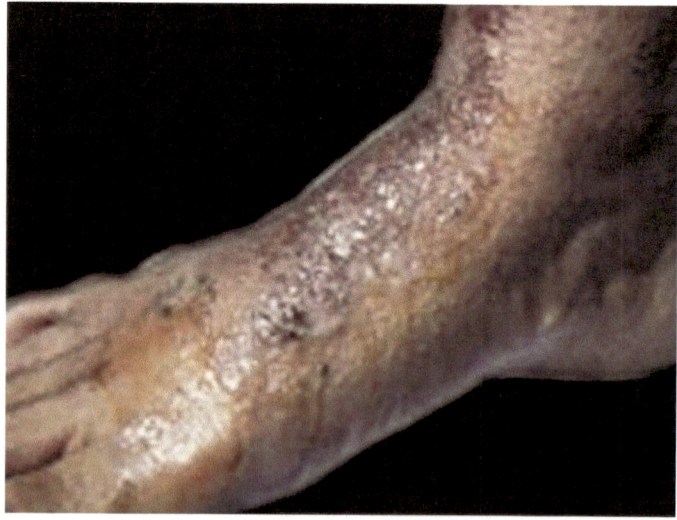

FIGURE 8.1. Acute eczema – note the oozing.

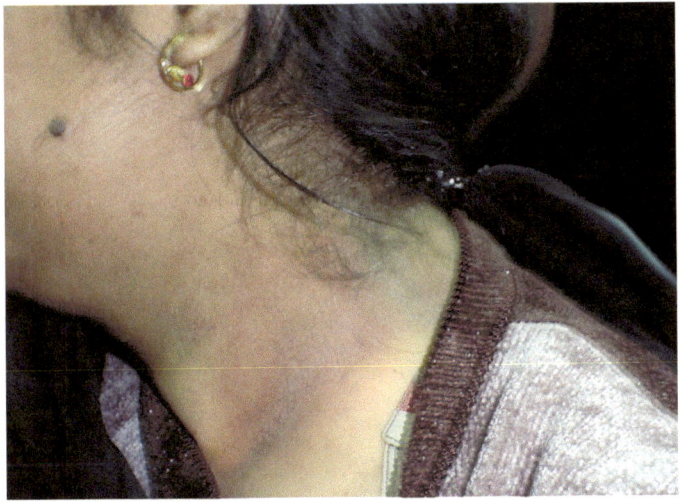

FIGURE 8.2. Subacute eczema – note the erythema and scaling.

edema). In the dermis, the blood vessels are dilated and there is a dermal infiltrate consisting mainly of lymphocytes.

8.2.2 Subacute Eczema

Clinically as the eczema becomes subacute, it becomes less vesicular and exudative, and more scaly. The edema diminishes and acanthosis develops (Fig. 8.2).

8.2.3 Chronic Eczema

This is characterized by thickening of the skin, lichenification, fissuring, and pigmentation (Fig. 8.3). Histologically there is increased thickness of the epidermis, the underlying edema is less marked. Vascular dilatation decreases and lymphocytic infiltration persists around the blood vessels. The skin lines become exaggerated, producing lichenification of the skin. Chronic eczema is associated with severe itching.

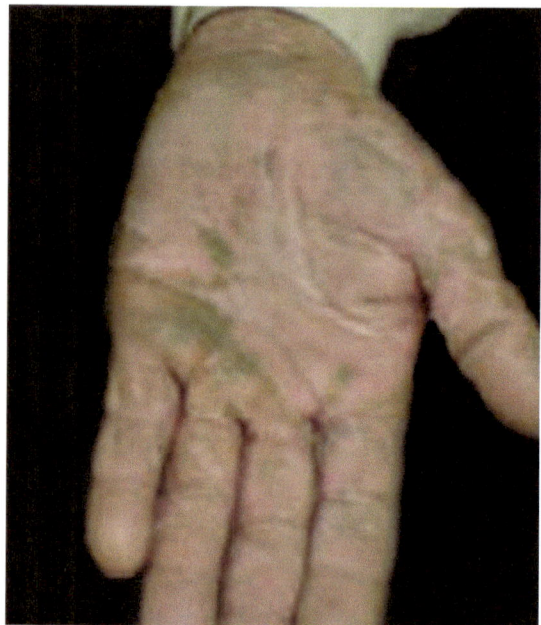

FIGURE 8.3. Chronic eczema – dry, thick, and fissured skin.

8.3 Treatment

Corticosteroids are used for the treatment of eczema; emollients are very effective for the dry skin of chronic eczema. The topical route is usually preferred in prescribing steroids for eczema, as the disease is localized and often chronic. The potency of steroid used depends upon the site affected; if a strong steroid is used, it should be gradually tapered to moderate strength, and then to low potency. This reduction should be gradual.

8.3.1 Topical Treatment

Topical steroids are the mainstay of treatment.

• Low potency steroids should be used on the face and groin.

- Medium potency steroids should be used on the body and extremities.
- Strong steroids are used in severely affected areas, and palms and soles.

In persistent cases, it may be advisable to resort to systemic steroids rather than to continue with potent topical steroids.

8.3.1.1 Acute Eczema

Rest is most important; all work should be stopped while treating hand eczema. Acute eczema is a moist, weeping eczema; it should be treated several times daily with wet soaks, such as 0.65% aluminum acetate solution, saline, tap water, or potassium permanganate soaks diluted to a light pink color. This is a soothing lotion; it also prevents secondary infection due to its anti-bacterial properties. These solutions, tend to reduce the weeping, but will cause dryness and cracking when used for a long time. The disadvantage of potassium permanganate solution is that it stains the skin and nails brown.

A steroid preparation is applied once a day; the strength depends upon the site and age of the patient. In general, 1% hydrocortisone is used for children and 0.025–0.1% betamethasone, or triamcinolone for adults.

8.3.1.2 Subacute Eczema

Wet dressings should be discontinued in treating subacute eczema; use of emollients will depend upon the dryness of the skin and the site affected. The strength of steroid lotions or creams depends upon the severity of the attack and the site of eczema. Topical antibiotics can be added if an infective element is present.

8.3.1.3 Chronic Eczema

As the eczema becomes chronic, the skin becomes dry and lichenified. Lubrication is an essential part of therapy; dry skin is more susceptible to further irritation and inflammation. Emollients soothe and hydrate the skin, as the effect of emollients is short-lived, these should be applied several times a day. Over-frequent bathing causes removal of skin lipids with subsequent dehydration of the keratin and this makes the eczema worse. The use of emollients should be continued for several weeks after the inflammation has subsided. Ointments are preferred to creams while treating chronic eczema.

8.3.1.4 Topical Steroids

Patients should be warned of the possible side effects; the weakest steroid preparation effective for a particular patient should be used. Steroids should generally be used once a day and not as a substitute for emollients. Patients who have failed to respond to treatment will often improve when hospitalized. Various tar preparations, zinc paste, or cream, PUVA are also helpful in chronic eczema.

The strength of the steroid is important; 0.5 or 1% hydrocortisone should be used on the face, infancy, and intertriginous areas and moderate strength steroids on the body and potent steroids are used in severe cases of eczema. Occasionally, occlusion of the skin after application can increase the effectiveness, but it also increases the risk of side effects. Very potent steroids should not be used for a long-term.

8.3.2 Systemic Treatment

Short course of systemic steroids may occasionally be used in very severe, persistent cases of acute and chronic eczema. Azathioprine is less commonly used. Antihistamines help at night. Systemic antibiotics may be required when there is super-added severe bacterial infection.

> *Use the weakest steroid that controls the eczema effectively.*
> *Regular check-up of patients to note for any side effects, and tachyphylaxis*

Avoid using potent steroids in the intertriginous areas, genitals, and the face. These areas should be treated with 0.5% or 1% hydrocortisone.
Eczematous plaques that become bright red on treatment with topical steroids may be infected.

8.4 Types of Eczema

8.4.1 Exogenous

8.4.1.1 Contact Dermatitis

This may be irritant or allergic.

- Irritant dermatitis accounts for 80% cases of contact dermatitis. It can occur at all ages and in both sexes. Irritant eczemas occur most commonly on the hand, as they are exposed most to irritants. Prolonged exposure to weak irritants is required for eczema to occur. A strong irritant can produce an immediate reaction, resulting in the formation of vesicles and bullae. Little is known about the pathogenesis of irritant dermatitis. Irritants probably cause direct injury to the keratinocytes, releasing mediators of inflammation. Irritant contact dermatitis is sharply localized to the area of contact with the irritant.

Primary irritant dermatitis causes an inelastic feeling of the skin; there is discomfort due to dryness and pruritus. Chronic exposure results in dry, thick, and fissured skin
The common irritants are soaps, detergents, acids, alkalis, solvents, and cutting oils.

- Allergic contact dermatitis is a manifestation of delayed hypersensitivity (type IV cell-mediated immunological reaction). Contact allergy is rare before the age of 15 years and in extreme old age, due to diminished cell-mediated immunity. Allergic contact dermatitis develops after weeks or years of exposure to the sensitizing agent. Once the individual is sensitized, further exposure will cause dermatitis within 48 h. The allergy is frequently transferred to other parts of the body, where an allergic rash appears.

Common sensitizers are nickel, paraphenylenediamine (found in hair dyes), rubber, cosmetics, medications, plants, and wood. A positive patch test is diagnostic of allergic contact dermatitis (Figs. 8.4a, b and 8.5).

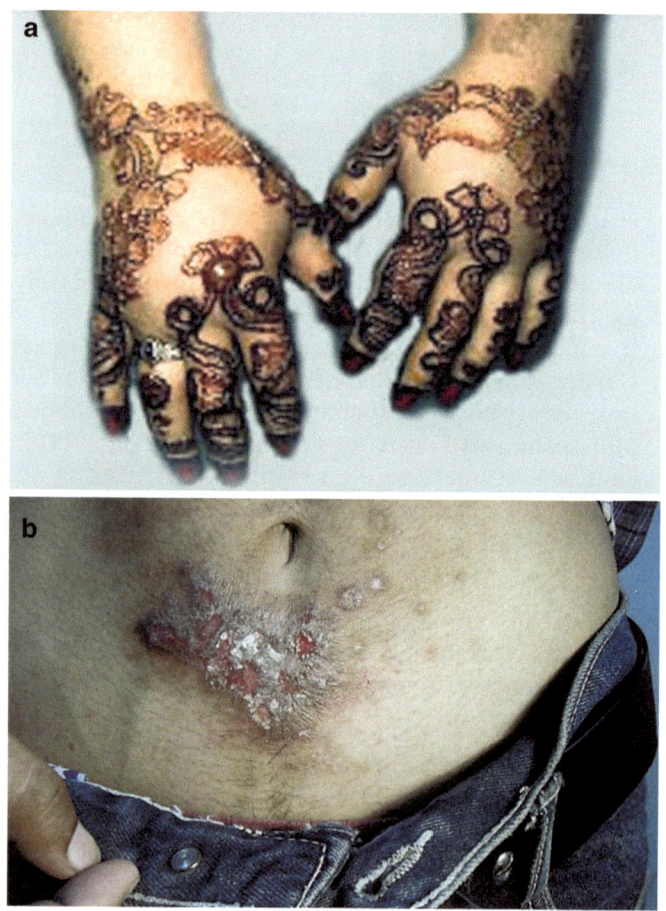

FIGURE 8.4.   (a) Contact dermatitis due to henna. (b) Nickle dermatitis.

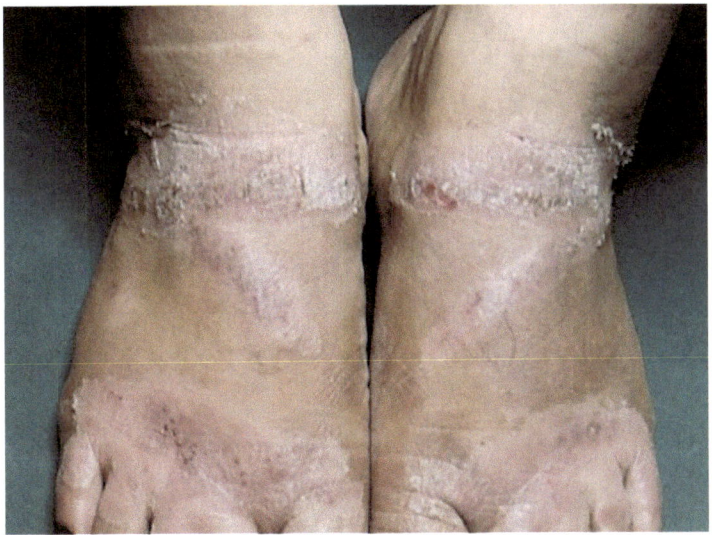

FIGURE 8.5. Shoe dermatitis.

Differential Diagnosis

Contact eczema of the hands should be differentiated from psoriasis, lichen planus, atopic dermatitis, climacteric keratoderma, and dermatophytosis

Treatment

Withdrawal of the offending agent is vital. Appropriate barrier creams, emollients, wearing cotton gloves inside rubber gloves for all wet and dirty tasks is recommended; appropriate occupational advice should be given to the patient.

Acute reactions require wet soaks and application of soothing creams and lotions. After vesiculation subsides, a topical corticosteroid cream or lotion should be applied.

Subacute and chronic dermatitis responds to topical steroids and systemic antihistamines. Liberal use of emollients should be emphasized. Tar preparations are a useful adjunct in chronic eczema. Bacterial infections, which are usually common, should be treated with topical and systemic antibiotics.

Hyposensitization may be required in patients who cannot avoid exposure to the substance causing contact dermatitis, dangerous adverse effects may occur with hyposensitization.

Patch test will help in finding the allergen in allergic contact dermatitis, this is then avoided.

Site of contact dermatitis	Common causative agents
Scalp	Shampoos, oil
Earlobe	Earring
Face	Cosmetics
Forehead	Bindi (Indian subcontinent)
Wrist	Watch, bangles, bracelet
Hands	Soaps, detergents, chemicals of occupation, henna (Indian subcontinent)
Fingers	Rings
Feet	Shoes
Flexures	Clothing, deodorants in axillae

8.4.1.2 Napkin Dermatitis

A common type of irritant eczema, it is due to the irritant affect produced by fecal enzymes and ammonia. It is seen in children when nappies are not changed for a long time and with the wearing of waterproof plastic pants. Napkin dermatitis is localized to the area covered by napkins; the skin folds are spared. Yeasts often aggravate the dermatitis.

Treatment

Most cases respond to improved hygiene, frequent change of nappies, and application of emollients. In severe cases, mild steroid preparation may be prescribed, often with a combination of anti-yeast preparations, because of the overgrowth of yeast in many cases.

8.4.1.3 Infective Eczema

This eczema can occur on any infection of the skin, e.g., it can superimpose on fungal infections, scabies, impetigo, etc. In such cases the underlying infection should be treated; the eczema clears when the infecting organism is eliminated.

8.4.1.4 Photosensitive Eczema

The eczema is localized to the areas exposed to the sun. On the face, the forehead, nose, cheeks, rim of the ears, and sides and back of the neck are affected. Sparing of the shielded areas is characteristic of photosensitive eruptions. These are the retroauricular folds, submental region, upper eyelids, and nasolabial folds. Photosensitive eczema is due to the effect of ultraviolet rays on the skin; the action spectrum is usually in the range of 290–320 nm.

Differential Diagnosis

Photosensitive eczema should be differentiated from other photosensitive disorders such as systemic lupus erythematosus, polymorphic light eruption, photosensitive drug eruptions, sun burn, and eczemas of the face such as seborrheic dermatitis and contact dermatitis.

Treatment

The patient should be advised to avoid exposure to ultraviolet light (particularly between 11.30 am and 4 pm), use sunscreens, wear protective clothing such as broad-brim hats, and long-sleeved clothing. Dark-colored clothes tend to absorb heat; these should be avoided. In severe cases chemical photoprotective agents such as chloroquine may be used.

8.4.2 Endogenous Eczemas

8.4.2.1 Atopic Dermatitis

A strong genetic component is obvious in many patients; there is often a family history of asthma, hay fever, urticaria, or atopic dermatitis in other members of the family. Atopic dermatitis generally begins in infancy but may be delayed until childhood or adult life. The distribution of the lesion varies with age, but dryness of the skin persists throughout life; the condition is very itchy.

Infancy – atopic dermatitis begins after the age of 3 months; it starts on the face, sometimes with a few patches of eczema on other parts of the body. The lesions in infancy are vesicular and weeping. The napkin area is often spared. In about 40% of cases, atopic dermatitis clears spontaneously by the age of 2–5 years.

Childhood – the eczema is mainly localized to the flexures, the knee, elbow, ankle, and wrist. It is dry, leathery, and excoriated due to excessive scratching. In most cases, the eczema remits spontaneously by the age of 10 years (Fig. 8.6).

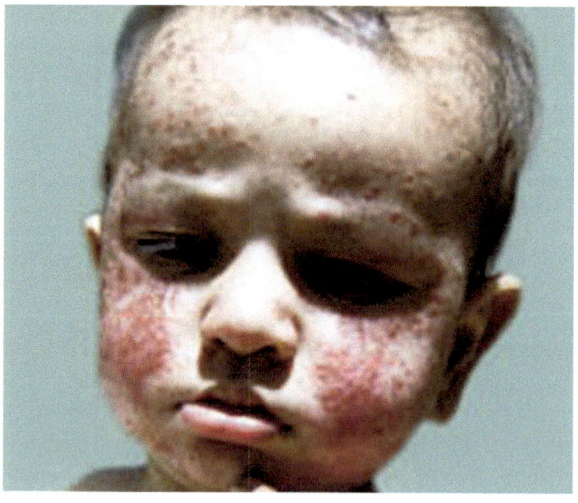

FIGURE 8.6. Atopic eczema – note the sparing of the nasolabial folds.

Adults – the eczema remains localized to the flexures, but the lesions may also be present on the hands, face, and trunk. The skin becomes thickened, pigmented, and lichenified.

The other features of atopic dermatitis are white dermographism; accentuation of palmar creases; keratosis pilaris; Dennie Morgan's folds; pallor around the eyes, nose, and mouth; pityriasis alba; early onset of posterior capsular cataract; and keratoconnus. Pruritus and dryness of the skin are cardinal features of atopic dermatitis. There is an increased tendency for the development of bacterial, fungal, and viral infections.

Major diagnostic criteria of atopic dermatitis:

- Pruritus and dryness of the skin
- Typical morphology in different age groups
- Family history of atopy
- Increased levels of IgE
- Fluctuating abnormalities in T cell immunity
- Chronic relapsing dermatitis

Complications

Secondary bacterial infections are common. Patients are also prone to viral infections such as molluscum contagiosum and warts. Infection with herpes virus can lead to eczema herpeticum; this is a serious and widespread infection with the herpes virus. Cataracts and keratoconus are more likely to develop in atopic patients.

Investigations

Prick testing though helpful for the diagnosis of asthma and hay fever is controversial for the diagnosis of atopic dermatitis for multiple positive reactions may occur. It may be used for testing inhalants and sometimes food allergens; indicating type I hypersensitivity. Total serum IgE levels are raised in 80% of individuals. RAST (radioallergoabsorbance test) may be positive for specific allergens. Swabs for bacterial and viral culture may be helpful in exacerbations.

Differential Diagnosis

Atopic dermatitis of infancy should be differentiated from infantile seborrheic eczema. In adults, atopic dermatitis should be differentiated from the lesions that involve the flexures such as fungal infection, seborrheic dermatitis, intertrigo, clothing dermatitis, and flexural psoriasis.

Treatment

Atopic eczema can be stressful for both the patient and the family. The principles of therapy are to keep the skin moist with emollients and to minimize itching with antihistamines.

The young patient is irritable and itchy. The family needs a lot of reassurance and explanation. Avoid exacerbating factors such as extremes of temperature, use of irritants (such as wearing woolen clothes next to the skin, soaps, detergents, etc.), stress, infections, airborne allergens (pollens, animal dander, house dust mite), and excessive washing of the skin without the use of lubricants. Moisturizers should be used frequently and copiously as the skin of atopics is very dry. Regular vacuuming of the room to reduce house dust mite will help, but removal of carpets in the house if indicated is more effective.

Acute flare-ups produced by surface proliferation with staphylococci can be treated with a course of oral antibiotics such as erythromycin.

Avoid allergens; do not keep pets to which there is an obvious allergy.

Topical steroids are the mainstay of treatment; use the weakest steroid that controls the eczema. As the eczema is recurrent, regularly check for local and systemic side effects of steroids therapy. Avoid the use of strong steroid in children.

New generations of topical steroids, such as fluticasone and mometasone have a better safety profile, i.e., they cause less adrenal suppression and less skin atrophy. Once daily applications are required.

Sedative antihistamines are helpful if sleep in affected.

Topical immune-modulators are useful when the patient has been on topical steroids for a long time and there is a possibility of developing side effects, when topical steroids are ineffective, when the patient is reluctant to use topical steroids, or when systemic treatment is considered.

Tacrolimus 0.1% and 0.03%, a macrolide immunosuppressant produced by spectromycete, has shown to be a successful treatment in atopic eczema. A slight tingling and burning sensation may be felt, but this fades with time. It is steroid sparing and atrophy of the skin does not occur. Local infection may occur, and there is a potential risk of development of skin cancer with long-term use.

Pimecrolimus 1%, is another immunosuppressant; it is a derivative of askamycin. Its action is similar to tacrolimus but weaker.

Ascomycin (cytokine inhibitor) a nonsteroidal ointment may shortly be available for treatment.

Occlusive dressings are helpful by reducing the ability to scratch.

Although the role of diet is debatable, it is beneficial to breast-feed an atopic child as long as permissible. Rigid dietary exclusions without evidence of allergy should be discouraged. They often causes anxiety, and seldom helps the patient.

In severe extensive disease, oral steroids are helpful to quickly control the eczema. However, they are not a good choice if prolonged treatment is required. In such cases cyclosporine, azathioprine, or narrow band UVB may be used.

Eczema herpeticum should be treated immediately with acyclovir. Antibiotics are frequently required for secondary bacterial infections.

> *Routine inoculations are permissible during the less active phases of eczema; patients allergic to egg should not be vaccinated for measles, influenza, and yellow fever.*
> *Patients with atopic dermatitis have a very dry, pruritic skin.*
> *There is a changing morphology in different age groups.*
> *Increased levels of IgE are present in most cases.*
> *Atopic patients are more prone to bacterial, fungal, and viral infections.*

8.4.2.2 Seborrheic Dermatitis

This dermatitis may be seen in the newborn, but is rare in children and the elderly. It is commonly seen between adolescence and middle age. A hormonal influence has been postulated (androgenic stimulation of the sebaceous glands). Areas rich in sebaceous glands are most affected, but hyper-secretion of sebum is not present.

The lesions are commonly seen on the scalp, face, chest, and back. The intertriginous areas may also be affected. The lesions may be yellowish and greasy, or dry and scaly. There may be extensive follicular papules or pustules on the chest and back, probably due to the close association of Malassezia furfur with seborrheic dermatitis.

Scalp

The lesions may be dry and scaly, or erythematous and greasy. The mildest form is pityriasis capitis (dandruff). The oily type (pityriasis steatoides), may spread to the upper border of the forehead.

Face

The eyebrows, glabella, nasolabial folds, and the cheeks are involved. There may be associated chronic blepharitis and otitis externa (Fig. 8.7).

Chest

The lesions are prominent in the interscapular and presternal areas. Seborrheic dermatitis on the chest may also present as follicular papules and pustules, due to Malassezia furfur.

Flexures

The lesions appear as a moist intertrigo, often secondarily infected with Candida albicans.

Seborrheic dermatitis in infants. In a newborn, seborrhiec dermatitis is due to maternal androgens. Oozing and crusting of the scalp (cradle cap) may be the sole manifestation, or the face, buttocks, napkin area, and the body folds may be affected. This should be differentiated from atopic dermatitis of infancy. In contrast to the atopic infant the baby with seborrheic eczema is rarely irritable or showing signs of an itchy skin.

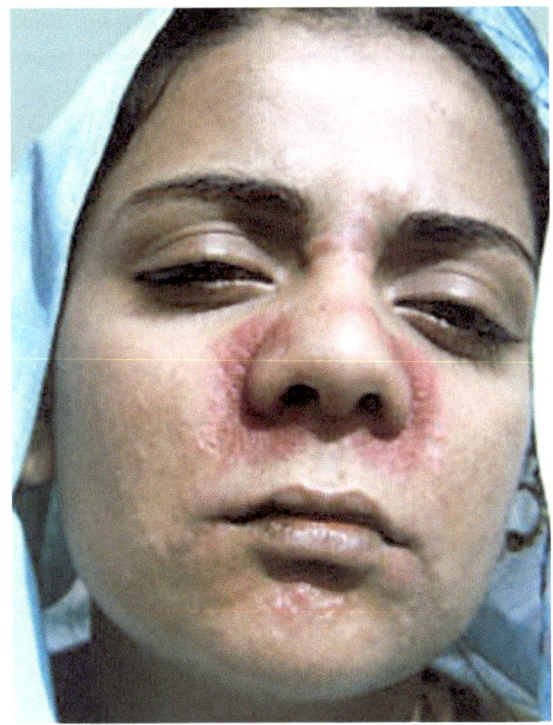

FIGURE 8.7. Seborrheic dermatitis.

Differential Diagnosis

On the scalp, seborrheic dermatitis should be differentiated from psoriasis, pediculosis, fungal infections, and other forms of eczema. On the face, it should be differentiated from atopic dermatitis, lupus erythematosus, rosacea, and contact dermatitis. On the chest it should be differentiated from pityriasis versicolor, pityriasis rosea, and psoriasis. In the flexures it should be differentiated from fungal infections, contact dermatitis, erythrasma, and flexural psoriasis.

A rash similar to seborrheic dermatitis occurs in young children due to Class 1 Histiocytosis X (Langerhans cell histiocytosis). Several entities have been included in this disorder, with a great deal of overlap between them. This is a rare disorder with cutaneous lesions similar to seborrheic dermatitis associated with purpura and hepatosplenomegaly. Diabetes insipidis may occur; there may be loss of teeth and alveolar bones. The disease is fatal in 20–50% of cases.

Treatment

Therapy is suppressive rather than curative. As seborrheic dermatitis is often associated with Malassezia furfur; topical imidazoles are often the first line of treatment.

Scalp

Mild seborrheic dermatitis is treated by medicated shampoos containing selenium sulphide, ketoconazole, or tar. Simple washing of the scalp daily is also therapeutic as it removes the surface lipids, which are a nutrient for the fungus (Malassezia furfur).

If the scales are prominent then a preparation of salicylic acid (2–5%, depending upon the scaling), is applied at night, and then wash the hair with a medicated shampoo the next morning.

Face and Flexures

These respond to combination of steroid-antifungal or steroid-antiseptic preparation. Tacrolimus ointment and Lithium succinate creams are also effective for the facial rash.

Infantile atopic dermatitis	Infantile seborrhoeic dermatitis
Begins 3 months after birth	Begins shortly after birth
Markedly pruritic	Asymptomatic
Presents as erythema, papules and vesicles	Presents as greasy scales on an erythematous base
Prominent on the cheeks and extensor surface of the limbs.	Prominent on the scalp, cheeks, eyebrows, nasolabial folds, and proximal flexures

Trunk

Treat as for the face, but cases which are follicular should be treated as for Malassezia furfur with topical imidazoles.

For severe and unresponsive cases, a short course of oral itraconazole may be effective.

A course of oral itraconazole 200 mg daily for the first week of the month, then first 2 days every month for 11 months, has helped patients with recalcitrant seborrhoeic dermatitis.

Recurrences are common and repeated treatment is often necessary.

8.4.2.3 Pompholyx

The eczema affects the palms and soles, and is characterized by the formation of vesicles and bullae. These appear in crops, which last for a few days, vesicles rupture to form crusts, and they then slowly desquamate (Fig. 8.8). The cause is unknown; it can be associated with stress, contact dermatitis, and atopy.

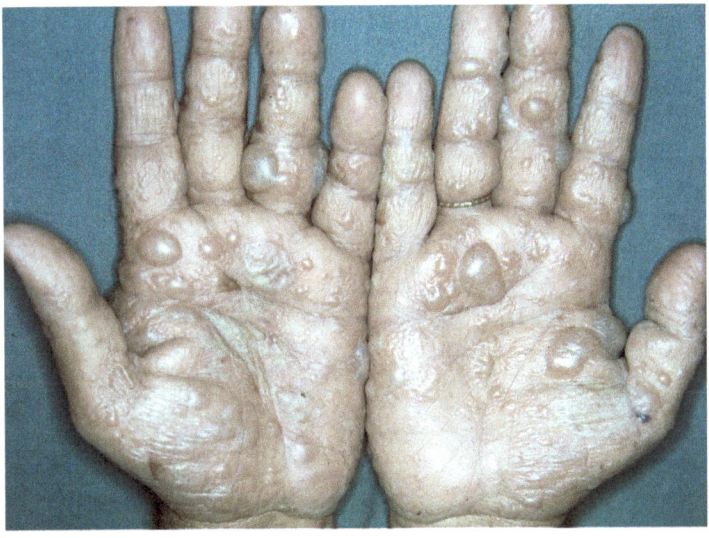

FIGURE 8.8. Pompholyx.

A fungal infection elsewhere in the body can produce a pompholyx eruption on the hands (pompholyx dermatophytid), and similarly bacterial foci anywhere in the body can also cause pompholyx. A sympathetic reaction can occur on the hands, if the feet are involved.

Treatment

It is similar to that of acute eczema. Large bullae should be drained. A potent steroid preparation should be applied after wet soaks. If the cause can be found it should be treated accordingly, e.g., an appropriate antibiotic for a bacterial infection, anti-fungal agent for tinea.

If a fungal infection is suspected then scrapings from the feet are taken, or from the roof of a blister for examination of hyphae.

Nummular eczema (discoid eczema)

This presents as round or nummular (coin shaped) lesions distributed mainly on the extensor surface of the extremities; less commonly the trunk is also involved. In most cases, the cause is unknown; infection, trauma, stress, drugs, and xerosis have been implicated as causative factors (Figs. 8.9 and 8.10).

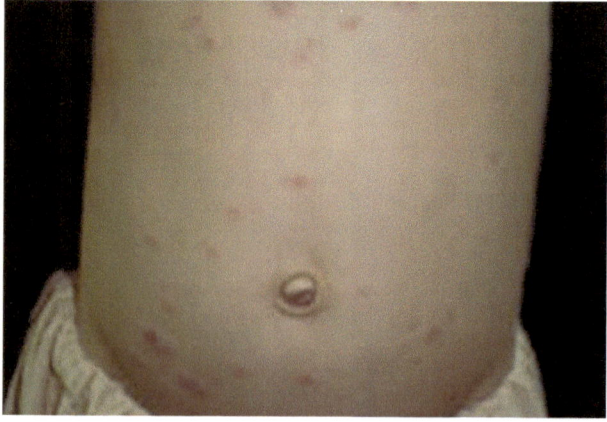

FIGURE 8.9. Nummular eczema.

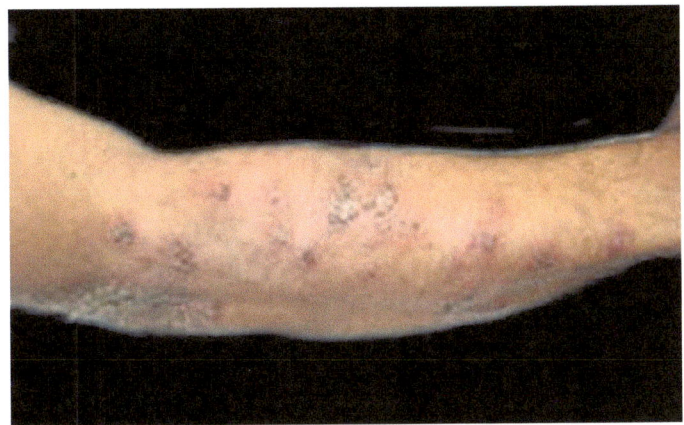

FIGURE 8.10. Nummular eczema.

Differential Diagnosis

Nummular eczema should be differentiated from tinea corporis, contact dermatitis, granuloma annulare, and psoriaisis. The edge of nummular eczema is broader and vesicular. A scraping for mycology will exclude a fungal infection.

Treatment

An emollient with a moderately potent steroid, with or without a combination of an antibiotic or anti-fungal preparation is needed. A combination of tar and steroids is effective in long-term management.

8.4.2.5 Pityriasis Alba

Usually seen on the face of children, the lesions are dry, scaly, and slightly hypopigmented. Excessive dryness followed by exposure to sunlight may be a contributory factor. All races are affected, but it is more common in dark-colored skin (Fig. 8.11).

Differential Diagnosis

These include postinflammatory hypopigmentation, leprosy, and vitiligo.

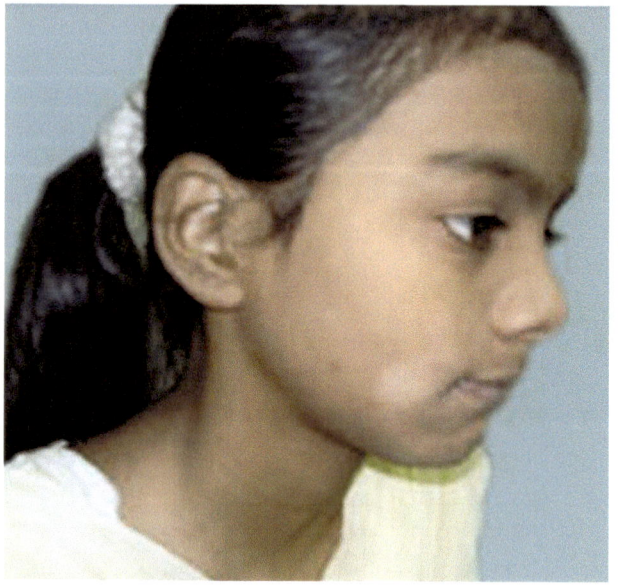

FIGURE 8.11. Pityriasis alba.

Treatment

Visual response to treatment is disappointing, as the repigmentation takes time to return. Emollient creams, 1% hydrocortisone ointment, and mild tar preparations are helpful. Sun exposure should be avoided as exposure to the sun makes the patches more obvious.

8.4.2.6 Asteatotic Eczema

This eczema is common in the elderly, and seen in the winter season. The lower limbs are most commonly affected; they appear dry, cracked, and fissured. There is a glazed "crazy paving" effect, giving it the name eczema craquele. Sun, wind, and low humidity are the predisposing factors. The condition may remain in this state for months, recurring every winter. In generalized asteatotic eczema, internal malignancy should be excluded. Pain rather than itching is the main complaint of this eczema (Fig. 8.12).

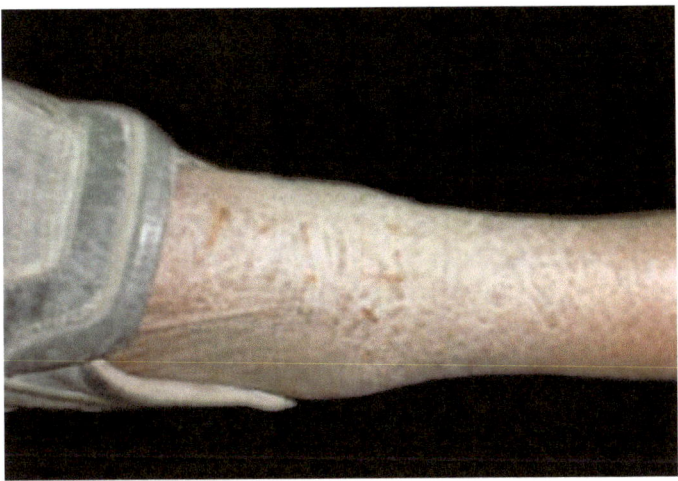

FIGURE 8.12. Asteatotic eczema.

Treatment

Emollients are the mainstay of treatment. Patient should be advised against excessive bathing; use of soap should be avoided. Urea-based emollients and weak corticosteroids are helpful. Topical steroids should be avoided in the elderly, as their skin is already thin and fragile.

8.4.2.7 Hypostatic Eczema (Varicose Eczema)

This results from venous hypertension. It may be related to venous valvular damage from deep venous hypertension, pregnancy, etc. Blood leaks from the capillaries into the surrounding tissues, depositing fibrin around the capillaries, thereby diminishing tissue perfusion, predisposing to inflammation and ulceration. The lower limb above the medial malleolus is commonly affected. The onset is gradual, with edema at the end of the day. Later, brown pigmentation develops on the inner aspect of the leg. The dermatitis may be weepy or dry, scaly and lichenified. Varicose veins are often present.

Treatment

The only effective way of treating venous hypertension is by external compression of the leg by bandaging or support stockings. This compresses the superficial veins so that the blood can flow to the deeper veins. The patient should use their calf muscles, so they need to be mobile and walking. When sitting, the feet should be raised on a stool to the level of the patient's chest, and dorsiflexed frequently.

Weak topical steroids should be applied twice daily, once before applying the bandage or stocking and once before going to bed. Any potent sensitizer should be avoided; local antiseptics are preferable to topical antibiotics for secondary infection.

8.4.2.8 Keratolysis Exfoliativa

This is a common chronic asymptomatic, noninflammatory peeling of the palms and soles of unknown etiology. The eczema is common in summer and is often associated with increased sweating of the palms and soles. Scaling starts simultaneously on the palms and soles that appear to have originated from ruptured vesicles, although the vesicles are never seen. The skin continues to peel and extend peripherally forming large circular areas. The scaling borders may coalesce.

Juvenile plantar dermatosis is a variant affecting the soles of children, who wear occlusive trainers for long periods.

Treatment

The condition often resolves by itself in 2–3 weeks, it requires no therapy other than lubrication.

8.4.2.9 Lichen Simplex Chronicus (LSC)

The skin damaged because of repeated scratching or rubbing, becomes thick, pigmented, and lichenified. The areas most accessible to scratching are affected, e.g., the ankles, nape of the neck, genitals, and wrists and forearms. There is often no underlying cause. The term neurodermatitis, for this eczema, indicates that increased itch is a pathogenic trigger, and stress

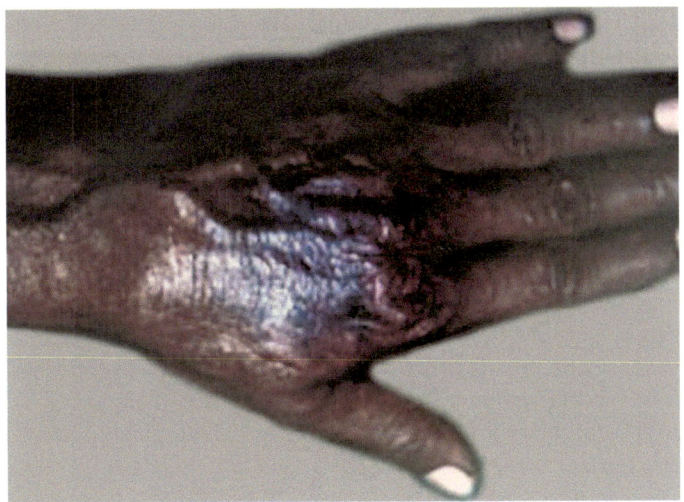

FIGURE 8.13. Lichen simplex chronicus.

may be responsible. Lesions resolve with treatment, but tend to recur (Fig. 8.13).

Differential Diagnosis

Lichen simplex chronicus should be differentiated from a plaque of psoriasis and lichen planus. A plaque of lichen planus will have papules of lichen planus at the periphery of the lesion, its purplish color and Wickham's striae are other differentiating points. A psoriatic plaque will be more scaly; there may be lesions of psoriasis elsewhere on the skin.

Treatment

This should be aimed at breaking the itch-scratch-itch cycle. The treatment consists of antihistamines to reduce pruritus, topical steroids to reduce inflammation and tar preparations for their antipruritic and antikeratolytic effects. Occlusive dressings including medicated paste bandages, help to prevent scratching, this can produce dramatic improvement.

In some cases where lichenification is intense, an intrale-sional injection of steroid is very helpful. Continued use of emollients helps to prevent recurrences.

8.4.2.10 Nodular Prurigo

This may be a variant of LSC; patients scratch and rub remorse-lessly to produce itchy nodules. The initial lesion is a dome-shaped papule, topped by a small vesicle, the vesicle soon ruptures. The disease is seen in middle-aged people. Prurigo-like lesions are seen in other conditions such as pregnancy (prurigo of pregnancy), atopic dermatitis (Besniers prurigo), in cold weather (winter prurigo), summer (Hutchinsons summer prurigo), or following insect bites (papular prurigo).

Nodular prurigo is most common on the extensor surface of the forearms and legs (Fig. 8.14). Histologically the lesions resemble LSC. The nodules are hard, and globular with a

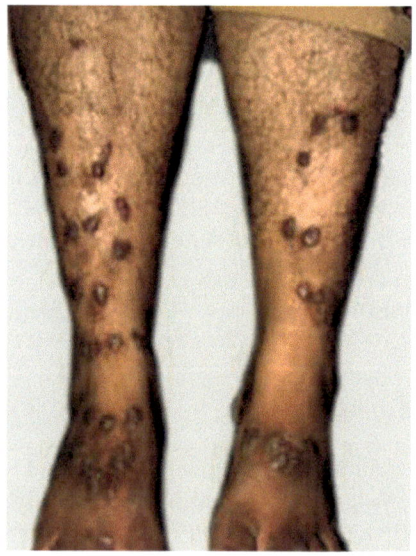

FIGURE 8.14. Prurigo nodularis.

warty surface. Pruritus is intense; occurring at intervals and lasting for from a few minutes to an hour or two. New nodules develop from time to time. Old ones take a long time to heal; the lesions healing with scarring.

Treatment

Treatment is difficult; intralesional steroids are helpful and so are steroids under occlusion. Thalidomide, PUVA, and benoxaprufen have also given favorable results. Many patients continue to suffer from intractable itching.

Ferdinand von Ritter Hebra (1816–1880)

Hebra was the founder of modern dermatology. His discoveries and teachings, together with his successor Kaposi, laid the foundations for modern day dermatology. He was the first to prove that skin diseases were due to agents acting on the skin. He experimented with local irritants and found that they produced eczema.

Chapter 9
Keratinizing and Papulosquamous Disorders

9.1 Psoriasis

Psoriasis is a chronic inflammatory disorder, characterized by the formation of well-defined raised erythematous plaques, with silvery white scales; that preferentially localize on the extensor surfaces.

9.1.1 Etiology

The etiology is unknown; various hypotheses have been put forward:

- It is an immune disorder and responds to immunosuppressive agents such as methotrexate and cyclosporine. Whether it is an autoimmune response or due to foreign antigens is not known. Autoantibodies have been found against the stratum corneum. A retrovirus has been considered as a causative agent in recent years. In AIDS a very active and aggressive form of the disease develops. Evidence of the presence of T lymphocytes in psoriatic lesions, and the treatment of psoriasis by cyclosporine, indicate a pointer toward cell-mediated immunity.
- The disease is hereditary; it is found in members of the same family. Twins have a high concordance for psoriasis, and it is associated with HLA B-13 and HLA B-17 antigens.

Z. Zaidi, S. W. Lanigan, *Dermatology in Clinical Practice*,
DOI: 10.1007/978-1-84882-862-9_9,
© Springer-Verlag London Limited 2010

A number of factors such as infections, drugs, stress, trauma, puberty, etc. can aggravate psoriasis.

Whatever the provocation, the result is an increased number of cycling cells recruited from the normal resting cell proportion. This leads to an increased number of dividing cells. Cellular turnover is increased sevenfold, and the transit time from the basal layer to the stratum corneum is reduced to 8–10 days from 52 to 75 days. Growth factors, especially transforming growth factor-α seem to mediate these events. The cell cycle time is not reduced.

9.1.2 Histopathology

The main pathological abnormalities in psoriasis are an increase in epidermal thickness, an increase in the inflammatory component and increased vascularity. The papillary capillaries are grossly dilated and tortuous; these abnormal capillaries are the last features to clear during resolution of psoriasis. The other characteristics are presence of polymorphonuclear cells in the stratum corneum (Munro's abscess), absence of the granular layer, elongation of rete pegs, and long, edematous, club shaped dermal papillae.

9.1.3 Clinical Features

Psoriasis is found principally on the extensor surface of the elbows, knees, lumbosacral area, and the scalp. The areas are sharply demarcated, raised, erythematous (salmon red), and covered with silvery white scales. On removal of the scales, bleeding points are manifest (Auspitz sign); Koebner's phenomenon is seen in active psoriasis, with development of psoriasis in injured or traumatized skin. Woronoff's ring is a concentric blanching of erythematous skin at or near the periphery of a healing psoriatic plaque. Reverse Koebner's phenomenon is also seen in psoriasis, i.e., clearing of psoriasis after trauma (Figs. 9.1–9.4).

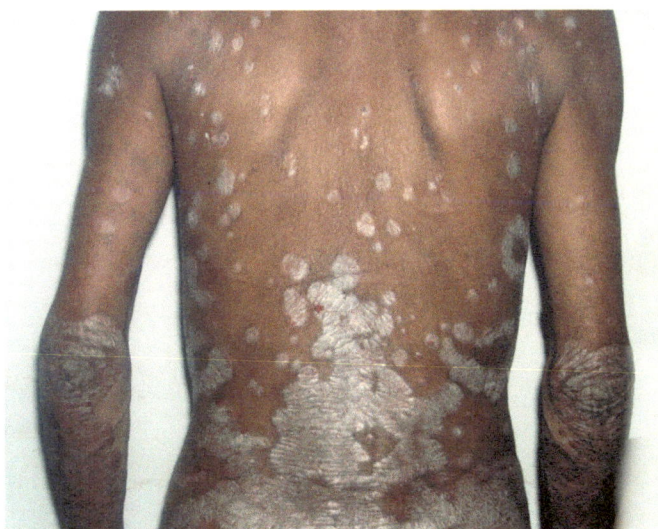

FIGURE 9.1. Psoriasis – note the silvery white scales.

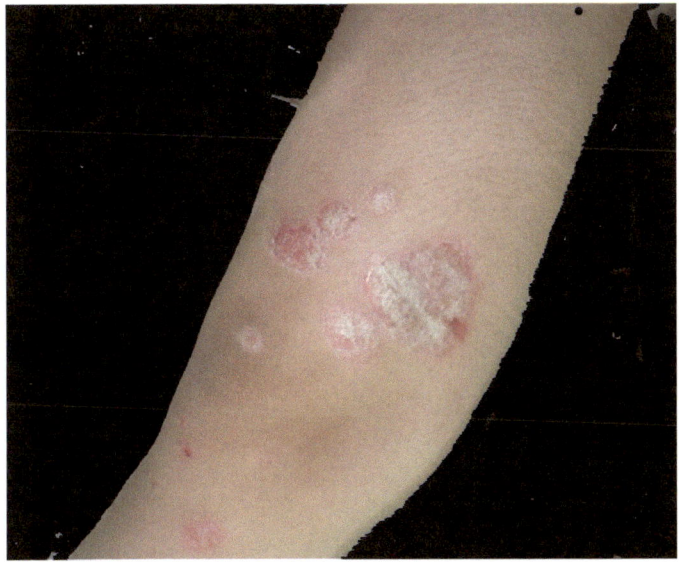

FIGURE 9.2. Psoriasis.

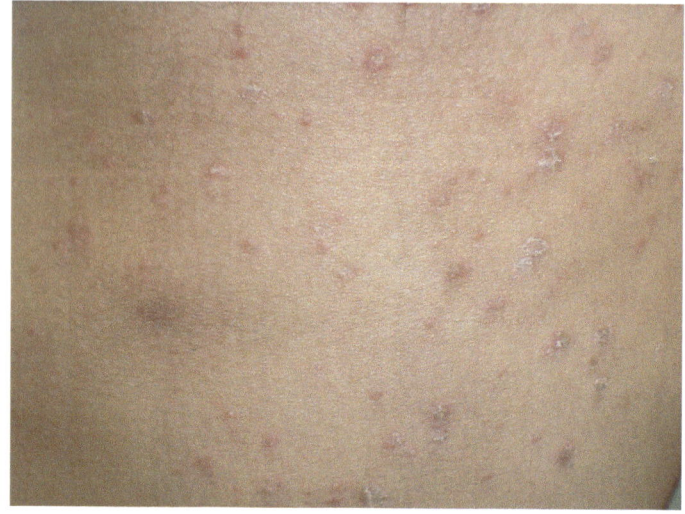

FIGURE 9.3. Guttate psoriasis.

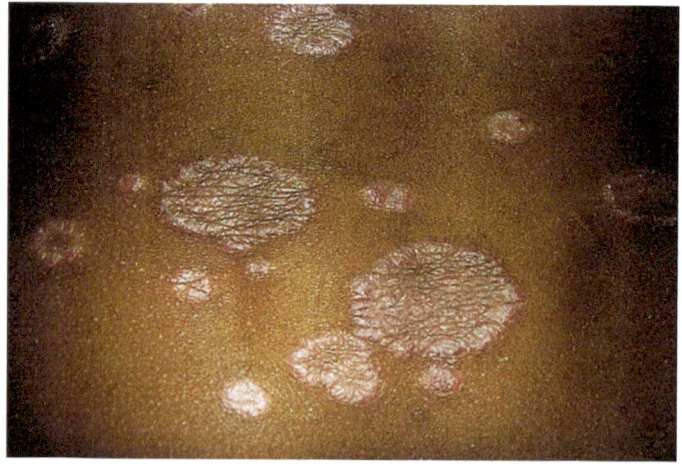

FIGURE 9.4. Annular psoriasis.

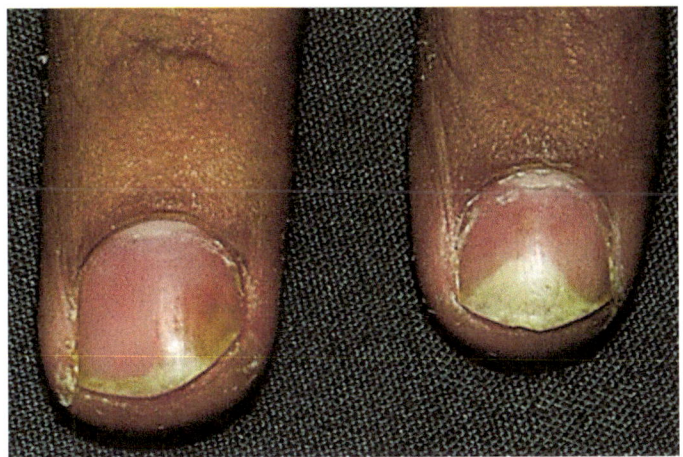

FIGURE 9.5. Psoriasis – note the pitting and onycholysis.

Psoriasis may also occur in various morphological forms, as it can be generalized, guttate, follicular, erythrodermic, flexural, annular, etc. Unstable psoriasis is the term used when the disease activity is marked and the course and immediate outcome of psoriasis is unpredictable. This type can rapidly worsen if irritants such as dithranol are used as treatment.

Nail involvement is demonstrated by pitting, onycholysis, subungul hyperkeratosis, and splinter hemorrhages (Fig. 9.5).

9.1.3.1 Psoriatic Arthritis

It affects the joints of the hands and the spine. The hand involvement includes distal interphalangeal arthritis (classic form), rheumatoid-like arthritis (this is seronegative), arthritis involving a few joints of both the above types (common type), axial arthritis such as spondylitis and/or sacroilietis, and arthritis mutilans which is a deforming arthritis of the hands or spine.

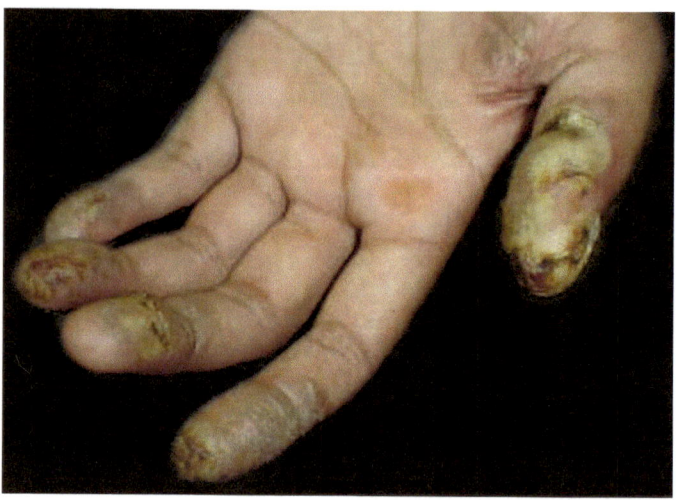

FIGURE 9.6. Pustular psoriasis of the palm-acrodermatitis continua.

9.1.3.2 Pustular Psoriasis

In this form, macroscopic pustules are associated with psoriasis; these pustules are sterile. It may be localized to the hands and feet, or is generalized. Its relationship with psoriasis is controversial in localized psoriasis. The psoriatic plaques are studded with pustules, or the pustules coalesce to form lakes of pus. The patient is acutely ill in acute generalized pustular psoriasis. Etretinate is often the treatment of choice in pustular psoriasis. Methotrexate is also helpful (Fig. 9.6).

Psoriasis-like eruptions can occur following the intake of drugs such as β-blockers, antimalarials, lithium, and interferon-α. Psoriasis may worsen after the withdrawal of systemic or potent topical steroids. Systemic steroids are therefore not given in generalized psoriasis.

9.1.4 Differential Diagnosis

Psoriasis of the scalp should be differentiated from seborrheic dermatitis. On the body it should be differentiated from discoid eczema, mycosis fungoides, secondary syphilis, and generalized lichen planus. Psoriasis of the palms and soles should be differentiated from dermatophytosis, eczema, and lichen planus. Tinea of the nails is often confused with nail psoriasis. In fungal infection of the nails, the neighboring skin may show signs of dermatophytosis, pitting is usually not seen, the nails are crumbly and break easily into a powdery form, and there may a number of uninvolved nails. A nail clipping for fungal hyphae will confirm the diagnosis.

Some diagnostic features of psoriasis are:

- Erythematous sharply defined plaques, covered with silvery white scales
- Extensor surface primarily involved such as the knees and elbows
- Auspitz's sign positive
- Koebner's phenomenon present in the active phase of the disease
- Woronoff's ring often present in the healing phase of the disease
- Characteristic histological features

9.1.5 Treatment

The natural history of psoriasis is as unpredictable as it was 150 years ago. The aim of treatment is to decrease epidermal proliferation and the underlying dermal inflammation. The type of treatment depends upon the extent of disease, duration, previous therapy, and psychological impact on the patient. First-line treatment is usually topical as the disease is chronic. Systemic therapy is indicated when topical treatment fails and in unstable psoriasis, acute generalized pustular psoriasis, and erythroderma.

9.1.5.1 Topical Therapy

Topical Steroids

These are both anti inflammatory and antimitotic. Steroids are used when there is limited involvement of the disease.

Potent steroids are effective, but they should be used on an intermittent regimen basis to avoid side effects. The response to steroids is rapid, tachyphylaxis (a progressive lack of effect with continual treatment), and rebound flaring of disease activity when stopping treatment can occur.

Topical Tar

Tars are hydrocarbons with antimitotic and antiinflammatory effects. The response is slow but more lasting and tachyphylaxis is less likely to develop. Tar is used for limited and generalized plaque psoriasis. Goekermann's regimen is still popular; the tar ointment is applied at night. In the morning after a tar bath, the patient is exposed to ultraviolet light.

Anthralin (Dithranol)

This is applied in the same way as tar, but anthralin is used instead (Ingram's regimen). As anthralin is irritating particularly when applied on noninvolved skin, face, and flexures, it is advisable to start with a low concentration of anthralin and gradually build it up until a response is obtained. To decrease spread of the drug it is applied in a thick paste (Lassar's paste). Concentrations are available from 0.025% to 1% and above. The other disadvantage of anthralin is that it stains the skin and clothing; the stains on clothing are permanent.

A 30-min short-term therapy with 0.5–3% diathranol is used. The preparation is washed off to decrease staining and irritation. The treatment is repeated daily until the lesions clear.

Calcipotriol

This is a vitamin D analogue with antimitotic activity. It is applied twice daily for several weeks. Some but not all patients respond. It can safely be used for long period.

Tazarotene (0.05–1%)

Tazarotene is a retinoid that promotes differentiation and inhibits proliferation. It is applied at bedtime. A steroid can be used in the morning; this can reduce irritant side effects. Tazarotene is teratogenic, so it should not be given to pregnant women; it is expensive and can cause irritation.

UVB

This can be used alone or with tar.

9.1.5.2 Systemic Therapy

The drugs used for the treatment of psoriasis are methotrexate, psoralens and UVA (PUVA), acitretin, and cyclosporine. The new biologic medications are used in unresponsive cases; these are alefacept, etanercept and infliximab.

Methotrexate

This is a folate antagonist, it blocks the formation of thymidine and thus DNA, and it inhibits cellular proliferation. The dose is 0.2–0.4 mg/kg given every 7–14 days; the dose is divided into three parts, given at 12 hourly intervals or as a single dose weekly. Complete blood examination and LFTs should be done prior to therapy. Clinical response is obtained in 1–2 weeks. Blood examination and LFT's, should be monitored regularly throughout therapy. A liver biopsy is done after every 1.5 g of methotrexate intake, liver toxicity can occur with methotrexate therapy. Measurement of serum procollagen N aminopeptidase may predict liver impairment. Methotrexate is a teratogen, it should not be given to pregnant women, and it also causes bone marrow suppression.

Psoralens and UVA (PUVA)

This is the least toxic of all the systemic medications, but requires frequent visits to the hospital for therapy. The psoralen intercalates between the DNA strands and binds to them during irradiation with UVA. When taken orally it enters all parts of the body, but only those parts that are exposed to UVA are affected. Eyes and the external genitals of male patients are shielded from the ultraviolet rays. If used over long period it can give rise to premature ageing and skin cancers.

Acitretin

This is a retinoid, especially effective in pustular psoriasis. It can also be used with PUVA; retinoids are given 2 weeks before the PUVA therapy (re-PUVA). Retinoids are teratogens and should not be used in pregnancy. Women with child-bearing potential, should use contraceptives when on acitretin therapy and for 2 years after stopping treatment. It is given in a dose of 1 mg/kg of body weight. Side effects include hyperlipidemia, dryness of the skin and mucosa and teratogenicity.

Cyclosporin

This drug decreases T cell proliferation in the dermis. It is given in a dose of 3–5 mg/kg daily in two divided doses. The major side effects are dose dependant hypertension and nephrotoxicity. Long term immunosuppression may increase the risk of skin cancer.

> *The younger the onset the worse is the prognosis of psoriasis.*
> *Psoriasis is life long disorder, subject to unpredictable remissions and relapses.*
> *In a psoriatic plaque the epidermal proliferation is increased sevenfold.*
> *When scaling is not prominent, it may be induced by light scratching of the skin, a useful sign when diagnosis is in doubt.*
> *The aim of therapy is to decrease epidermal proliferation and underlying dermal inflammation.*

9.2 Parapsoriasis

The word parapsoriasis was introduced by Brocq in 1902. Brocq described a group of diseases which had the features of erythema, pityriasiform scaling, long duration with no systemic symptoms and resistance to topical treatment.

Parapsoriasis was later grouped into four disorders: pityriasis lichenoides chronica, pityriasis lichenoides et varioliformis acuta, small and large plaque parapsoriasis. The former two are now considered as a form of immune complex vasculitis.

Chronic superficial scaly dermatitis (Small plaque parapsoriasis. Digitate dermatosis, Brocq's disease). The disease is characterized by oval or digitate patches, less than 5 cm in diameter, present on the trunk and proximal extremities.

Large plaque parapsoriasis is characterized by plaques greater than 10 cm in diameter, present on the trunk and extremities. Some plaques may show a poikilodermic change; often referred to as poikiloderma vascular atrophicans. This has a good prognosis. However some plaques may undergo a malignant change towards a lymphoma, indicating a close relationship to mycosis fungoides.

9.2.1 Treatment

Simple emollients help in controlling the scaling. A course of UVB may be required for clearing the lesions. A close follow-up is required for patients with large plaque psoriasis to monitor for any malignant change. UVB and PUVA are helpful in giving symptomatic relief; steroids should be used with care because of the atrophic nature of the disease.

9.3 Lichen Planus

This is an inflammatory disease characterized by the formation of flat, purple, pruritic papules. The sites of predilection are the flexural aspect of the wrists, forearms and immediately above the ankles.

9.3.1 Etiology

The etiology is unknown; it is probably an immune mediated disease. The basic process is thought to be an immunological attack on the epidermal basal layer. The changes in the epidermis are secondary to the damage in the basal cells.

9.3.2 Clinical Features

The primary lesion is a flat (plano), purple, pruritic, polygonal papule (5 Ps of lichen planus). The surface of the papule has reticulated white striae (Wickham's striae); these are areas of focal epidermal thickening. These striae can be easily seen if a drop of oil is put on the lesion. The papules are found on the flexural aspect of the wrist, forearms, above the ankles and the lumbar region. Some patients complain of intolerable pruritus. In males, the papules may also be found on the penis. In most cases there is spontaneous resolution within a year. Some cases become chronic particularly if involving the lower leg. Postinflammatory hyperpigmentation is common after healing; this persists for many months to years especially in darker skinned patients (Figs. 9.7–9.9).

Involvement of the mucous membrane is common; it may even be the only manifestation of the disease. A white reticulated

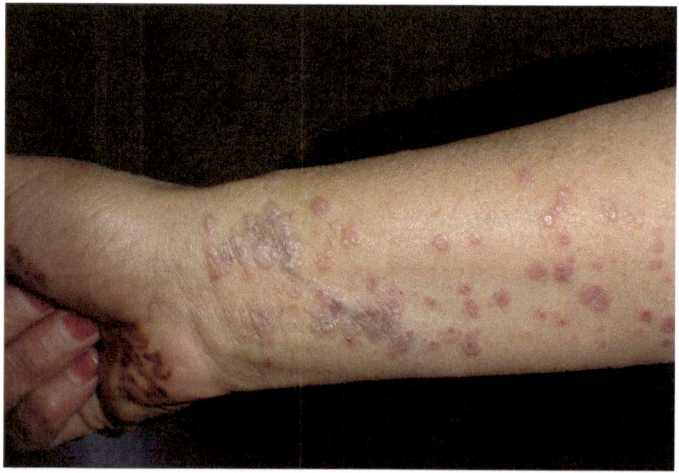

FIGURE 9.7. Lichen planus.

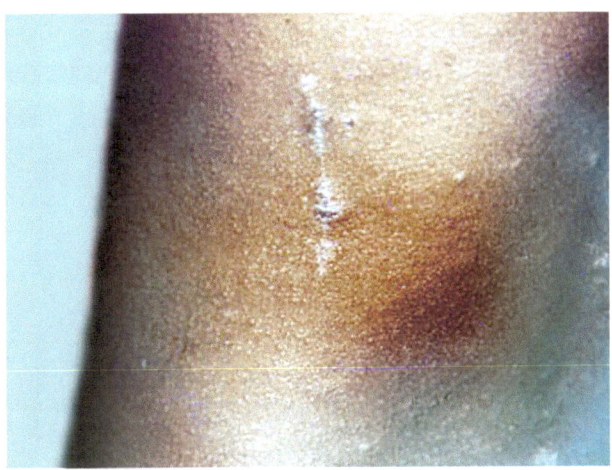

FIGURE 9.8. Lichen planus – note the Koebner's phenomenon.

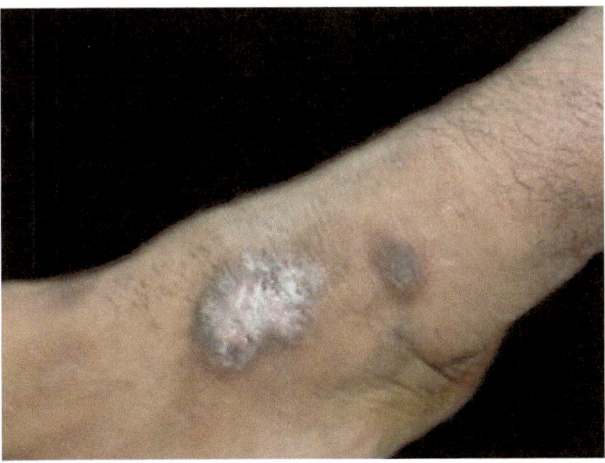

FIGURE 9.9. Hypertrophic lichen planus – note the papules at the periphery.

pattern is seen in the oral mucosa, in some cases bullae and erosions occur, these are very painful. Oral lichen planus may be associated with dental amalgam fillings, the patients often benefit by amalgam removal (Figs. 9.10 and 9.11).

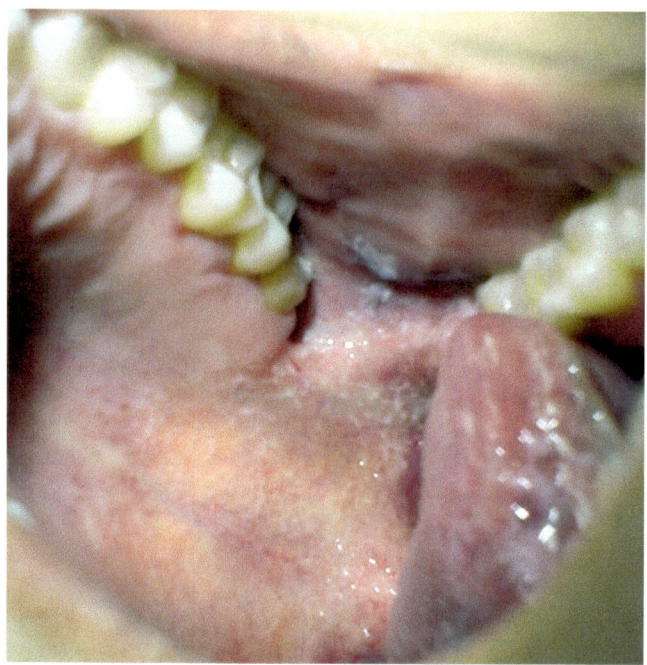

FIGURE 9.10. Lichen planus – oral cavity.

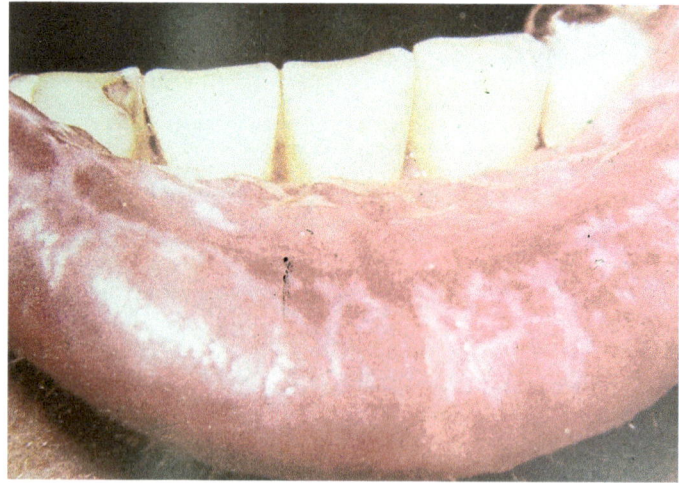

FIGURE 9.11. Lichen planus – note the reticulate appearance.

Nails are involved in 10% of cases; the nails are thin, dystrophic with longitudinal grooves and ridges. Pterygium formation is common.

In the tropics, actinic lichen planus is common. The lesions appear as hyperpigmented patches surrounded by a hypopigmented halo; the lesions are present in the sun exposed areas of the body, especially the face. Lichen planus pigmentosus is also common in the tropics; it may or not be associated with lichen planus. Macular hyperpigmentation is usually generalized, but prominent on the face, neck and upper back. There are no preceding papules. Colour varies from slate gray to brownish black. Mucous membrane, palms and soles are not involved (Fig. 9.12).

If the hair follicles are affected, then scarring alopecia occurs. Koebner's phenomenon occurs in active lichen planus. Palms and soles when affected are thickened and yellowish in color; ulcerated lesions are very difficult to treat.

The lesions can become generalized, and bullae can appear within the papules of lichen planus (bullous lichen planus). Papules can coalesce and form hypertrophic plaques; these should be differentiated from the plaques of lichen simplex chronicus when present above the ankles.

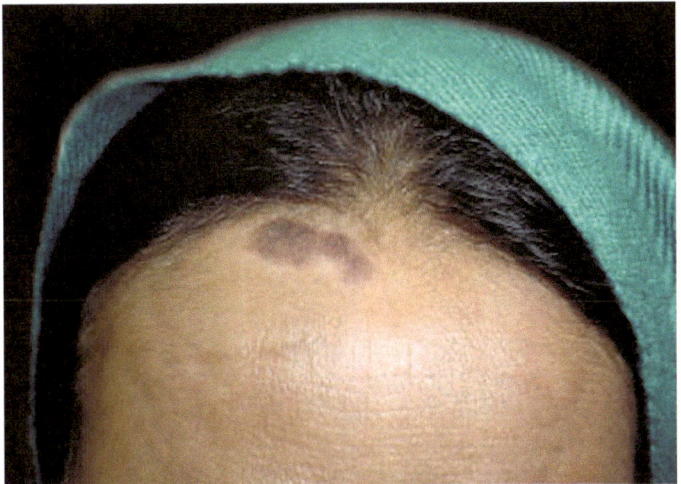

FIGURE 9.12. Actinic lichen planus.

Lichen planus like eruptions can occur after drug intake such as β-blockers, non steroidal anti inflammatory agents, gold and other heavy metals, antimalarials, diuretics, pencillamine, phenothiazine and methyldopa. Lichen planus like eruptions can also occur in graft versus host reaction and reaction to photographic developing chemicals.

9.3.3 Histopathology

Histology shows liquefaction necrosis of the basal layer and incontinence of melanin. A band like accumulation of lymphocytes is present near the dermo-epidermal junction. Because of the damage to the basal cells, the rate of mitosis is slow; there is pseudoacanthosis, irregular hypergranulosis and adhesiveness of the stratum corneum.

Diagnosis is easily made in typical cases, biopsy may be required in atypical cases.

9.3.4 Differential Diagnosis

Lichen planus should be differentiated from other pruritic disorders such as scabies. Hypertrophic lichen planus should be differentiated from lichen simplex chronicus, and a hypertrophic plaque of psoriasis. Generalized lichen planus should be differentiated from guttate psoriasis, secondary syphilis, lichenoid drug eruptions, and pityriasis lichenoides. Lichen planus of the palms and soles should be differentiated from psoriasis, eczema and fungal infection.

Some characteristic features of lichen planus are:

- Lichen planus is characterized by plane, purple, polygonal, pruritic papules.
- These are chiefly found on the flexures of the wrist and ankles.
- Wickham's striae may be present.
- The oral mucosa is involved in 50% of cases.
- Koebner's phenomenon is present in active disease.

9.3.5 Treatment

Potent topical steroids are the mainstay of treatment. Intralesional steroids are required for hypertrophic lesions. Oral steroids, acitretin, azothioprine, or cyclosporine may be used for generalized cases, and in severe progressive nail atrophy or progressive alopecia. Antihistamines are used for pruritus.

For oral lesions, steroids in orabase or cyclosporine mouthwashes in resistant cases are prescribed.

Erasmus Wilson first described lichen planus in 1869, and attributed its cause to stress. Wilson was a wealthy man and a philanthropist. He contributed a sum of £10,000 in the transportation of Cleopatra's Needle from Egypt to its present site on the Thames Embankment.

Lichen planus is a very itchy disorder.

5P's of Lichen planus are flat-topped (plano), pruritic, purple, polygonal, papules

9.4 Pityriasis Rosea

(Pityriasis means bran-like scale, rosea means rose-like).This is an acute self-limiting disorder of unknown origin. The disease affects young adults and has a seasonal variation, being least common in summer.

The generalized eruption is preceded by the appearance first of a single lesion the "herald patch." This is the largest of the lesions, it is about 2–5 cm in diameter, round or oval, pinkish in colour and covered with bran-like scales. Multiple lesions follow the herald patch; these are smaller, similar to the herald patch, follow the lines of cleavage and are arranged in an inverted Christmas tree like manner on the back. The scales in a mature lesion are located near the border of the lesion with their free edge pointing inwards (centripetal scaling) (Fig. 9.13).The patients generally feel well; a slight itching may be the only symptom. The rash fades in about 6 weeks.

Diagnosis is clinical; skin biopsy which is rarely needed is nonspecific.

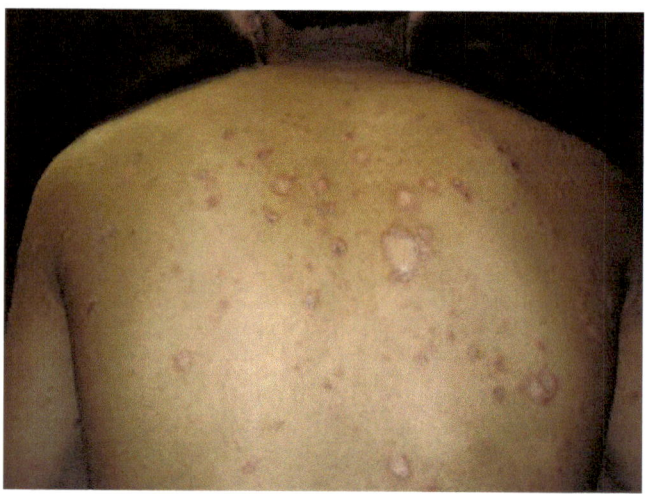

FIGURE 9.13. Pityriasis rosea.

9.4.1 Differential Diagnosis

The "herald patch," should be differentiated from tinea corporis; and the secondary lesions from other papulosquamous diseases such as psoriasis, lichen planus, seborrhoeic dermatitis, pityriasis versicolor, syphilis, parapsoriasis and nummular eczema.

Diagnostic criteria of pityriasis rosea:

- The "herald patch."
- Secondary lesions are distributed parallel to the rib lines, radiating away from the spine.
- The individual lesions have a fine peripheral "collarette" of scales.

If the rash lasts for more than 3 months, then the rash is probably not pityriasis rosea, and the diagnosis should be revised.

9.4.2 Treatment

Is symptomatic, moisturizers are required for dryness and antihistamines for itching if present.

9.5 Pityriasis Rubra Pilaris (PRP)

Is a rare chronic disease of unknown origin, with a unique combination of features: erythematous plaques, follicular papules and skip spots in the generalized form of the disease. It can occur in adults or in children.

Adult PRP begins in the fifth or sixth decade, characterized by the formation of red scaly plaques on the face and upper part of the body. The eruption then slowly involves the whole body surface. A characteristic feature of PRP is that areas of normal skin "skip spots," can be seen through the erythematous skin.

The hair follicles are also involved; the follicular papules are most prominent on the dorsal aspect of the proximal phalanges, elbows, neck and trunk. The follicular papules coalesce to form plaques. The scales are coarse on the lower half of the body and fine on the upper half.

The palms and soles are thickened, and yellowish in colour, painful fissures may develop. The nails show yellowish brown discolouration with subungal hyperkeratosis.

There is no pruritus but the thick, tight scales may be painful. Eighty percent of the cases clear in about 3 years.

Childhood PRP has a similar appearance but is more resistant to treatment and seldom clears on its own.

9.5.1 Differential Diagnosis

PRP should be differentiated from psoriasis, especially when PRP is localized on the knees and elbows. The follicular erythema in the islands of uninvolved skin and follicular plugging within the plaques, are pointers towards PRP. A biopsy of PRP shows follicular plugs, increased granular cell layer and epidermal thickening.

9.5.2 Treatment

Topical treatment is with moisturizers and keratolytics. In adult, the disease responds well to oral retinoids. Methotrexate in a dose 2.5–7.5 mg for 3 doses/week; alternatively, a single dose of 10–25 mg/week is also effective.

> *Areas of normal skin "skip spots" in generalized erythroderma are characteristic of PRP.*
> *Follicular papules are prominent on the dorsal aspect of the phalanges.*
> *Adult PRP clears in about 3 years, childhood PRP is resistant to treatment and does not remit on its own.*

9.6 Parapsoriasis

Parapsoriasis is now grouped under four disorders, small and large plaque parapsoriasis, pityriasis lichenoides varioliformis acuta, and pityriasis lichenoides chronica. The small and large plaque parapsoriasis are a group of maculopapular scaly disorders of slow evolution; they are chronic in nature and resistant to treatment. They look like psoriasis but do not have well defined borders; the scales are not silvery white. The small plaque is less than 5 cm in diameter and the large plaque is larger than 10 cm or more. The large plaque psoriasis may change into a lymphoma; so a very vigilant follow up is required.

PUVA is the treatment of choice. Potent steroids may be tried, but they should be used with care because of side effects.

> *Pityriasis lichenoides varioliformis acuta and pityriasis lichenoides chronica are discussed in the Chap.9*

9.7 Follicular Keratoses

These are a group of disorders in which the abnormality of keratinization lies in the pilosebaceous follicle. A number of diseases show follicular keratinization such as lupus erythematosus, pityriasis rubra pilaris, Darier's disease, etc.

9.7.1 Keratosis Pilaris

The disease often inherited as an autosomal dominant, is usually seen in childhood. Small follicular papules are found on the upper arm and thigh; the lesions are erythematous or appear grayish, occasionally the papules become infected. The condition is often associated with xerosis and is common in atopic children; it can also be seen in patients with ichthyosis vulgaris. In severe cases, the disease is widespread.

The disease should be differentiated from phrynoderma (deficiency of Vitamin A); it can also result from deficiency of other vitamins.

Keratosis pilaris is treated by moisturizers, which are the mainstay of treatment. They act by supplying an oily film to the epidermis, which prevents the evaporation of water. An oil bath deposits a film of lipid on the skin surface; this is helpful in generalized cases. Resistant cases can be treated with topical tretinoin or keratolytics (Fig. 9.14).

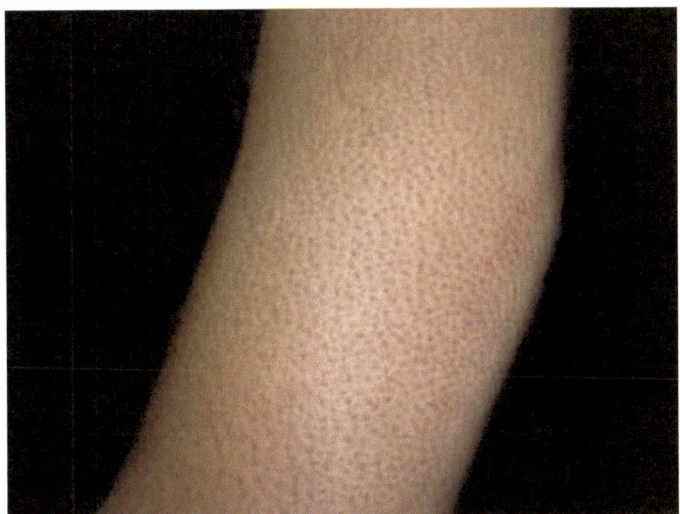

FIGURE 9.14. Keratosis pilaris.

9.7.2 Lichen Spinulosis

This is also more common in children, characterized by the formation of minute horny filiform spines that protrude from the follicular openings. They appear as grouped lesions on the abdomen, limbs, buttocks, knees and elbows. Histology shows inflammatory changes.

The condition is treated with keratolytics, topical tretinoin, and lactic acid.

9.8 Hyperkeratosis of the Palms and Soles

This can be congenital or acquired. Acquired hyperkeratosis of the palms and soles is seen in a number of cutaneous disorders such as psoriasis, lichen planus, fungal infections, contact dermatitis, Darier's disease, pityriasis rubra pilaris, etc. .

Congenital hyperkeratosis may have different morphological features; it can be generalized on the palms and soles (tylosis), punctuate, linear, and progressive, when the keratosis extends beyond the palms and soles to the forearms, legs, knees, elbows, etc (Fig. 9.15).

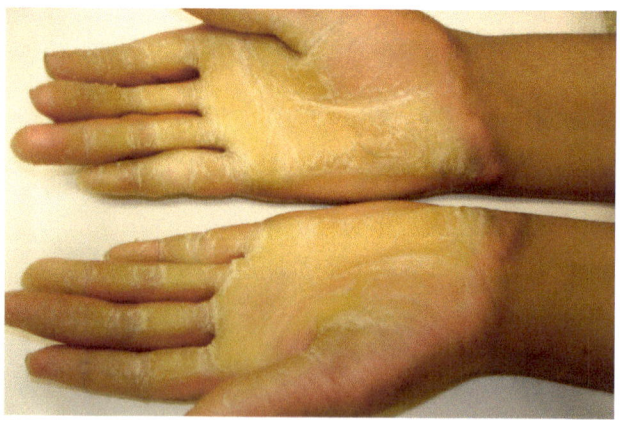

FIGURE 9.15. Keratoderma – palm.

9.8.1 Treatment

Keratolytics are the drugs of choice, as the concentration of keratin is higher on the palms and soles than elsewhere, so the concentration of keratolytics is also high, e.g. 20–25% of salicylic acid, and urea 20% is often combined with it. In extreme cases, oral retinoids are used. Emollients should be used regularly.

9.9 Corns

Corns are localized thickenings of the epidermis, secondary to chronic pressure or friction. Repeated pressure from ill-fitting shoes is the main cause for the formation of corns. Corns are commonly found on the back of toe joints and on the soles under prominent metatarsal bones. Corns consist of a conical wedge of hyperkeratosis that penetrates in the dermis; if it presses on the nerve endings it will cause pain (Figs. 9.16 and 9.17).

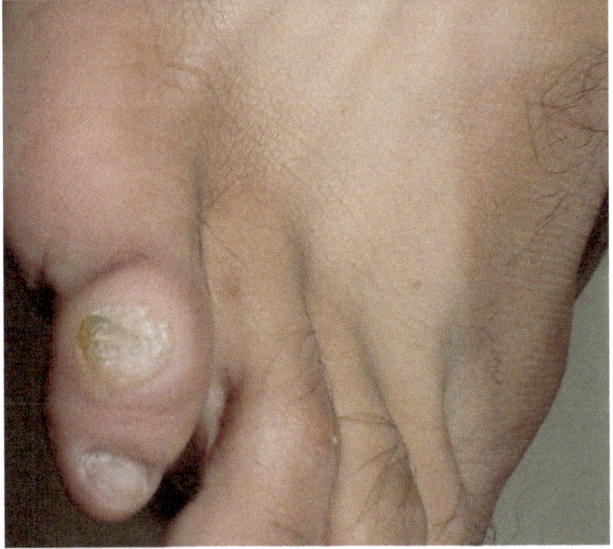

FIGURE 9.16. Corn.

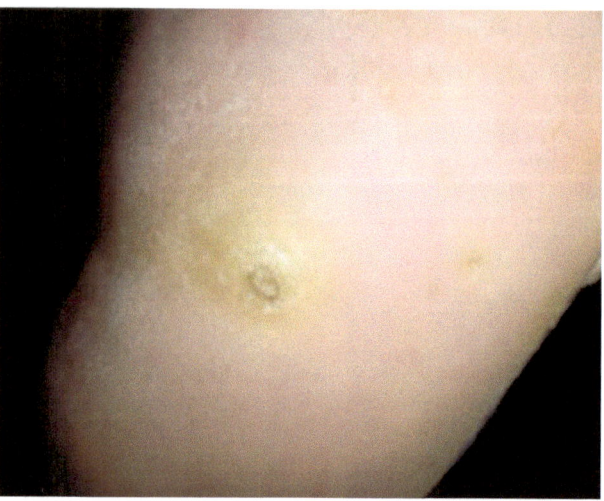

<small>FIGURE 9.17.</small> Corn.

Soft corns are found between the third and fourth toe clefts, they occur due to the pressure caused by tight shoes, when the toes are pressed together; these corns are often macerated. Corns should be differentiated from a fungal infection. Sometimes corns are formed by intrinsic pressure from an exostosis or anatomical skeletal defects.

Callosities occur where the intermittent pressure on the skin is spread over a large area; they do not cause pain and have no penetrating core of hyperkeratosis.

9.9.1 Differential Diagnosis

Corns should be differentiated from warts. Warts show tiny bleeding points when pared representing thrombosed capillaries. Skin markings are present on a wart but absent from a corn. Pinching a corn is painless, while lateral pressure on a wart causes pain.

A corn consists of a central core of whitish material composed of degenerated cells and cholesterol, and encircled by a narrow area of hyperkeratosis. The main histological feature of a wart is vacuolation of cells in and below the stratum granulosum, these cells are called koilocytes.

9.9.2 Treatment

The appropriate treatment is to remove the pressure that was responsible for the formation of the corn. Changing of ill-fitting shoes and shielding the pressure sites with pads, or orthotic devices reduces mechanical trauma.

Corns require 40% salicylic acid plaster, for 48 h, the plaster is then removed, and the superficial skin is cleaned and scraped, a new plaster reapplied. The process is repeated until the corn is gone. Duofilm can also be used. In difficult cases the corn can be removed surgically. For intrinsic defects, an orthopaedic surgeon should be consulted.

> *Corns in diabetic patients and those with ischaemic changes of the foot need special care, because of the greater risk of infection and ulceration.*

9.10 Congenital Disorders of Keratinization

9.10.1 Darier's Disease

This is an autosomal dominant. Inherited disorder of keratinization. The disease usually appears in adolescence, often after exposure to sunlight. It presents as brownish, greasy horny papules in the seborrhoeic areas of the body. The papules are easily infected due to decrease in cell-mediated immunity. Other features of the disease are hyperkeratosis of the palms and soles, palmar pits (these are pathognomonic of Darier's disease), and nails showing red and white striations with a nick at the free border of the nail.

The disease is due to a loss of adhesion between the keratinocytes above the basal layer. These acantholytic cells then keratinize prematurely, in which eosinophilic bodies (corps ronds) are formed, these later become basophilic and the cell shrinks (grains). Grains are found in the upper part of the epidermis (Fig. 9.18).

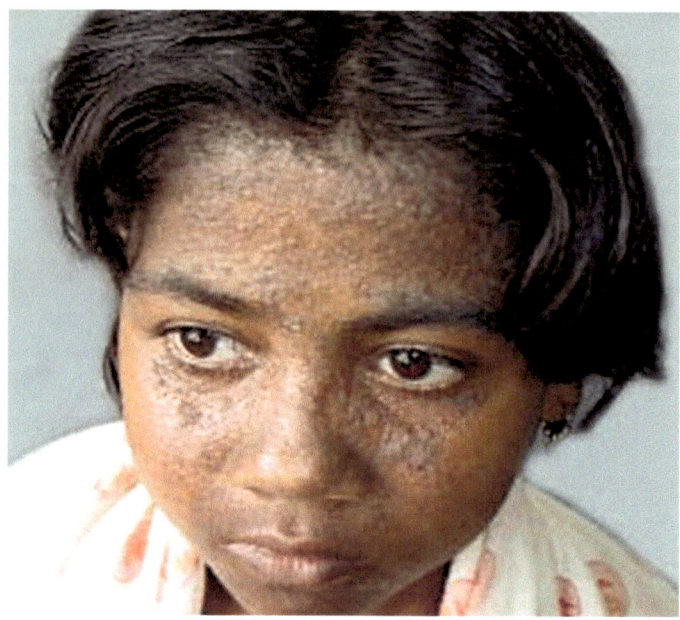

FIGURE 9.18. Darier's disease.

The disease should be differentiated from seborrhoeic dermatitis and acne. There are no comedones in Darier's disease; the papules are greasy, crusted and warty. The palms, soles and nails are involved in Darier's disease, these are normal in seborrhoeic dermatitis.

9.10.1.1 Treatment

In mild cases topical keratolytics are prescribed, severe cases require oral retinoids. The disease relapses on stopping the drug.

9.10.2 Ichthyosis

Generally, this is the name given to a group of hereditary generalized noninflammatory disorders of keratinization giving rise to excessive scaling of the skin. These disorders may be autosomal dominant, autosomal reccesive or x-linked recessive. Ichthyosis can also be acquired. It can occur in severe nutritional deficiency, leprosy, malignancies such as Hodgkin's disease, and hypothyroidism. Drugs such as nicotinamide and clofazamine can also cause dryness and scaling of the skin.

9.10.2.1 Ichthyosis Vulgaris

This is an autosomal dominant disorder; it is the mildest form of ichthyosis. Fine, white, scales cover the body, the flexures are spared. Keratosis pilaris is present on the outer aspect of the arms and thigh. The granular layer is absent and there is a decrease in the histidine rich protein fillagrin (Figs. 9.19 and 9.20).

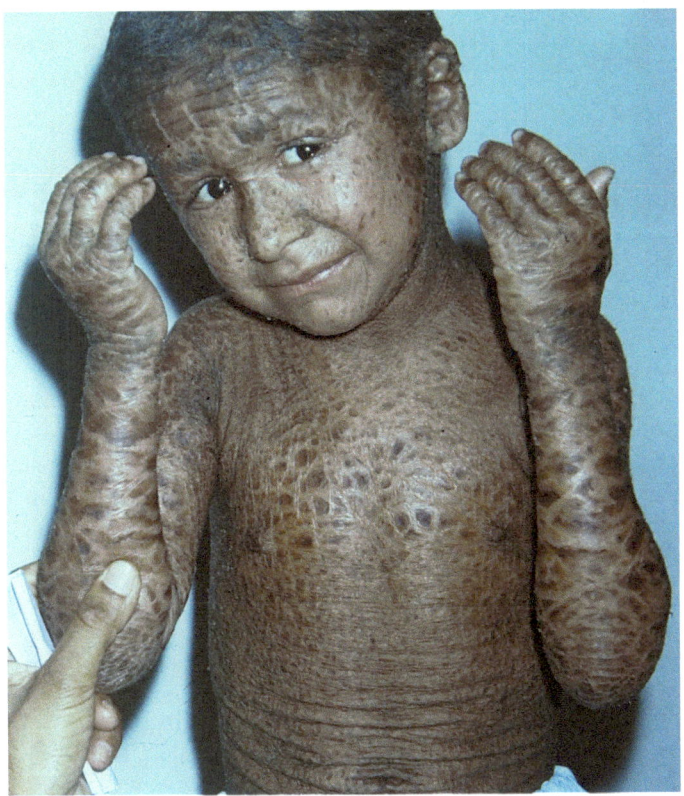

FIGURE 9.19. Ichthyosis.

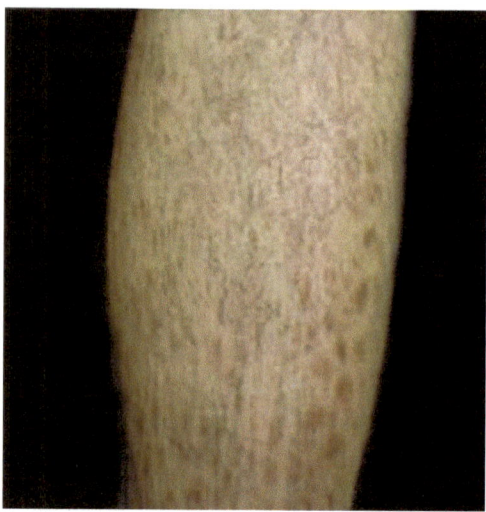

FIGURE 9.20. Acquired ichthyosis.

9.10.2.2 X-Linked Recessive Ichthyosis

The disease is seen in males, females being carriers. The body is covered with dark coloured scales except the palms and soles which are spared. The patients often have cryptorchism, corneal opacities, and mental retardation.

Biochemically the affected males show a steroid sulphatase deficiency. For diagnostic purposes fibroblasts, lymphocytes or epidermal cells are tested, the steroid sulphatase deficiency results in excessive quantities of cholesterol sulphate in the stratum corneum and with a decrease in free cholesterol.

9.10.2.3 NonBullous Ichthyosiform Erythroderma

This is an autosomal dominant disorder; affected children are often born enclosed in a collodion membrane. These patients also often have ectropion and crumpled ears. The entire body is erythematous and covered with fine white scales. The erythema gradually becomes less with age, but the scaling persists.

9.10.2.4 Bullous Ichthyosiform Erythroderma (Epidermolytic Hyperkeratosis)

This is an autosomal dominant disorder; the infant may be born in a collodion membrane as in nonbullous ichthyosiform erythroderma. Blistering is associated with erythema and scaling. The scales are fine and white. The blisters and erythema decrease with age, but there is excessive hyperkeratosis especially at the flexures and palm and soles. Maceration at the flexures gives a foul smell. It is the most recalcitrant form of ichthyosis. The pathognomonic histological feature of epidermolytic hyperkeratosis is a reticulate degenerative change in the epidermis.

9.10.2.5 Lamellar Ichthyosis

This is an autosomal recessive disorder; the child may be enclosed in a collodion membrane. There is ectropion and crumpled ears as in the ichthyosiform erythrodermas. The scales are dark brown in colour, thicker than those of x-linked ichthyosis.

9.10.2.6 Collodion Baby

Infants are sometimes born with a tough, inelastic, collodion-like membrane covering the body. The membrane over a period of time fissures and peels off. Collodion babies are often seen with congenital ichthyosiform erythroderma or lamella ichthyosis. Affected babies are often dehydrated and in danger of hypothermia. Mortality is high (Fig. 9.21).

9.10.2.7 Harlequin Foetus

This disorder is of autosomal recessive inheritance; the skin is covered with thick heavy armour-like plates covering the skin. The ears are rudimentary or absent, eclabium is present. The infant is often premature and of low birth weight, the child may be still born, or may die soon after. There is no effective treatment although some cases of recovery following treatment by etretinate have been reported (Fig. 9.22).

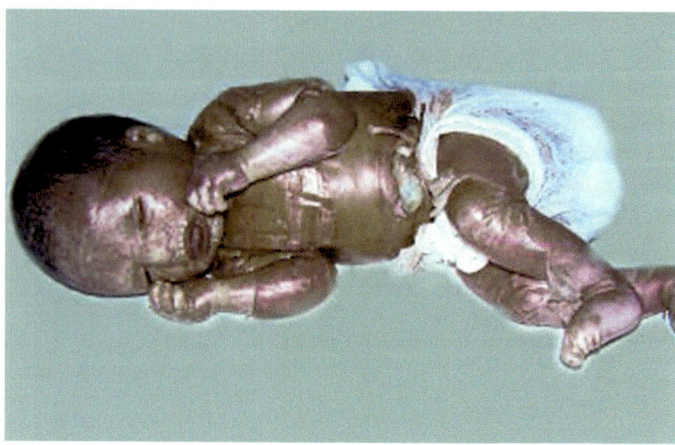

FIGURE 9.21. Collodoin baby.

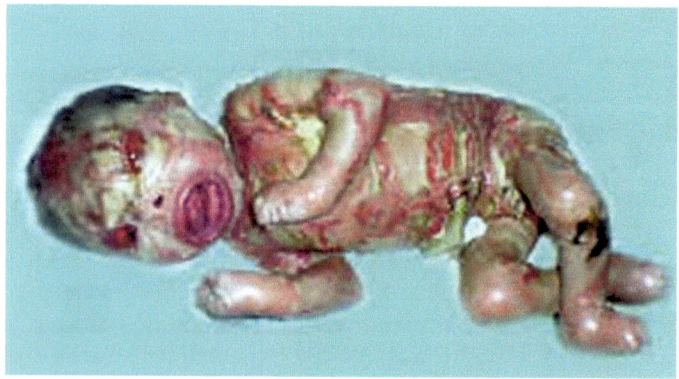

FIGURE 9.22. Harlequin fetus.

9.10.3 Treatment of Ichthyosis

The aim of treatment is to hydrate the skin and the use of keratolytics to remove the scales. Emollients occlude the skin surface with a lipid film, which prevents the evaporation of water from the surface, and it hydrates the stratum corneum.

Keratolytic agents such as salicylic acid, lactic acid, glycolic acid, pyruvic acid, and retinoic acid remove the scales. In severe cases where topical treatment fails oral retinoids are given. These children should be monitored very carefully due to the side effects of premature epiphysial closure, hyperostosis, and hyperlipidemia.

Chapter 10
Diseases of Connective Tissue

Lupus erythematosus, scleroderma, and dermatomyositis are frequently referred to as autoimmune collagen disorders. They are all associated with a high incidence of circulating autoantibodies, and with widespread fibrinoid degeneration of collagen fibers occurring in mesenchymal tissues.

10.1 Lupus Erythematosus

The disease may range from purely cutaneous (discoid lupus), through involvement of a few organs (subacute lupus) to a severe multisystem disease (systemic lupus erythematosus).

10.1.1 Chronic Discoid Lupus Erythematosus (CDLE)

This is the most common form of lupus erythematosus. The disease is localized to the skin; it affects the exposed areas of the body. The lesions may be few or many. The disease is characterized by the formation of erytematous scaly plaques, with follicular plugging. When the scale is lifted follicular plugs are seen on the undersurface; this is the "carpet tack sign." As the disease progresses the center shows areas of atrophy and

Z. Zaidi, S. W. Lanigan, *Dermatology in Clinical Practice*,
DOI: 10.1007/978-1-84882-862-9_10,
© Springer-Verlag London Limited 2010

scarring, these areas appear white and hypopigmented, with a peripheral erythematous scaly border, which later becomes hyperpigmented. These lesions are very typical of CDLE (Figs. 10.1 and 10.2).

Lupus profundus affects the subcutaneous fat; it produces deep nodular swelling which later causes depression of the skin due to fat atrophy. The skin surface may be clinically normal. On the scalp CDLE results in cicatricial alopecia. There is no evidence of systemic involvement. Blood tests are usually normal, occasionally ANA is positive, showing a diffuse pattern.

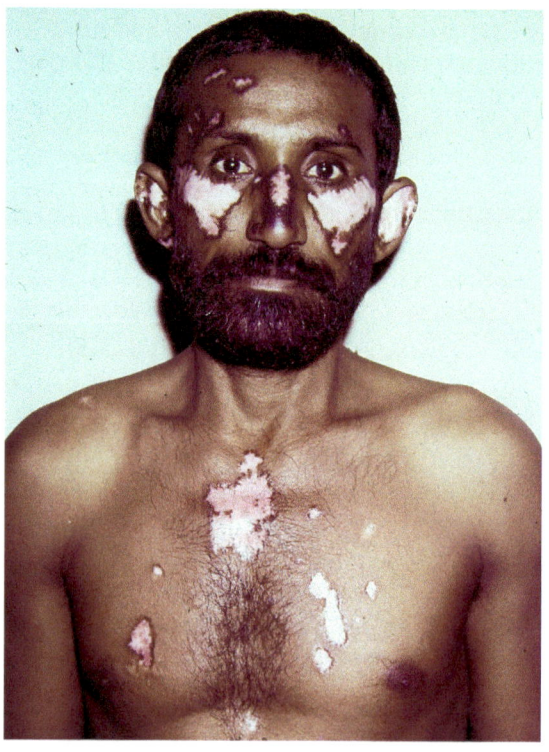

FIGURE 10.1. Chronic discoid lupus erythematosus.

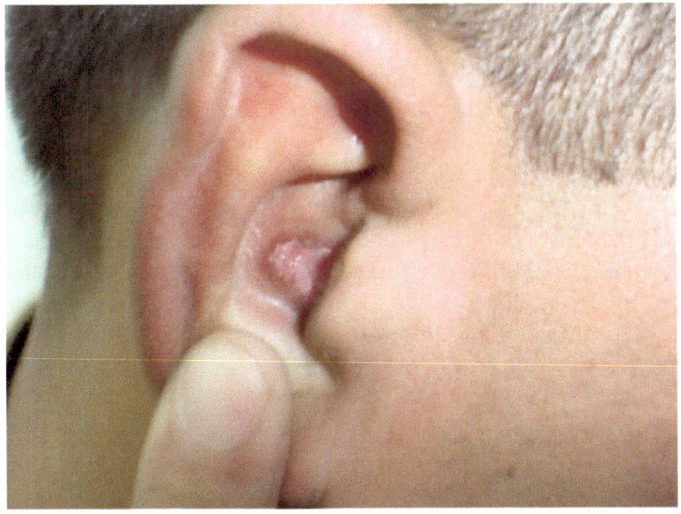

FIGURE 10.2. Chronic discoid lupus erythematosus.

10.1.2 Subacute Cutaneous Lupus Erythematosus (SCLE)

The lesions are most prominent on the face, upper part of the chest, and back. The lesions appear as erythematous scaly plaques or are annular; these may have a wavy outline. The lesions are slow to heal, but do not show scarring. SCLE runs a mild course; renal, vascular, and CNS complications are rare. Many patients have antibodies to cytoplasmic antigen Ro (SS-A).

10.1.3 Systemic Lupus Erythematosus

This is the most severe form of lupus erythematosus: affecting women more than men. The disease can be transient, recurrent, or continuous. It affects the skin and multiple systems of the body.

10.1.3.1 Cutaneous Manifestations

The patient has a characteristic scaly erythematous plaque on the face in the butterfly distribution, on the cheeks and nose. Other dermatological signs are periungul telangiectasia, palmar erythema, erythematous plaques on the dorsum of the hand; digital ischemia leading to digital infarcts, livido reticularis, and Raynaud's phenomenon present in 60% of cases. Typical CDLE-like lesions may also be present. Generalized nonscarring alopecia can occur; the hairs on the frontal margin are thin, dry and brittle, often called the lupus hair. Ulcers may be present in the oral mucosa (Figs. 10.3–10.5).

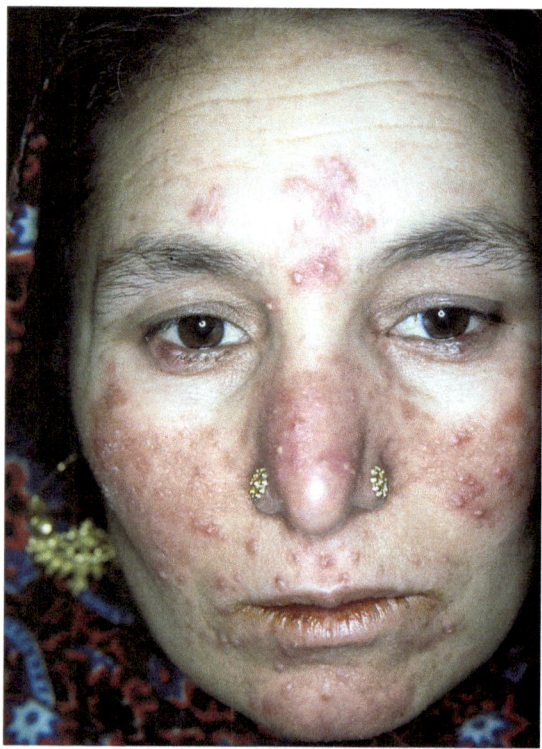

FIGURE 10.3. Lupus erythematosus – butterfly rash.

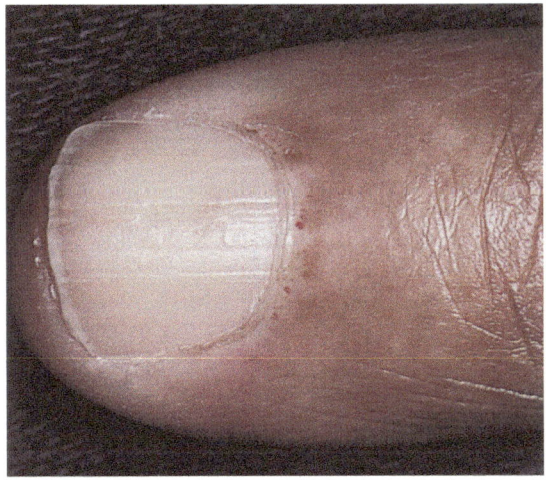

FIGURE 10.4. Periungal telangiectasia.

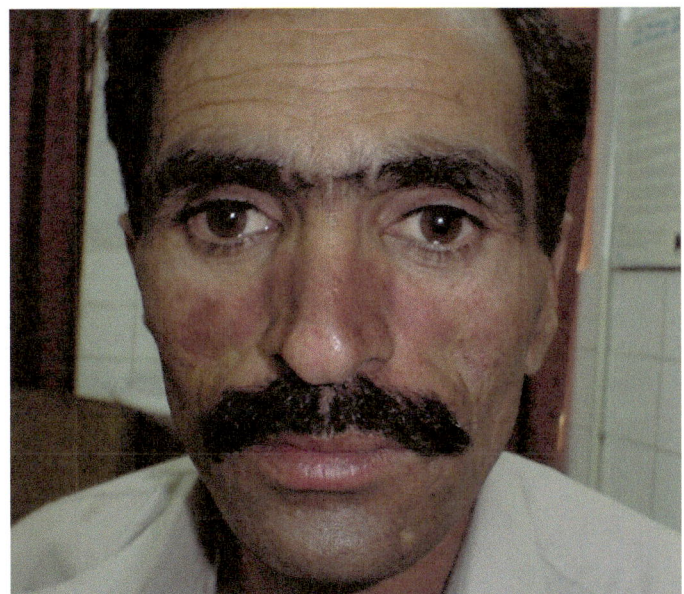

FIGURE 10.5. Lupus erythematosus – butterfly rash.

10.1.3.2 Systemic Manifestations

These include fever, weakness, malaise, arthralgia, arthritis, myalgia, and myositis.

Cardiovascular abnormalities include myocarditis, pericarditis, and Libmann Sach endocarditis. Central nervous system manifestations include migraine, nerve palsies, meningitis, fits, and stroke. Psychiatric disturbances range from depression to psychosis. Gastrointestinal involvement is rare, ascites may be present, and hepatitis is often drug-induced. Pleurisy is common. Fifty percent of the patients have renal involvement leading to albuminuria, hematuria, and hypertension. Renal and CNS involvement indicates a poor prognosis. The disease is characterized by pancytopenia.

A large number of antibodies are present in the patient's serum such as ANA, Ds DNA, anti-La; anti-Ro. Serum compliment levels are low.

Skin biopsy shows liquefaction degeneration of the basal layer, and a lymphocytic infiltration around the blood vessels and skin appendages.

ARA criteria for the diagnosis of SLE (at least four required for diagnosis):

- Butterfly rash
- Discoid plaques
- Photosensitivity
- Ulcers in the oral cavity
- Arthritis
- Serositis
- Renal involvement
- Neurological disorder
- Hematological disorder
- Immunological disorder
- Antinuclear antibodies (ANA)

10.1.4 Diagnosis

The following investigations are helpful in the diagnosis of SLE:

- Hematology – pancytopenia, raised ESR.
- Urine examination – proteinuria or hematuria.

- Blood tests for autoantibodies, a number of antibodies are present, the ones generally tested for are: ANA, Ds DNA, anti-Ro for subacute SLE.
- Skin biopsy – degeneration of basal cells, epidermal thinning, inflammation around the appendages.
- Skin immunofluorescence – this shows a "lupus band" of immunoglobulins and complement at the dermo-epidermal junction, in the involved and uninvolved skin.

10.1.5 Differential Diagnosis

CDLE on the scalp should be differentiated from other scarring alopecias; on the face it should be differentiated from psoriasis, lupus vulgaris, and Jessner's lymphocytic infiltration. Subacute lupus erythematosus should be differentiated from annular psoriasis, tinea corporis, annular erythemas, and the generalized form of CDLE. SLE is a great imitator of other disease due to its widespread involvement of other organs. On the face, it should be differentiated from other photosensitive disorders including rosacea, and seborrheic dermatitis. The generalized lesions of SLE should be differentiated from rheumatoid arthritis and other collagen disorders.

10.1.6 Treatment

CDLE

- Avoid sunlight; sunscreens should be applied half an hour before going out in the sun.
- Tablet hydroxychloroquine 400 mg daily or b.i.d. Eyes should be examined periodically; monthly for 6 months and then every 4–6 months.
- Local application of corticosteroids, potent corticosteroids are effective. In resistance cases intralesional steroids can be used.
- In resistant cases, oral retinoids and thalidomide have been reported to be helpful.

SCLE

- The treatment is similar to CDLE, oral retinoids, and corticosteroids are indicated especially if the disease is widespread.

SLE

- The treatment of SLE is to maintain optimal function with minimum of therapy. In acute cases bed rest is required; undue exposure to sun should be avoided. Mental and physical stress should be minimized and, secondary infection should be prevented.
- The symptoms should be controlled with acetyl-salicylic acid derivatives; if this is not effective then anti-malarial drugs should be added. Treatment with corticosteroids depends upon the severity of the illness; this can be judged by the severity of the symptoms, serum C3 complement levels and anti-DNA titres. Prednisolone 60 mg daily is the steroid of choice. Once the disease is under control, the dose is gradually reduced to 10–15 mg daily. Immunosuppressive drugs are used for patients not responding to corticosteroids. Plasmapheresis may be helpful in small number of cases.
- Intermittent intravenous infusion of gamma globulin has shown some good results.
- Long-term and regular follow-up of the patient is necessary.

Severe cases of SLE should be started on steroids before waiting for laboratory results.

Lupus erythematosus was first recognized as a cutaneous disorder for many years; the systemic form of the disorder was unknown. Kaposi in 1871 was the first to recognize the systemic component of the disease.

10.2 Dermatomyositis (DM)

As the name suggests the disorder affects both the skin and muscles. Females outnumber males, as in SLE. DM affects two age groups; adults and children. Adult dermatomyositis is often associated with malignancy of the GIT, prostate, ovary, and blood. The cause is unknown, but an autoimmune etiology is likely. Autoantibodies to striated muscle are found.

10.2.1 Adult Dermatomyositis

10.2.1.1 Cutaneous Signs

This is manifested by violaceous erythema of the face and hands. On the face the eyelids are affected first due to involvement of the orbicularis oculi; the eyelids are swollen and have a purplish color (called heliotrope, because of the color of the flower); and are tender to touch (Fig. 10.6). Erythema and edema over the cheeks is followed by erythema of the neck and presternal area. Linear erythema occurs on the dorsum of the digits. Flat-topped papules are present over the knuckles; known as Gottron's sign. It is said to be pathognomonic of dermatomyositis (in SLE the plaques

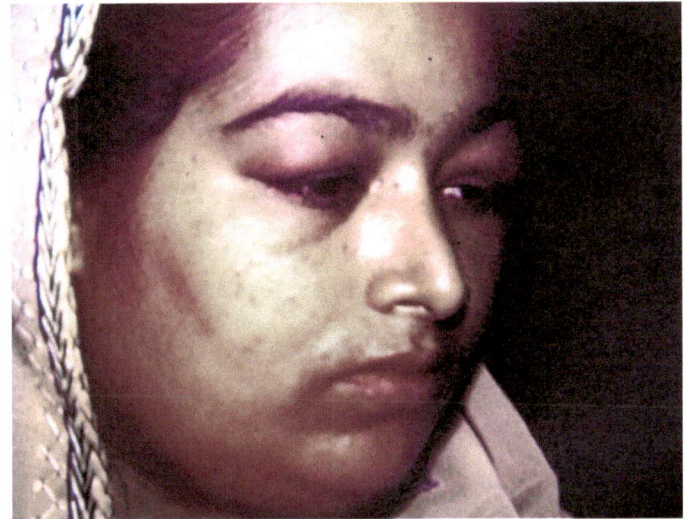

FIGURE 10.6. Dermatomysitis – note the erythema and edema around the eyelids.

are present on the digits between the knuckles). Telangiectasia is present on the posterior nail folds. The cuticles are ragged. On the knees and elbows calcified nodules may occur.

10.2.1.2 Muscle Involvement

Muscles of the proximal extremities of the upper and lower limb are affected first. Patients find it difficult to comb their hair or to climb stairs. Later the pharyngeal, esophageal, and cardiac muscles are involved. Myositis may lead to permanent weakness and immobility. Some patients die from severe and progressive myopathy.

Toxoplasmosis may cause a dermatomyositis-like syndrome. Thirty percent of adults with DM may have an undiagnosed malignancy. DM improves when the tumor is removed.

10.2.2 Childhood Dermatomyositis

Internal malignancy is not associated with childhood dermatomyositis. The disease may be progressive and rapid or it may be benign and slow to progress. It is associated with vasculitis and calcinosis cutis.

10.2.3 Diagnosis

Electromyography (EMG), elevation of serum aldolase, creatinine phosphokinase (CPK), lactic dehydrogenase, and amino transferase may help to confirm the diagnosis. Biopsy of the affected muscles shows inflammation and destruction of the muscles.

10.2.4 Treatment

Bed rest is essential during the acute phase. For muscle pain aminosalicylic acid two tablets four times a day are given. Oral corticosteroids 60 mg/day give symptomatic relief; the dose is reduced as remission occurs. Persistent cases respond to cyclosporine or methotrexate. Azathioprine is added to control the disease and reduce the dose of steroids. In severe muscle involvement, physiotherapy is an adjuvant to drug therapy. Gamma globulin infusions appear promising.

To prevent muscle from destruction a maintenance regimen is needed for several years. Serum levels of CPK can help to monitor disease activity and can help to distinguish between relapse and steroid myopathy.

> *Investigate for internal malignancy in adult dermatomyositis. Edema of the eyelid with, heliotrope discoloration, and Gottron's signs are specific for dermatomyosistis.*

10.3 Scleroderma

The disease may be localized (morphea) or generalized (systemic sclerosis). The disorder is characterized by sclerosis of the connective tissue, which makes the skin hard and tight. The cause of the disease is unknown; it is thought that an abnormality of the endothelium of the blood vessels, is the initial target of the disease, followed by fibrosis.

Lesions similar to systemic sclerosis are also seen in graft versus host reaction, polyvinyl chloride workers, ingestion of adulterated rapeseed oil, and in cases of prolonged untreated porphyria cutanea tarda.

10.3.1 Morphea

This is localized scleroderma. A patch of skin becomes hard due to fibrosis. The hair follicles and sweat glands are destroyed. The affected area of the skin is initially purplish in color, as the fibrosis increases; the skin becomes white, smooth and shiny, often surrounded by a violaceous halo. The overlying skin is dry and without hair. Plaques of morphea may be nummular, linear, or guttate. Prognosis is slow, fibrosis slowly clears leaving slight depression and hyperpigmentation. Generalized morphea has a poor prognosis with spontaneous resolution unlikely.

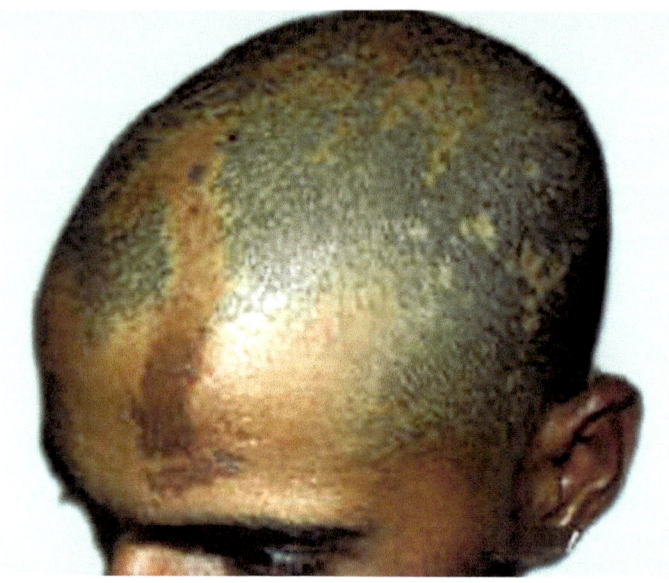

FIGURE 10.7. Morphea.

Linear morphea is a rare type of morphea; plaques of cutaneous sclerosis follow a linear pattern along a limb, scalp, or face (Fig. 10.7). It may lead to arrest of growth of the underlying bones causing facial hemiatrophy or shortening of a limb.

Lymes borreliosis may be associated with morphea in Europe.

10.3.1.1 Treatment

It is difficult and the response is slow. Potent topical steroids are used; in some cases, intralesional steroids are preferred. Hydroxychloroquine may be used in selected cases.

If steroids fail or side effects occur, then calciprotriol, NSAIDS, or PUVA may be tried.

Pencillamine is said to be helpful in a few cases. Phenytoin sodium may be used for the treatment of linear morphea.

10.3.2 CREST Syndrome

The acronym stands for *C*alcinosis, *R*aynaud's phenomenon, o*E*sophageal dysmotility, *S*clerodactyly, *T*elangiactasia. Anticentromere antibody is considered to be specific for CREST syndrome. The prognosis is generally good.

10.3.3 Systemic Sclerosis

This is the generalized form of scleroderma, with involvement of the skin and internal organs. The skin involvement may be acral; involving the face and extremities, or it may be generalized.

10.3.3.1 Cutaneous Manifestations

The skin of the face and hands, have a characteristic appearance. The face is mask-like, with limited or no facial expression. The nose is beaked and the mouth shows radial furrowing. Multiple mat-like telangiectasia are seen on the face. The skin is hide-bound.

On the hands, the fingers are tapered and hardened. Fingertip ulcers are due to vasculitis. This may lead to gangrene and absorption of the digits. Nail telangiestasia are prominent. Calcinosis cutis is seen on the hands and feet (Fig. 10.8).

The generalized form of the disease is very disabling, where the movement of the joints is limited and the patients have difficulty in breathing.

10.3.3.2 Systemic Manifestations

Raynaud's phenomenon is the usual presenting symptom. Systemic sclerosis affects almost all the organs of the body. GIT is involved in almost all the cases. The esophagus is involved in about 90% of cases leading to dysphagia and reflex esophagitis. Disturbance of bowel movement, constipation, colicky pain, and abdominal distension are some of the signs of

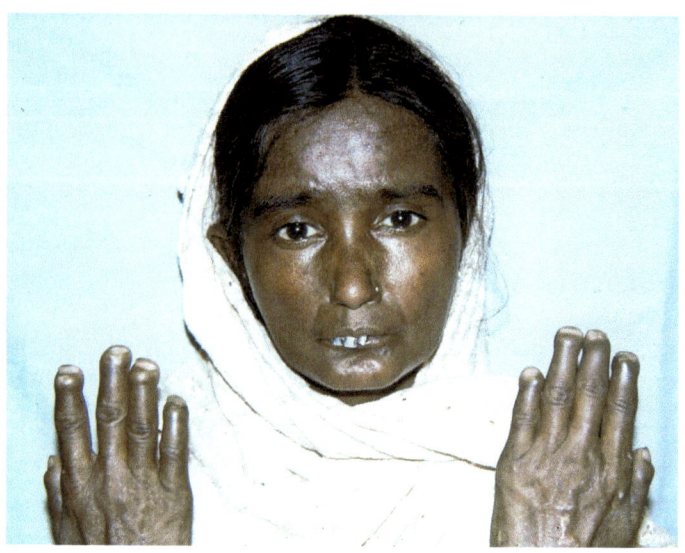

FIGURE 10.8. Systemic sclerosis.

GIT involvement. Pulmonary involvement leads to pulmonary fibrosis, dyspnea, and pulmonary hypertension. Cardiovascular involvement manifests as conduction block and left ventricular diastolic dysfunction. Renal involvement from malignant hypertension is late but has a grave prognosis.

10.3.3.3 Diagnosis

The characteristic features of the face and hands are diagnostic of systemic sclerosis. This is confirmed by the presence of ANA, anti-Scl-70 and anti-centromere antibodies. A barium swallow shows loss of esophageal peristalsis; this is not recommended as obstruction may follow poor evacuation of the contrast medium.

10.3.3.4 Differential Diagnosis

Systemic sclerosis should be differentiated from other causes of Raynaud's phenomenon. Sclerosis should be differentiated from widespread morphea, porphyria cutanea tarda, mixed connective tissue disorder, eosinophilic fasciitis, and diabetic sclerodactyly.

10.3.3.5 Treatment

There is no specific therapy but symptomatic treatment and management are important. Well-planned general exercises, regular massage, warmth, protection from trauma are beneficial, and exposure to cold should be minimized and smoking should be prohibited. Patients with esophagitis should avoid lying flat, the patients may benefit from H2 receptor antagonists and metoclopramide. Electrically heated gloves and socks, and vaso-active drugs may help digital ischemia.

Drugs used in scleroderma are the immunemodulators, vasoactive drugs and the antifibrotics. Ten to fifteen milligrams of prednisolone daily may be used. Corticosteroids do not offer any lasting benefit, but the patient feels better and the joint symptoms may be ameliorated. A variety of vasoactive drugs may be used. Thirty milligrams of nifedipine, captopril 150 mg daily, 2.5 mg/kg of prostacyclin infused I/V in 24 h. In some cases D-pencillamine in doses of 150–300 mg daily may be used; it inhibits the synthesis of collagen cross-links. Other antifibrotic agents are cyclofenil, colchicine, etc. Griseofulvin in a dose of 750 mg daily inhibits the proliferation of fibro-blasts. Azathioprine and cyclophosphamide may also be used to reduce the inflammatory changes of scleroderma.

Recently phototherapy with ultraviolet A-1 (340–400 nm) has shown some promising results.

Mask-like face, mat-like telangiectasia, and sclerodactyly help in the diagnosis of systemic sclerosis.

Sjogrens syndrome – The syndrome consists of a triad of dry-ness of the cornea and conjunctiva, xerostomia, and rheumatoid arthritis. Rheumatoid arthritis may be replaced by other con-nective tissue disorders. The cutaneous symptoms consist of palpable purpura, urticaria, and erythema multiforme. The patients are prone to lymphoreticular malignancies.

10.3.4.1 Treatment

This is directed against the vascular manifestations of connective tissue disease. Artificial lubricants are used for oral, anal, and vaginal dryness. Artificial tears are used for dryness of the cornea.

10.3.5 Mixed Connective Tissue Disorder

This is an overlap between SLE with either one or other collagen diseases (dermatomyositis, scleroderma, and occasionally rheumatoid arthritis). The most striking laboratory finding is the presence of ANA in a speckled manner. As in SLE, females are more affected than males.

It usually presents with swollen hands, and sclerodactyly; skin lesions of SLE may be present. Alopecia is mild and mimics telogen effluvium. About 25% of patients will have small vessel vasculitis; many show Raynaud's phenomenon. The disorder is chronic and usually develops into one of the other known collagen diseases.

10.3.5.1 Treatment

There is no specific treatment, but depends upon which organs are involved and which disease predominates. Usually systemic steroids are needed, as in SLE. Immunosuppressive agents help to lower the dose of steroids. NSAIDS are used for malaise and arthralgia.

10.4 Miscellaneous Disorders of Connective Tissue

10.4.1 Keloids

A keloid is an excessive connective tissue response to injury; it extends beyond the site of tissue damage. The common sites of

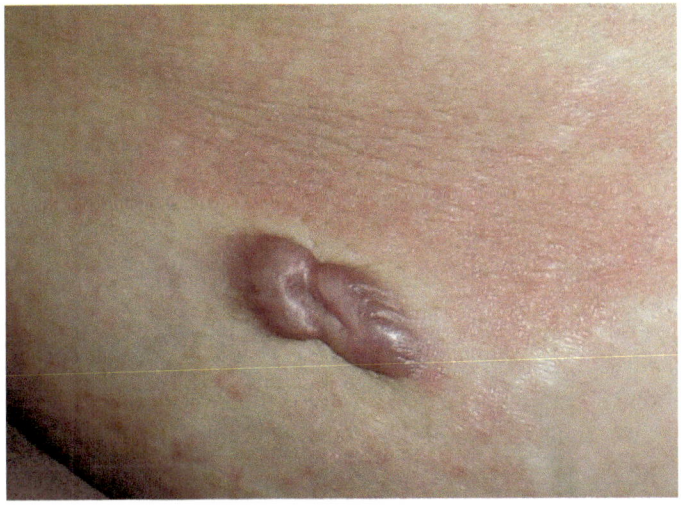

FIGURE 10.9. Keloid.

keloid formation are the chest, upper back, and shoulders. Keloids appear as firm reddish plaques, with finger-like projections; later the color changes to brown (Fig. 10.9). Keloids may be painful, tender, or pruritic. Occasionally they can become inflamed. Neuropeptides contribute to the pain and mast cell mediators are responsible for the itching felt in keloids. Keloids tend to be familial and are common in Negroes.

10.4.1.1 Prophylaxis

Nonessential surgery should be avoided at the sites where there is a tendency for keloids to occur. If surgery is essential then simple excision with sutures without tension should be applied. Preoperative and postoperative steroid injections should be given. Preoperative radiotherapy is also used in some cases. Precautions should be taken to avoid secondary infection. Electrocoagulation and caustic chemicals should be avoided at such sites.

10.4.1.2 Treatment

Intralesional injections of corticosteroids are used for early keloids. Forty milligrams per milliliter of triamcinolone is injected in the keloid; the treatment is repeated every 6–8 weeks. Several injections may be required. Prior freezing with liquid nitrogen before the injection causes edema, softens the keloid, and helps in the injection within the keloid. A dermo-jet can be used for keloid injection.

If surgical removal is required then preoperative and post-operative injection of triamcinolone should be given in a dose of 10 mg/mL. Surgical excision and control with metho-trexate have given good results. Methotrexate is given orally 15–20 mg in a single dose and repeated every 4 days, starting a week before surgery and for about 4 months after surgery.

Colchicine, which prevents fibrous tissue formation, has also been used in the treatment of keloids.

A cream containing 20% of silicon acid applied under occlusion has also been used for the treatment of keloids. Topical retinoic acid applied daily may be helpful in some cases. Pulsed dye laser therapy will reduce scar redness and pruritus. Systemic retinoids can enhance keloid formation.

10.4.2 Knuckle Pads (Holoderma)

These are well-defined fibrous thickenings on the extensor surface of the proximal interphalangeal joints of the fingers. The toes are seldom involved. It is said to have an autosomal dominant inheritance. The age of onset is variable and is commonly seen after the fourth decade. The growth is rapid initially; it grows to a diameter of 10–15 mm and then persists permanently. Knuckle pads are skin-colored or slightly brownish in color, freely movable over the underlying structures (Fig. 10.10). They are often associated with Dupuytrens contracture and other fibromatous lesions.

Treatment is unsatisfactory. Excision is often followed by keloid formation. Intralesional steroids may be beneficial.

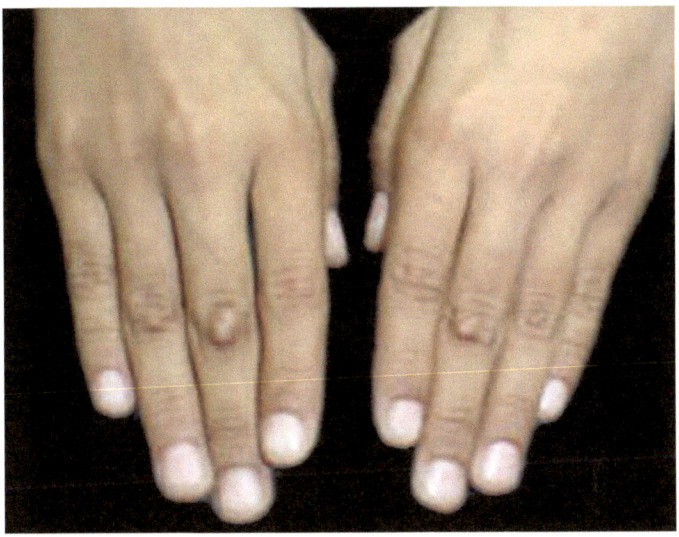

FIGURE 10.10. Knuckle pads.

10.5 Hereditary Disorders of Connective Tissue

10.5.1 Pseudoxanthoma Elasticum

This is an inherited disorder of connective tissue, characterized by elastorrhexis of the dermis, blood vessels, and Bruch's membrane of the eye. Calcium is deposited in the abnormal elastic tissue. The disease appears in childhood, and is usually present before the age of 30 years.

Cutaneous changes consist of small, yellowish papules in a linear or reticular pattern, most prominent in the neck, resembling plucked-chicken skin (Fig. 10.11). Other sites affected are the axillae, groin, perineum abdomen, and the thighs. Mucous membranes are also affected; the oral lesions resemble Fordyce spots.

Systemic manifestations. The arteries throughout the body are affected resulting in intermittent claudication, decreased

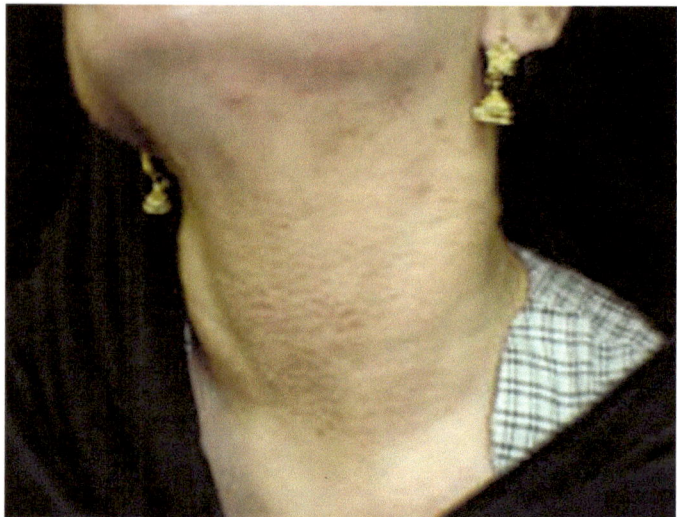

FIGURE 10.11. Pseudoxanthoma elasticum.

peripheral pulses, cardiac myopathy, and hypertension. Rupture of Bruch's membrane causes angoid streaks of the retina.

No definite therapy is available.

10.5.2 Cutis Laxa

The disorder is due to the generalized loss of elastic fibers in the dermis. The disease may be autosomal dominant, recessive, or acquired. The skin hangs in folds; the face and neck are most affected. The abdomen is also a site of large pendulous folds.

In the recessive variety of Cutis laxa, both skin and systemic manifestations are seen. Pulmonary changes include emphysema, tracheobronchomegaly, and fibrosis. Cardiac involvement results in cor-pulmonale; gastrointestinal involvement results in esophageal dilation, dyspepsia, gastric ulcers, intestinal diverticulae, and rectocele.

The acquired variety may be secondary to urticaria, angiodema, systemic lupus erythematosus, syphilis, multiple myeloma, etc.

No definite therapy is available; plastic surgery for cosmetic purposes may be helpful.

10.5.3 Ehlor Danlos Syndrome

This is a generalized disorder of connective tissue, characterized by increased fragility of the skin and blood vessels, hyperextensibility of the skin, and joint hypermobility.

The skin can stretch out like rubber and then snap back with equal resiliency. Minor trauma may give rise to gaping wounds and hematoma formation.

Systemic manifestations include intestinal hemorrhage and perforation, intestinal diverticulae, intraocular hemorrhage, keratoconus, and aortic aneurysm.

Pregnancy should be avoided because of the risk of uterine rupture.

Treatment is unsatisfactory.

Chapter 11
Bullous Disorders: Autoimmune and Childhood Bullous Dermatoses

Vesicles and bullae can be formed in a number of cutaneous disorders, ranging from simple infections such as impetigo, eczema, insect bites, and lichen planus to autoimmune disorders such as pemphigus and systemic bullous lupus erythematosus.

There are a number of reasons for blister formation, some of these are:

- Intercellular edema (spongiosis) as seen in contact dermatitis
- Epidermal cells necrosis, e.g., viral infections such as herpes simplex
- Loss of intercellular adhesion (acantholysis) as in pemphigus
- Basal cell damage, e.g., epidermolysis bullosa simplex
- Damage to the dermo-epidermal junction, e.g., bullous pemphigoid
- Dermal damage, e.g., some porphyrias, dermatitis herpetiformis

In pemphigus and pemphigoid, there are impaired adhesions between the cells of the epidermis (pemphigus), and in the basement membrane (pemphigoid). In dermatitis herpetiformis, the exact mechanism of bulla formation is still unclear, but probably the deposition of IgA in the dermal papillae produces inflammation, which separates the epidermis from the dermis. Previously some of the autoimmune disorders were fatal, but with the introduction of steroids and other

Z. Zaidi, S. W. Lanigan, *Dermatology in Clinical Practice*, 233
DOI: 10.1007/978-1-84882-862-9_11,
© Springer-Verlag London Limited 2010

immunosuppressive drugs, the mortality and morbidity have been considerably reduced.

Bullous diseases can be diagnosed by a skin biopsy and immunofluorescence; this may be direct, using skin, or indirect, using patient's blood. The skin biopsy is taken from the edge of a fresh lesion. For direct immunofluorescence two biopsy specimens are taken, one from the edge of a fresh lesion for histology and the second from the skin near the lesion to establish the diagnosis. Direct immunofluorescence gives the level of blister formation. Indirect immnuofluorescence is used to detect the presence of tissue-bound and circulating antibodies.

11.1 Pemphigus

This is an autoimmune disorder, in which the antibodies are formed against the proteins within the desmosomes of the stratum malpighian. It is a disease of middle-aged people, although in the Indian subcontinent cases of pemphigus have been reported in the third decade. Deposits of IgG are directed against epidermal cadherins, a family of calcium-dependent cell-to-cell adhesion molecules, in the demosomes. Pemphigus can occur secondary to drugs such as penicillamine, captopril, rifampicin, and cephalosporin. It is also seen with thymoma and myasthenia gravis.

Bullae in pemphigus are formed intraepidermally due to the loss of cohesion between the epidermal cells; these cells (acantholytic cells) are rounded, with a large basophilic nucleus, with a rim of eosinophilic cytoplasm. The bullae are very fragile as they are superficial and rupture easily. A little pressure over the bulla causes the bulla to spread laterally due to the loss of adhesion within the epidermis (bulla spreading sign), and a mild twisting pressure on the skin separates the epidermis from the level of acantholysis (Nikolsky sign).

11.1.1 Clinical Features

The site of blister formation in the epidermis will determine the clinical features.

In pemphigus vulgaris and pemphigus vegetans, the site of blister formation is above the basal layer. *Pemphigus vulgaris* is the most common form of disease and the one with the worst prognosis. The bullae form on normal or erythematous skin. They are very fragile, ranging in size from 1 to 10 cm; these rupture within 24 h of formation to form painful erosions. The erosions are painful and often offensive. They show no tendency to healing. Bullae are also formed in the oral mucosa in 50–70% of cases; sometimes this can be the only manifestation of the disease. Mucous membrane of the conjunctiva, pharynx, larynx, and genitals may also be affected. *Pemphigus vegetans* is characterized by the formation of vegetating erosions in the flexures; it is more inflammatory in nature (Figs. 11.1 and 11.2).

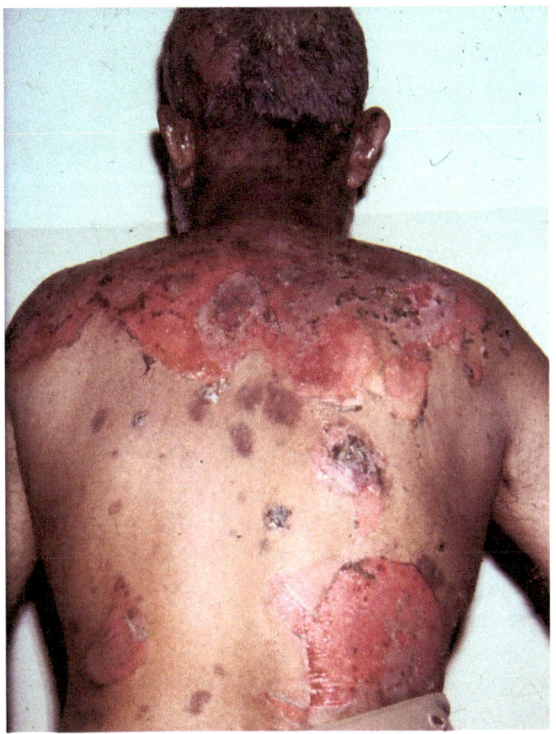

FIGURE 11.1. Pemphigus.

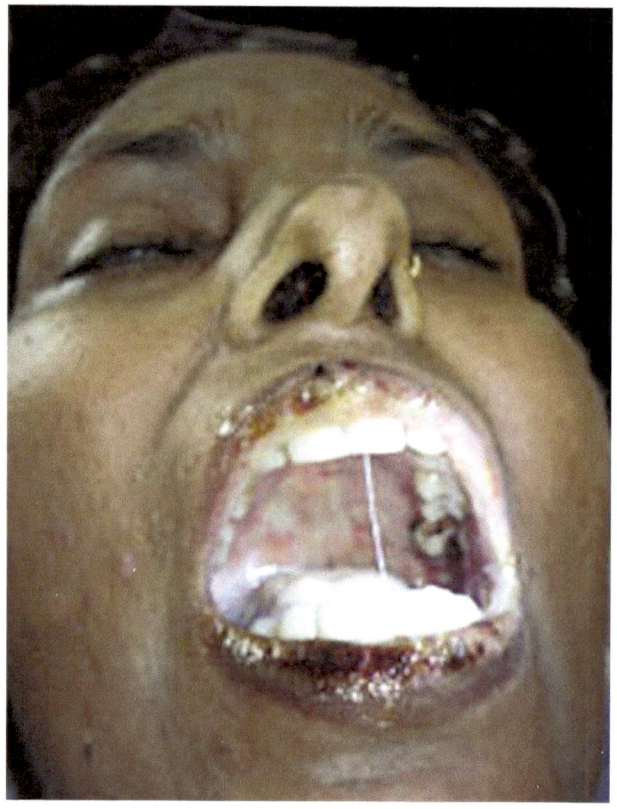

FIGURE 11.2. Pemphigus vulgaris – lesions of the oral cavity.

In *pemphigus foliaceus* and pemphigus erythematosus, the bullae are formed high in the epidermis. These superficial blisters are extremely fragile; many patients give a history of erosions rather than bullae formation. The involvement of the mucous membrane is rare. The prognosis is better than pemphigus vulgaris. In *pemphigus erythematosus*, the lesions are present on the face; they may spread to the chest and back in a seborrheic distribution. The lesions on the face resemble systemic lupus erythematosus and immunofluorescence may be positive for systemic lupus erythematosus. The histology is similar to systemic lupus erythematosus and pemphigus.

11.1.1.1 Paraneoplastic Pemphigus

This form of pemphigus is associated with a variety of underlying neoplasms such as B cell lymphomas, thymomas, sarcomas, and carcinomas. The clinical features are an overlap of erythema multiforme, and lichen planus pemphigoides. This form of pemphigus is refractory to all treatment, most patients deteriorate and death is due to sepsis, gastrointestinal bleeding, and multiple organ failure or the malignancy itself.

11.1.2 Diagnosis

The diagnosis is confirmed by a skin biopsy taken from a fresh lesion near the margin of the blister, Tzanck's test, and immunofluorescence. Direct immunofluorescence confirms the site of blister formation, it shows the deposition of IgG in the intercellular space and indirect immunofluorescence gives the level of antibodies in the serum.

11.1.2.1 Tzanck's Test

The surface of a fresh bulla is removed, the base of the bulla is gently scraped, and the contents put on a slide. This is then stained with Giemsa's stain, which shows the presence of acantholytic cells.

11.1.3 Differential Diagnosis

Pemphigus should be differentiated from other bullous disorders such as pemphigoid and dermatitis herpetiformis. Widespread erosions should be differentiated from impetigo, ecthyma, and epidermolysis bullosa. The bullae are very flaccid in pemphigus and rupture easily and oral ulcerations are often present.

When oral lesions are the only manifestations of pemphigus then it should be differentiated from apthae, herpes simplex, and other oral ulcers.

11.1.3.1 Diagnostic Points

The following points help in diagnosing pemphigus vulgaris:

- Bullae appear in middle-aged persons.
- Bullae appear on normal skin or on an erythematous base.
- Bulla is flaccid and ruptures easily.
- There is no sign of self-healing of these bullae.
- Nikolsky's sign is positive.
- Bulla spreading sign is positive.
- Oral mucosa is usually involved.
- Disease should be confirmed by a Tzanck's test and by immunofluorescence.

11.1.4 Treatment

Corticosteroids have greatly reduced the mortality and morbidity of pemphigus. All precautions should be taken to prevent secondary infection by using potassium permanganate baths and applying topical antiseptic applications. Good oral hygiene is important.

Pemphigus vulgaris and pemphigus vegetans require a high dose of steroids about 80–120 mg/day. Because of this high dose of steroids there are two schools of thought of initiating the treatment. According to one it is best to start with steroids and a steroid-sparing drug at the beginning of treatment. Azathioprine is often the drug of choice. The other mode of treatment is to add the steroid-sparing drug after a few weeks of treatment, depending upon the response of the patient. The dose of steroid should be monitored with the patient's condition and progress of the disease. Once the lesions are controlled (there are no new eruption and the previous lesions start healing) then the steroids should be gradually reduced. If the lesions progress in spite of treatment then the dose of steroids should be increased or else an immunosuppressive agent such as cyclosporine, azothioprine, or methotrexate should be added. Often a maintenance therapy of steroids is required which may vary from 5 to 40 mg daily. Opportunistic infections are frequently the cause of death in immunosuppressed persons.

The control of infection is a very important aspect of treatment. Monitor the patient closely while on steroid therapy.

Pemphigus foliaceus and pemphigus erythematosus may respond to topical steroids; if control is inadequate then prednisone in a dose of 20–40 mg/day may be required.

The newer antimetabolite mycophenolate mofetil is used to treat difficult cases of pemphigus. Immunoglobulin and plasmaphoresis are also used to treat pemphigus as used in other autoimmune disorders. Tetracycline and prednisolone have also shown a good response in controlled studies.

> *Blisters are very fragile; they rupture soon after formation, leaving erosions and crusts.*
> *Acantholytic cells can be seen by a Tzanck's test.*
> *High dose of steroids are required for treatment.*

11.2 Pemphigoid

This is a disease of the elderly. The site of disruption is at the dermo-epidermal junction. Deposits of IgG and C3 are present in the basement membrane zone (lamina lucida). Pemphigoid is often self-limiting.

11.2.1 Clinical Features

The lesions of pemphigoid begin as urticarial plaques or as an eczematous rash; a diagnosis of urticaria is often made at this point. The plaques then turn red or cyanotic and blisters appear on the surface. The disease gradually becomes generalized. The most common sites involved are the lower abdomen, groin, and the flexures. As the bullae are formed below the epidermis, they are firm and rupture after a few days. The bullae are often hemorrhagic. Nikolsky's sign is absent. Pemphigoid can occur secondary to drugs such as frusemide, spironolactone, and penicillin; it can also occur with multiple sclerosis and malignancy of the stomach (Fig. 11.3).

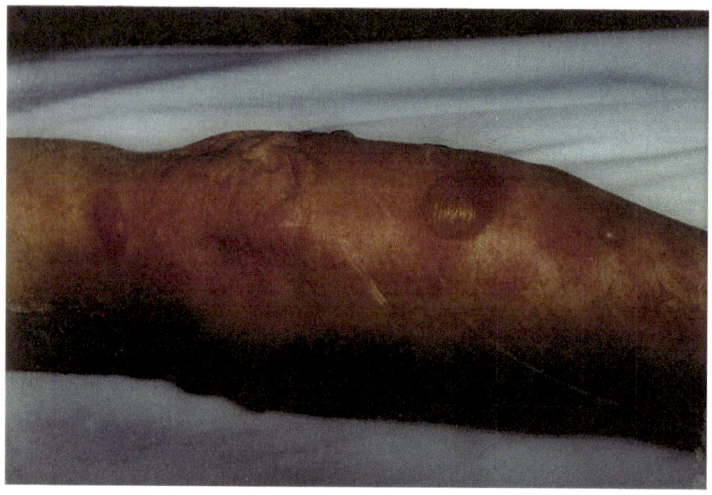

FIGURE 11.3. Pemphigoid.

11.2.1.1 Pemphigoid Nodularis

The patient presents itchy nodules suggesting a diagnosis of prurigo nodularis. Blisters are rarely recorded. The eruption can be generalized or localized to the shins. Treatment is difficult.

11.2.1.2 Localized Forms of Pemphigoid

The lesions are localized; the lower legs are the commonest site of involvement. The lesions may be vesiculobullous or vegetative, and the lesions heal with scarring. *Mucous membrane pemphigoid (Cicatricial pemphigoid)* involves the oral mucosa, eyes, and vulva. The lesions of the eyes have a poor prognosis; they leads to corneal ulcers, adhesions, impairment of vision, and even blindness. Topical steroids are ineffective in the eye; dapsone, oral steroids or cyclophosphamide are preferred.

11.2.2 Diagnosis

Histology of the lesion shows a sub-epidermal blister. Direct immunofluorescence shows the deposition of IgG and C3 along the basement membrane.

11.2.3 Differential Diagnosis

Pemphigus should be differentiated from acquired epidermolysis bullosa, linear IgA disease, and bullous lupus erythematosus. Linear IgA disease can occur in children or adults. In adults the disease is similar to pemphigoid; the extensor surfaces of the body are usually involved and, as the name implies, it is associated with linear deposition of IgA and C3 at the basement membrane.

11.2.3.1 Diagnostic Points

The following features are characteristic of pemphigoid:

- Bullae appear in the elderly.
- Bullae appear on an erythematous or urticarial base.
- Bullae are tense.
- Bullae may contain hemorrhagic fluid.
- Bullae heal with time without treatment.
- Oral mucous membrane is occasionally involved.
- Direct immunofluorescence shows deposition of IgG and C3 along the basement membrane.

11.2.4 Treatment

Patients with bullous pemphigoid are elderly and usually on many medications, so they are susceptible to adverse drug reactions and side effects. Topical steroids are the mainstay of treatment. Oral prednisolone is used when topical steroids fail or the disease is very extensive with multiple blisters at presentation. A dose of 20–50 mg/ a day is given depending upon the severity of the disease; the drug is then gradually withdrawn as the patients go into a remission. Oral steroids should be carefully monitored in an elderly patient; all measures should be taken to prevent osteoporosis and other adverse effects. Immunosuppressive drugs are best avoided due to the age of the patient; azathioprine is the best choice if required. Localized variants usually respond to topical steroids.

Tetracycline and niacinamide may help some patients.

Bullae are tense; they rupture after a few days.
Most common autoimmune bullous disorder in Western Europe.

11.3 Dermatitis Herpetiformis (DH): Duhring Brocq Disease

Dermatitis herpetiformis is a very pruritic disorder characterized by the formation of grouped papules and vesicles on an erythematous base, or the lesions may be isolated. The disease is associated with gluten-sensitive enteropathy. The enteropathy is always present; it involves the proximal part of the small intestine, but most patients are asymptomatic. Absorption of gluten leads to the formation of circulating immune complexes, which become deposited in the skin. Deposits of IgA are present in the dermal papillae; these are slowly cleared once gluten is removed from the diet.

11.3.1 Clinical Features

In the skin the common sites of the eruption are the knees, elbows, buttocks, and over the scapulae. The eruptions are grouped vesicles and so the name herpetiform is used. These lesions are often excoriated due to scratching. Sometimes the patients may show only grouped excoriations due to scratching with no vesicles present. The age range for DH is 20–55 years (Fig. 11.4).

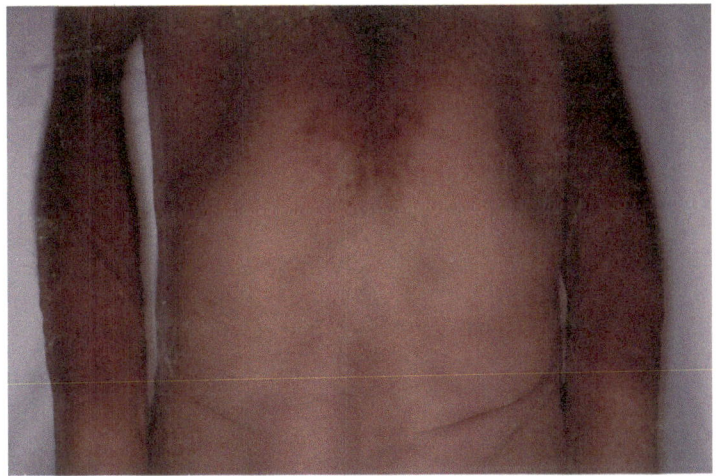

FIGURE 11.4. Dermatitis herpetiformis.

DH may be associated with other autoimmune disorders; the most common association is with diseases of the thyroid gland. There is an increased incidence of lymphomas in patients with DH.

11.3.2 Diagnosis

The presence of IgA antiendomycial antibodies (IgA-EmA) is a useful diagnostic marker for the enteropathy. Granular deposits of IgA and C3 are seen in the dermal papillae. A subepidermal blister is found on biopsy with neutrophilic abscesses in the dermal papilla.

11.3.3 Differential Diagnosis

DH should be differentiated from other pruritic disorders; in particular, scabies and neurodermatitis.

11.3.3.1 Diagnostic Points

The following are some of the diagnostic features:

- Very itchy papulovesicular eruption arranged in a group.
- Common sites are the elbows, knees, scapulae, and the buttocks.
- Vesicles and bullae are tense if not excoriated.
- Age group is between 20 and 55 years.
- All patients are associated with a gluten-sensitive enteropathy. Symptoms may be present in only 20% of cases.

Diagnosis can be confirmed by a skin biopsy, direct IF test, and biopsy of the jejunal mucosa.

- IgA deposits are found in the dermal papillae. A biopsy shows subepidermal blister and microabscess in the dermal papillae, which is pathognomonic for dermatitis herpetiformis.
- Hematology may show iron and folic acid deficiency due to gluten-sensitive enteropathy.

11.3.4 Treatment

The rash of dermatitis herpetiformis can be controlled by dapsone. The mechanism of action is unknown, but it probably acts by lysosomal enzyme stabilization. The dose varies from one person to another; it may be as high as 300 mg/a day, or as little as 50 mg twice a week. The drug is started at 50 mg a day and then increased up to 100–200 mg daily. The clinical response is so specific that it may be used as a therapeutic test for dermatitis herpetiformis. Dapsone is not without side effects, the most serious of which is hemolytic anaemia, and it produces methemoglobinemia. Regular blood checks are necessary when the patients are on dapsone, to check for hemolysis. Weekly blood examination for the first month and then every 2 weeks for 3 months, then monthly for 6 months should be performed. (The drug should not be given to patients with glucose 6 phosphate dehydrogenase deficiency.)

Other drugs that may control the condition are sulphapyridine in a dose of 0.5–1 g/day and sulphamethoxypyridine. These are useful if dapsone is not tolerated.

The disorder can be controlled by a gluten-free diet; the bowel changes revert quickly to normal, but IgA deposits remain in the skin, for a long time. Adherence to a gluten-free diet can be monitored by measuring the titres of antiendomysial antibody, which should fall if gluten in the diet is strictly avoided.

The effects of dapsone are quick, and the effect of gluten-free diet is slow. Combine the two at the start of treatment, and then slowly decrease the dose of dapsone. Tetracycline and nicotinamide have also been advocated for patients with dermatitis herpetiformis who cannot tolerate dapsone.

> *The disease is intensely pruritic; because of scratching sometimes only excoriations are seen.*
> *Dapsone is the treatment of choice; it also helps in confirming the diagnosis.*
> *Dapsone works quickly and a gluten-free diet is slow to act. Combine the two at the start of treatment; gradually reduce the dose of dapsone.*

11.4 Acquired Epidermolysis Bullosa (Epidermolysis Bullosa Acquisita)

This occurs later in life, it is an autoimmune disorder, with antibodies against collagen type VII. Epidermolysis bullosa acquisita is associated with a number of disorders such as amyloidosis, inflammatory bowel disease, lung cancer, SLE, and multiple myeloma. The defect of cleavage lies below the lamina densa, and the disease can be diagnosed by immuno-electron microscopy. Blisters heal with scarring and milia formation. Mucous membranes may or may not be involved.

Treatment is unsatisfactory and most cases are resistant to steroid therapy.

Differentiation of pemphigus, pemphigoid, and dermatitis herpetiformis

Characteristics	Pemphigus	Pemphigoid	Dermatitis herpetiformis
Blister	Flaccid, ruptures within 24 h	Tense does not rupture easily	Tense vesicles occurring in groups
Distribution	Generalized	Face and scalp usually spared	Elbows, knees, scapula, buttocks commonly affected
Oral cavity	Affected	Occasionally involved	Rarely affected
Prodomal phase	None	Eczematous or urticarial	None
Age of onset	Middle age	Elderly	20–55 years
Pruritus	Present	Common	Severe
Gluten sensitivity	Absent	Absent	Present
Resolution	No sign of resolution	Self-limiting	Healing in course of time
Nikolksy's sign	Present	Absent	Absent
Bullae spreading sign	Present	Absent	Absent

11.5 Congenital Bullous Disorders

11.5.1 Epidermolysis Bullosa

The disease can be congenital or acquired. Congenital epidermolysis bullosa are a group of genetically determined disorders, which have a tendency to form blisters on slight trauma. The type depends upon the level of the skin, where the genetic abnormality occurs.

In *epidermolysis bullosa simplex* the defect is in the basal layer. Blisters form on sites of trauma particularly as knees, elbows, hands, feet, buttocks, and other pressure sites. The bullae heal without scar formation. The oral mucosa, teeth, and nails are usually not affected (Fig. 11.5).

In *junctional epidermolysis bullosa*, the defect is in the dermo-epidermal junction. The blisters show a very poor

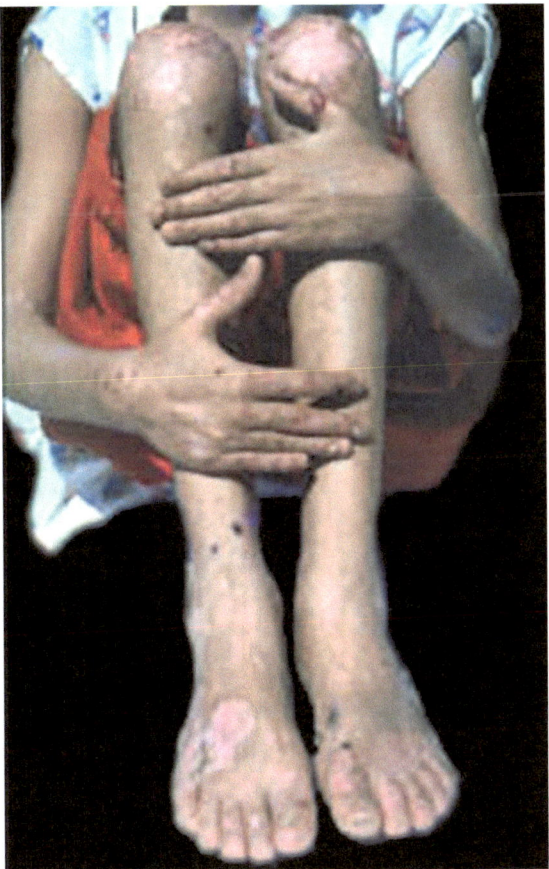

FIGURE 11.5. Epidermolysis bullosa simplex.

tendency to heal, leaving large raw areas of erosion. The mucosa is affected, resulting in difficulty in swallowing and eating. This type is called epidermolysis bullosa lethalis. The condition is lethal due to septicemia and failure to thrive due to severe mucosal ulcerations.

In *dystrophic epidermolysis bullosa*, the defect is in the anchoring fibers. The blisters heal with scar formation. The recessive variety is severe, with involvement of the mucosa, nails, and teeth. Carcinoma of the esophagus may occur due

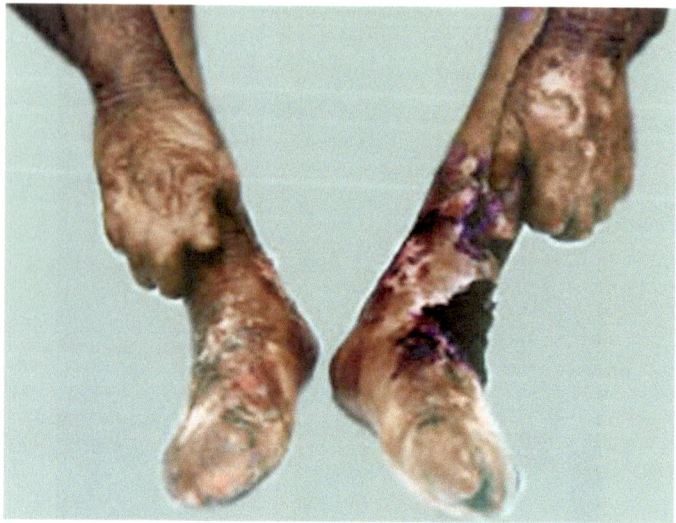

FIGURE 11.6. Dystrophic epidermolysis bullosa.

to repeated trauma and scarring. The hands and feet are fused to form a useless club-like fist or foot (Fig. 11.6).

11.5.2 Treatment

Patients with epidermolysis bullosa should have genetic counseling, as prenatal diagnosis is now possible. All efforts should be made to reduce trauma to the skin and mucosa, e.g., drinking bottles should have soft nipples with slightly larger holes to make sucking easy, and food should be soft. Elastic diapers should be avoided, knees and elbows should be padded to avoid trauma, and footwear should be soft and well-ventilated.

Suitable employment should be considered; those jobs prone to trauma should be avoided. Farming, mechanical work, typing, and sports should be avoided especially in the dystrophic type of epidermolysis bullosa.

Once blistering has occurred, blisters should be drained followed by the application of topical antibiotics. In severe junctional type of epidermolysis bullosa, fluid and electrolyte balance should be maintained; treatment of sepsis is most important in this type of disease, as septicemia is the most important cause of death.

In severe recessive forms of epidermolysis bullosa, phenytoin is rapidly becoming the mainstay of treatment. Phenytoin works by inhibiting the synthesis and secretion of collagenase from the dermal fibroblasts. It is started in a dose of 2–3 mg/kg body weight in two divided doses and then gradually increased until the blood levels exceed 8 mg/mL. Steps must be taken to keep the blood levels under 20 mg/mL, as lethargy, dizziness, and nystagmus are common at higher levels.

Surgical treatment of syndactaly may be required to restore the function of the hands with fused digits. Because of the high incidence of carcinoma of the esophagus, annual examinations beginning in early adolescence have been recommended in recessive dystrophic epidermolysis bullosa.

Hopes for the future include gene therapy. Adding the normal gene to the epidermal stem cells and then laying these onto the denuded skin.

> *Acquired epidermolysis bullosa looks like pemphigoid, but the blisters appear in response to trauma on a normal skin.*
> *Milia formation is a feature of the healing lesions in acquired epidermolysis bullosa.*

11.5.3 Chronic Bullous Disease of Childhood (Childhood Linear IgA Disease)

This is a rare self-limiting bullous disorder of children, average age of onset is about 5 years, and it remits by the age of 13 years. The initial attack is more severe than the subsequent recurrences. A linear band of IgA is present at the basement membrane. Patients are HLA B8 positive.

Three distinct clinical lesions characterize this disease: large tense bullae as seen in bullous pemphigoid, grouped vesicles as seen in dermatitis herpetiformis, or lesions similar to those seen in erythema multiforme. One lesion type may predominate, or a combination of the three may be found. Bullae arise on normal skin; they are often arranged in a rosette; as new bullae cluster around the older lesions, they form a "cluster of jewels" arrangement. Healing is rapid with hyperpigmentation, but without scarring.

Common areas involved are the inner thighs, the groin, and pelvic areas, and the central facial area around the mouth. Mucous membranes are commonly involved. Pruritus is mild or may be absent.

11.5.3.1 Treatment

Dapsone in a dose of 20–125 mg daily or sulphapypridine 250 mg–3 g daily usually controls the condition. In those who do not respond to the above treatment, corticosteroids may be added. A conservative approach should be followed, as the disease is a self-limiting disorder.

Most of the IgA dermatoses respond to dapsone.

11.5.4 Acrodermatitis Enteropathica (AE)

Acrodermatitis enteropathica is a rare autosomal recessive disorder due to the failure of the intestinal tract to absorb zinc. The condition is also seen in adults who are on long-term parental therapy without zinc supplements.

The basic lesion in AE is a bullous, occurring typically on the hands and feet, and around the periorificial skin. The lesions become eroded, crusted, and sharply marginated. The other characteristics are alopecia, nail dystrophy, gastrointestinal disturbances particularly diarrhea with exacerbations and remissions, and a peculiar apathy during periods of exacerbations. If left untreated patients can become mentally impaired (Figs. 11.7 and 11.8).

AE has a number of findings similar to epidermolysis bullosa (EB); particularly the bullous nature of the disorder and the acral distribution led many early investigators to classify AE with EB of the dystrophic type.

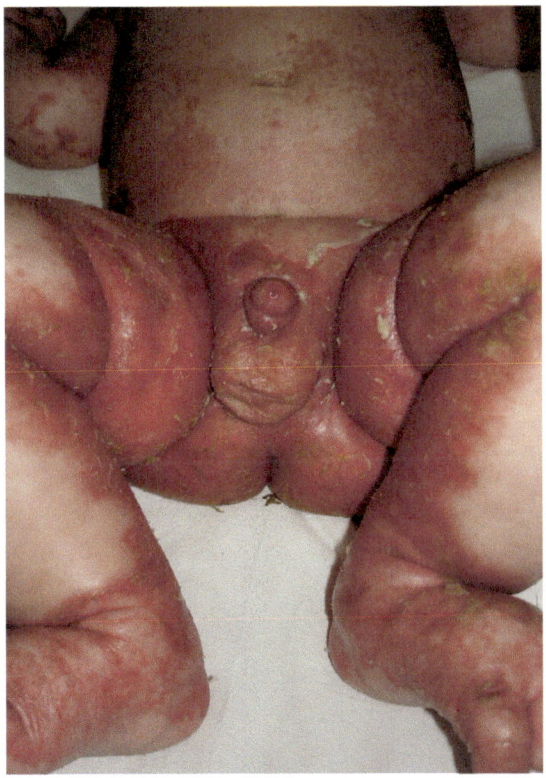

FIGURE 11.7. Acrodermatitis enteropathica.

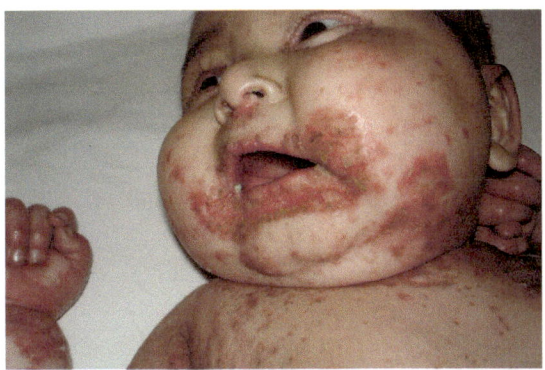

FIGURE 11.8. Acrodermatitis enteropathica – perioral lesions.

11.5.4.1 Diagnosis

The disease is diagnosed by examining the blood levels for zinc. Serum zinc levels are below 50 μg/100 mL. Decreased zinc levels are found in RBC, hair, and urine.

11.5.4.2 Treatment

Oral zinc gluconate or sulphate in doses of 5 mg/kg/day in two to three divided doses bring about complete remissions; symptoms respond in 1–2 weeks before zinc reaches normal levels.

Bullous ichthyosiform erythroderma is described in Chap. 9
Porphyrias are described in Chap.18
Bullous impetigo in Chap. 4

Chapter 12
Vasculitis, Common Erythemas, and Lymphatic Disorders

Vasculitis is a term applied to inflammation and necrosis of the blood vessels; the blood vessels may be small, medium, or large. Vasculitis may be purely cutaneous, or associated with systemic disease. The cause may be immunological or secondary to infection, drugs, collagen disorders, malignancy, etc. It is important to know the underlying diagnosis before initiating therapy, the type of vessel involved, and the extent of damage.

In small vessel involvement, the vessels affected are the arterioles, capillaries, or small venules. The cutaneous manifestation is palpable purpura; the common sites are the dependent areas of the body, the lower legs in mobile patients, and the back in immobile patients. The purpura appears as raised papules, rather than petechiae or ecchymosis. The lesions are palpable due to inflammation and edema. These purpuric papules may be symptomless or painful. The three "P"s of small vessel vasculitis are *P*ainful *P*ruritic *P*apules. Severe inflammation leads to necrosis and ulceration.

In medium-sized vessel involvement, the visceral vessels are affected, including renal, hepatic, and coronary arteries. In large vessel involvement, the aorta and its great vessels are affected; there are obvious clinical signs; necrotizing livido reticularis, or multiple site gangrene.

Vasculitis, which is confined to the skin, and when an underlying cause cannot be found is called "hypersensitivity vasculitis." This is a common form of vasculitis, but is a diagnosis of exclusion.

Z. Zaidi, S. W. Lanigan, *Dermatology in Clinical Practice*,
DOI: 10.1007/978-1-84882-862-9_12,
© Springer-Verlag London Limited 2010

12.1 Approach to a Patient with Vasculitis

A complete history and physical examination is performed which includes history of drug intake, evidence of collagen vascular disease, any foci of infection, internal malignancy, etc. Serious infections such as Rocky Mountain spotted fever and meningococcemia should always be excluded, for these diseases can be fatal if treatment is delayed while waiting for investigations.

Lesions of cutaneous vasculitis are often limited to the lower extremities and generalized in cases of systemic disease. In Rocky Mountain Spotted Fever the purpuric papules are first seen on the wrist and ankles; they then involve the palms and soles, the lesions later become generalized. In gonorrhea, the purpuric papules are acral in distribution; lesions are both pustular and purpuric.

12.2 Diagnosis

The diagnosis is confirmed by biopsy. The histological features include swollen endothelial cells, fibrinoid necrosis of the vessel wall, presence of neutrophils with leukocytoclasis (destruction of neutrophils leaving nuclear dust), and hemorrhage.

Laboratory tests should be done to detect any systemic disease and for the extent of disease involvement, e.g., ANA for SLE, urine examination, complete blood examination, X-ray chest, etc.

12.3 Treatment

Treat the underlying cause when found. If the diagnosis of an infection is suspected, the treatment should be immediate, not waiting for culture reports, e.g., in meningococcemia; a delay of a few hours may result in a fatal outcome rather than a favorable one. The same holds true of Rocky Mountain spotted fever. For a drug reaction, the drug should be stopped. Purpuric reactions associated with viral infections such as measles remit spontaneously.

Most other forms of vasculitis are treated by prednisolone or immunosuppressive therapy. Other drugs that can be used include colchicine and dapsone.

12.4 Leucocytoclastic Vasculitis

This is the most common form of small vessel necrotizing vasculitis. The disease may be purely cutaneous, it may involve many organs, or it may be a manifestation of other diseases such as collagen disorders.

12.4.1 Cuteneous Manifestations

The cutaneous lesions arise in dependent areas such as the lower extremities in ambulatory patients and buttocks and flanks in bedridden ones. Palpable purpuric papules; are seen that may coalesce to form plaques. Nodules and urticarial lesions may also be found. Severe form of inflammation leads to necrosis, hemorrhage and cutaneous ulceration (Fig. 12.1). Lesions usually occur in crops lasting for 1–4 weeks.

12.4.2 Systemic Manifestations

The disease is associated with prodromal symptoms such as fever, malaise, arthralgia, and myalgia. The kidneys are the most common organs affected, with the development of hematuria and proteinuria. Involvement of peripheral nerves leads to paresthesias. Abdominal pain, nausea, and vomiting indicate gastrointestinal involvement. Cardiovascular involvement leads to arrhythmias and congestive cardiac failure.

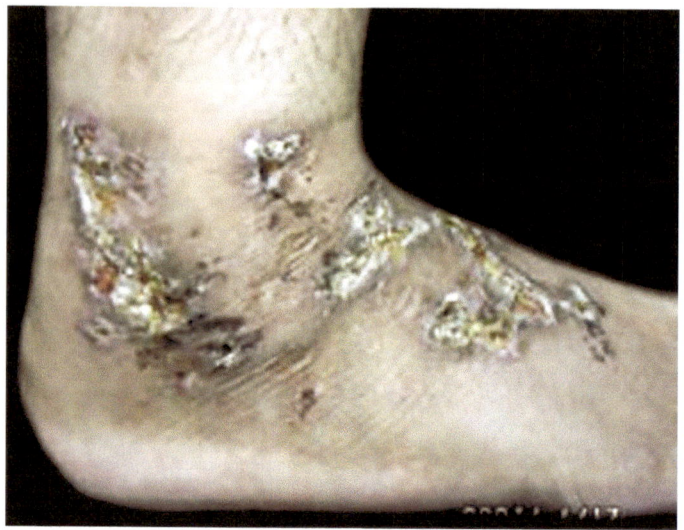

FIGURE 12.1. Cutaneous vasculitis.

12.4.3 Treatment

In many cases, treatment is unnecessary, as the disease is self-limiting. Effort should be made to minimize stasis by the use of compression hosiery and elevation of the dependent areas. Prednisone 30–80 mg/day controls systemic symptoms and cutaneous ulcerations in active disease. The drug should be tapered slowly to prevent rebound flare-up of the disease. Nonsteroidal antiinflammatory agents are used for fever and myalgias. Other immunosuppressants can be used if the condition fails to respond to steroids.

12.5 Henoch–Schonlein Purpura (HSP)

This is the most common form of leukocytoclastic vasculitis that occurs in children, although it may also be seen in adults. IgA plays an important role in the pathogenesis of HSP; there are increased levels of IgA in the blood, and immune complexes are deposited in the vessel walls. HSP involves the skin, kidneys, and the gastrointestinal tract. Palpable purpura, abdominal pain, gastrointestinal bleeding, arthralgia, hematuria, and proteinuria characterize the disease. The disease is self-limiting, but some patients may have one or more recurrences.

An upper respiratory tract infection often precedes the purpura by 1–3 weeks in children. Drugs, underlying malignancy and food are also responsible agents for the production of HSP. In many cases, the cause is not known. The purpura is most common on the lower extremities and buttocks (Fig. 12.2). Other parts of the body may be affected; the trunk is often spared. Lesions fade more rapidly with bed rest and reappear on ambulation. A skin biopsy for immunofluorescence to detect IgA is helpful in predicting nephropathy.

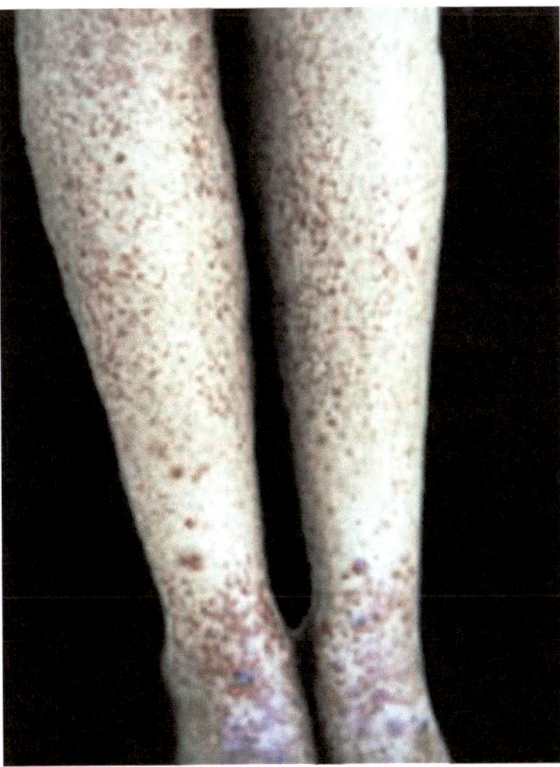

FIGURE 12.2. Purpura.

12.5.1 Treatment

Remove any offending factor when found. Corticosteroids, analgesics, and nonsteroidal antiinflammatory therapy are the mainstays of treatment.

> *Always examine the urine in leukocytoclastic vasculitis to exclude renal involvement.*

12.6 Polyarteritis Nodosa

This is a necrotizing vasculitis of medium-sized blood vessels. It is a disease of middle age, usually affecting men. The disease may be purely cutaneous or it may involve other organs. The kidneys and visceral vasculature are most often affected. The systemic illness is associated with fever, malaise, tachycardia, leukocytosis, and a high ESR. Death from renal disease is common.

The skin changes are mainly seen on the lower legs; the lesions appear as stellate patches of purpura, palpable subcutaneous nodules, livido reticularis, purple necrotic plaques, hemorrhagic bullae or deep punched out ulcers. Peripheral gangrene may also occur (Fig. 12.3).

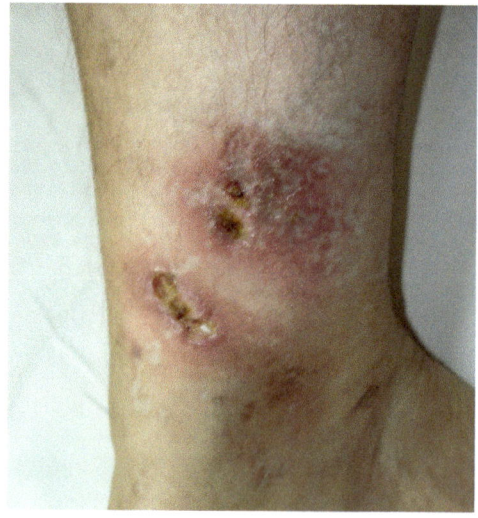

FIGURE 12.3. Polyarteritis nodosa.

12.6.1 Treatment

Low dose systemic steroids are usually sufficient for purely cutaneous forms. In systemic involvement steroids are used in higher dose; cyclophosphamide and fibrinolytic therapy are also helpful.

12.7 Pyoderma Gangrenosum

This is also a necrotizing vasculitis. It presents as a furuncle like nodule, pustule, or as a hemorrhagic bulla. The nodule breaks down to form an ulcer, which has an undermined purplish margin and surrounding erythema. The ulcer may extend rapidly and there may be more than one lesion. The ulcer heals forming a thin atrophic scar. It occurs mainly on the lower limbs or the trunk (Fig. 12.4).

Pyoderma gangrenosum can be associated with a number of underlying diseases. The commonest are: ulcerative colitis, Crohn's disease, rheumatoid arthritis, systemic lupus erythematosus, chronic active hepatitis, multiple myeloma, leukemia, and various paraproteinemias.

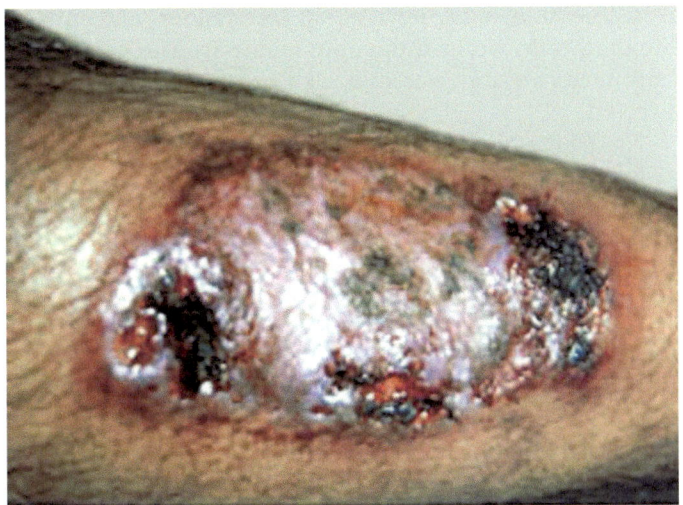

FIGURE 12.4. Pyoderma gangrenosum.

Pyoderma gangrenosum should be differentiated from deep fungal infections, atypical mycobactrium disease, necrotizing fasciitis, and tertiary syphilis.

12.7.1 Treatment

Treatment is with systemic steroids or cyclosporin. Other immunosuppressive agents can help in resistant disease. Cases associated with inflammatory bowel disease can improve if the bowel disease is controlled.

12.8 Giant Cell Arteritis

The disease affects large and medium-sized arteries, particularly those of the head and neck. Typical symptoms include pain and morning stiffness, involving the neck and shoulders. Cutaneous involvement is uncommon. The most common cutaneous finding is painful nodules over involved superficial arteries. It usually affects the elderly; the classical site of involvement is the temporal arteries. These become tender and pulseless, and are associated with severe headaches. Tender red nodules are seen on the scalp in the temporal area. The skin over the scalp is red, tender, and inflamed. Blindness may occur if the ophthalmic arteries are involved. Coronary, mesenteric, and celiac arteries can also be affected.

The ESR is significantly raised during the acute phase, and its level can be used to guide treatment. Steroids should be used as soon as the diagnosis is made to avoid complications such as blindness. The patients may need to continue treatment for a year or two.

12.9 Erythema Multiforme

This is an immunologically mediated disorder, probably triggered by circulating immune complexes. A number of etiological agents can cause this reaction, such as drugs; herpes simplex and other viral infections; bacterial infections; pregnancy; inflammatory disorders; and malignancy. Herpes simplex is the most common cause of recurrent erythema multiforme.

The disorder ranges in severity. In the mild form of the disease, the rash is most prominent on the forearms, legs, palms, and soles. As the name implies the lesions are varied, there are papules, plaques, and vesicles. The characteristic lesion is the "target" lesion. This consists of three zones. A dark central area or a blister; this is surrounded by a paler edematous zone and a peripheral rim of erythema. As a new lesion begins at the same site as the previous one, the two concentric plaques look like a target (Fig. 12.5).

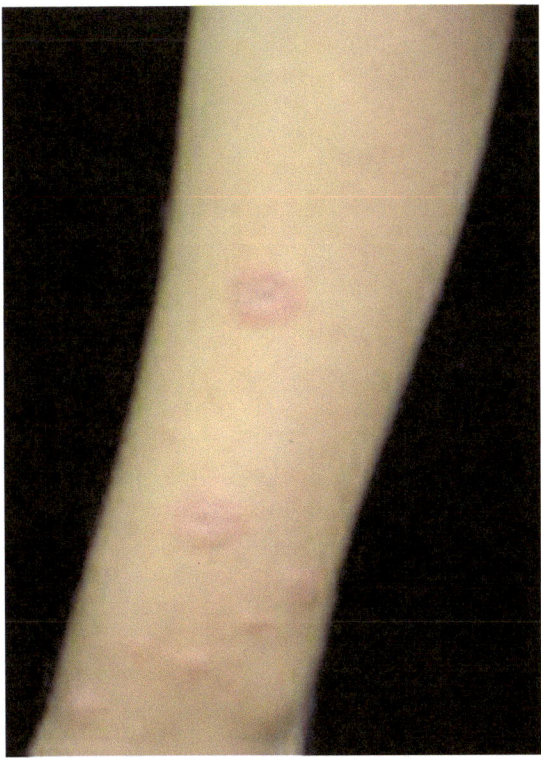

FIGURE 12.5. Erythema multiforme – note the target lesion.

In the severe form of the disease the mucous membranes are also involved and lesions are generalized. The oral mucosa, eyes, and the lips are most often affected. The patient looks and feels ill. There is fever and malaise (Steven Johnson's syndrome). In the most severe form of erythema multiforme, there is extensive denudation of the skin; the condition overlaps with Toxic Epidermal Necrolysis.

Complications occur when the mucosa is involved. Eye involvement can lead to corneal ulcers, anterior uveitis, panophthalmitis, and even blindness. Specialist ophthalmological advice should be sought early in the disease if there is a possibility of ocular involvement. Genital ulcers may lead to urinary retention, phimosis, or vaginal strictures. It is always best to involve other speciality consultants early in severe cases of erythema multiforme.

12.9.1 Investigations

Most cases are secondary to viral infections or drugs. A search for other infectious agents, malignancy, endocrine causes, or collagen disease is required when the course is prolonged.

12.9.2 Treatment

There is no convincing evidence that medical therapy can alter the course of the disease once it is established. Discontinue promptly any responsible drug. If erythema multiforme is due to recurrent herpes simplex, a course of acyclovir is given. Recurrent erythema multiforme associated with recurrent herpes simplex can be prevented by maintenance therapy with acyclovir.

The use of steroid is controversial. Nevertheless, systemic steroids 40–80 mg/day are still frequently used in severe cases. Supportive measures are important, such as maintaining water and electrolyte balance; I/V fluids are needed when there is severe oral involvement. Local therapy with antiseptics is needed to prevent secondary infection.

Patients with Toxic Epidermal Necrolysis should be referred to a burn ward for treatment.

Herpes simplex infection should be suspected in recurrent or continuous erythema multiforme.

Target lesions are characteristic of erythema multiforme; palms are commonly involved.

12.10 Erythema Nodosum (EN)

This is an inflammation of the subcutaneous fat, due to a hypersensitivity response to a variety of antigens. Evidence suggests that immune complexes mediate EN; the relative sluggish circulation of the lower extremities predisposes to the deposition of immune complexes in these blood vessels. EN may be secondary to bacterial infections, fungal infections, sarcoidosis, lymphomas, and drugs. The most common cause is streptococcal infection in children and sarcoidosis in adults. In Western and Southwestern United States, coccidioidomycosis is the most common cause.

Legs (shins) are the most common sites involved. The lesions appear as red, tender, and subcutaneous nodules. The patient has fever and arthralgia, most commonly affecting the knee and ankle joints. The course is usually self-limited, lasting from 3 to 6 weeks. As the lesions of EN evolve, the color changes mimic a bruise progressing to bluish or purple, and then to yellow. The nodules of EN do not ulcerate (Fig. 12.6).

12.10.1 Investigations

A complete history should be taken, in all cases of EN to find out the cause of this eruption. Physical examination, a chest X-ray, throat swab, antistreptolysin (ASO) titre, and a Mantoux test are required.

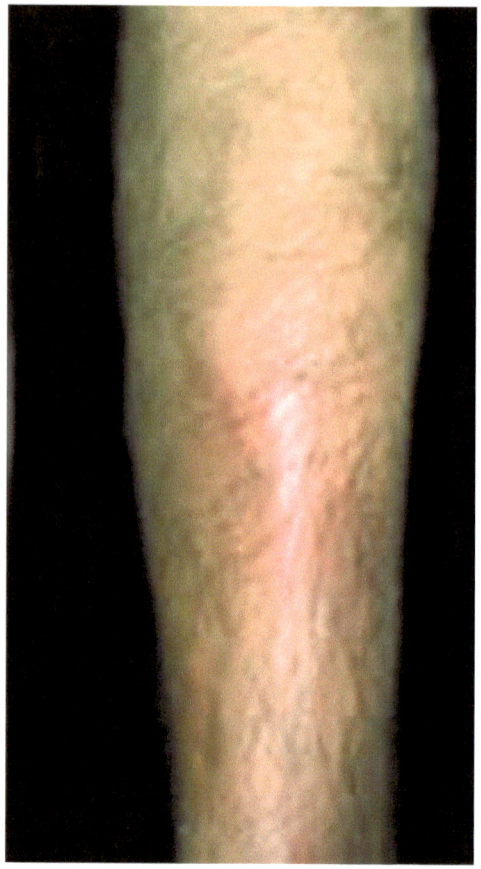

FIGURE 12.6. Erythema nodosum.

12.10.2 Differential Diagnosis

In nodular vasculitis, the nodules are smaller, harder, and more persistent. They are often asymmetrical. In erythema nodosum leprosum, the lesions are present in other parts of the body and other signs of leprosy are present. Thrombophlebitic plaques affect the side of the lower leg and hand; they are hard, irregular, and fibrotic. Erythema induratum affects the back of the legs and is seen in patients with erythrocynotic circulation.

12.10.3 Treatment

Therapy is directed towards the underlying disease. Symptomatic treatment with aspirin or nonsteroidal inflammatory drugs and bed rest is usually sufficient. In the resolving stage when the patient is ambulant supportive bandages may be used.

In patients with extensive involvement and marked discomfort, potassium iodide five drops in orange juice is started, the dose is increased by one drop daily until the patient responds. Other drugs that can be used are colchicine, prednisone, hydroxychloroquine, and dapsone.

12.11 Common Localized Erythemas

12.11.1 Flushing and Blushing

Flushing is a transient vasodilatation of the face that may occur in normal persons due to heat, exercise, or emotion (blushing). Flushing is also produced by ingestion of alcohol, or after hot drinks. Hot beverages increase the temperature of the blood draining the oral cavity.

The mechanism of alcohol-induced flushing is uncertain. It is probably related to acetaldehyde levels. Flushing is also seen in alcoholics after taking chlorpropanamide and disulfiram. It is thought that endogenous opiods such as encephalin may play a role in chlorpropanamide-induced ethanol flushing.

Flushing is a feature of rosacea, carcinoid syndrome, and the menopause. Systemic diseases associated with flushing include dumping syndromes and various forms of malignancy. It is probably due to release of prostaglandins. Pheochromocytoma may also induce flushing.

Flushing may also occur after taking monosodium glutamate; this is often called "Chinese restaurant syndrome." Drugs producing flushing include calcium channel blockers and vasodilators such as amylnitrate.

12.11.2 Erythema Palmare

This is usually most marked on the hypothenar eminence. It is associated with carcinoma of the pancreas, cirrhosis of the liver, pregnancy, graft versus host reactions, chemotherapy, and systemic lupus erythematosus. Erythema Palmare may be hereditary in some cases.

12.12 Generalized Nonspecific Erythemas

12.12.1 Scarlatiniform Erythema

The rash consists of two elements; a diffuse erythema on which are superimposed punctate areas of increased redness, but either of these two elements may be absent. The punctate lesions are about the size of goose pimples, but in a coarse rash they may be larger and the erythematous element indistinct. The rash resembles that of scarlet fever, but does not have the associated symptoms.

12.12.2 Morbilliform Erythema

This is a generalized maculopapular eruption with a characteristic blotchy appearance, resembling the rash of measles.

Scarlatiniform and morbilliform erythemas are often seen in drug eruptions, viral infections, etc.

12.13 Pigmented Purpuric Dermatosis (PPD)

This is a term used for capillaritis with characteristic histological features. Pathologically the disease is characterized by narrowing of the capillary lumen, due to swelling of the endothelial cells, accompanied by a perivascular T cell infiltration. There is extravasation of the red cells and hemosiderin deposits are seen in the macrophages. Capillaritis of unknown etiology is perhaps related to long hours of standing, or playing strenuous games. PPD may occasionally be due to drugs, mycosis fungoides, and rheumatoid arthritis.

12.13.1 Schamberg's Disease

Schamberg's disease is the most common PPD. This is a purely local inflammatory process in the skin, in which pigmented purpuric lesions appear on the legs. The lesions appear as irregular patches or plaques of orange or brown pigmentation due to deposit of hemosiderin, characteristic "cayenne pepper" spots occur within or at the edge of the lesion. The condition is often asymptomatic, but usually persistent. There may be occasional clearing in some cases (Fig. 12.7).

The disease is resistant to any form of therapy; simple support hosiery is the most appropriate approach. Topical steroids may be given for itchy lesions.

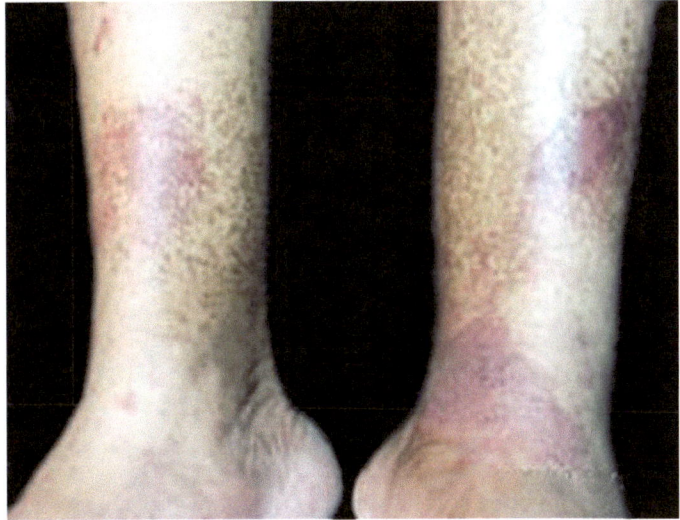

FIGURE 12.7. Schamberg's disease.

12.14 Lymphatic Disorders

12.14.1 Lymphangitis

Lymphangitis is defined as an inflammation of the lymphatic vessels. Infection spreads along the lymphatics to the regional lymph nodes. The infection is usually due to Group A β-hemolytic streptococci. It can occur secondary to wounds, abrasions, or as a complication of an infection such as cellulitis or an abscess. Lymphangitis may be recurrent as in cellulitis. Lymphangitis can also occur after extensive surgery such as radical mastectomy, or removal of a vein for coronary bypass operation.

Lymphangitis is seen clinically as red streaks, corresponding to the inflamed lymphatic vessels. In the lower limb, the diagnosis is not as clear as it is associated with edema. Lymphangitis appears as diffuse erythema, which should be differentiated from cellulitis. It is often associated with systemic symptoms such as chills, fever, loss of appetite, and malaise. The regional lymph nodes may be enlarged and tender.

When lymphatic insufficiency exists and the local lymphoid tissue fails in its host defense function, recurrent infection is likely to occur. Lymphatics act as a second line of defense, preventing onward spread of infection. Clinically this lymphatic insufficiency is seen as cellulitis/erysipelas. In fact, any person who has recurrent attacks of cellulitis in one leg almost certainly has a compromised lymphatic damage in that leg, whether lymphoedema is present or not. Permanent obliteration of the lymphatics may follow severe or recurrent lymphangitis.

12.14.1.1 Complications

Lymphangitis can spread within hours; locally it may lead to necrosis and ulceration. Lymphangitis caused by Group A β-hemolytic streptococci may lead to bacteremia, sepsis, and death.

12.14.1.2 Investigations

Complete blood picture shows a leukocytosis. Culture of the aspirate from the primary source of infection, and a blood culture to exclude septicemia have to be carried out.

12.14.1.3 Treatment

Hospital admission is usually necessary. Therapy is with a suitable intravenous antibiotic, e.g., benzyl penicillin; alternatively a broad-spectrum antibiotic may be used. This should be started before the culture results are available. The prognosis of a patient with uncomplicated lymphangitis is good.

12.14.2 Lymphoedema

Lymphoedema is edema due to inadequate lymphatic drainage. It may be primary or secondary. It is most frequently found on the lower limbs secondary to infections such as cellulitis , chronic venous ulcer, and filariasis. Lymphoedema develops secondary to penetration of silica dust, which damages the lymphatic vessels; a condition found in developing countries where people often walk barefooted. It may be seen secondary to inflammation such as in rosacea or acne. Lymphoedema may follow lymphatic blockage by tumors, and destruction of lymphatics by surgery. Primary lymphoedema is seen at adolescence, it is usually unilateral without any other findings (lymphedema praecox); or it involves both legs associated with ascites and pleural effusions (Milroys syndrome). Swelling of the limb as a result of lymphatic obstruction, followed by thickening of the skin and subcutaneous tissue is called elephantiasis.

Lymphoedema is nonpitting, and the overlying skin may be hyperkeratotic. The defect in the lymphatic system can be detected by lymphangiography or radiolabelled lymphoscintigraphy.

12.14.2.1 Complications

Swelling and infection are the common complications of lymphoedema. The swelling may restrict movement; this can be especially troublesome if there is associated scarring and fibrosis. Malignancy and some rare disorders such as necrotizing fasciitis, and toxic epidermal necrolysis can also occur.

12.14.2.2 Treatment

Patients with lymphoedematous limbs should be taught meticulous skin care, to prevent secondary infection. Good antiseptics following abrasions and minor trauma are important measures to be taken. Tight bandaging, massage, bed rest, and elevation of the affected limb, may help to control lymphoedema.

Lymphoedematous skin is at risk of repeated infection especially cellulitis. If the attacks are more than once a year then long-term prophylaxis is recommended, usually by phenoxymethyl penicillin.

Prompt diagnosis and treatment of bacterial cellulitis is important in preventing further lymphatic drainage and worsening of the existing elephantiasis.

Drug therapy is generally disappointing. Diuretics alone have little benefit in lymphoedema, because their mode of action is to limit capillary filtration, by reducing the blood volume. Improvement by diuretics suggests that the predominant cause of edema was not lymphatic. The benzopyrone group of drugs have been advocated for lymphoedema, but their clinical effects seem to be small.

Surgery may be of value in a few patients, in whom the size and weight of the limb inhibit its use and mobility. Relief may be obtained by removal of excessive tissue, but recurrences are common, unless new lymphatic drainage is established. Lifelong nonsurgical measures such as hosiery must be continued postoperatively.

Generalized specific erythemas and hypersensitivity syndromes discussed in Chapter 13
Lymphangioma described in Chapter 24

Chapter 13
Exanthems and Hypersensitivity Syndromes

13.1 Exanthems

Exanthem means a skin eruption that bursts forth or blooms. These eruptions are widespread, symmetrical, erythematous, discrete or confluent, and do not scale initially. The lesions erupt as macules or papules; other lesions such as vesicles, pustules or petechiae may form later. Oral lesions accompany some exanthematous diseases; the oral lesions are called enanthems. Common exanthematous diseases are discussed below.

13.1.1 Measles (Rubeola, Morbilli)

Measles is a contagious viral disease, spread by droplet infection. The patient is infectious from slightly before the prodromal period to 4 days after the appearance of the rash.

Prodromal symptoms consist of fever, cough, coryza (nasal congestion and symptoms of a "head cold"), conjunctivitis, and photophobia. Fever appears 3–4 days before the eruption of the rash. Koplik's spot are bluish white spots surrounded by a red halo appearing on the buccal mucous membrane, opposite the premolar teeth. They appear 24–48 hours before the exanthem and remain for 2–4 days. The rash begins on the face, behind the ears; it soon spreads to the trunk and extremities. Rashes reach maximum intensity in about 3 days, and then fade in 5–10 days. The affected child is usually miserable.

Z. Zaidi, S. W. Lanigan, *Dermatology in Clinical Practice*, DOI: 10.1007/978-1-84882-862-9_13, © Springer-Verlag London Limited 2010

The rash is characteristic; it is a maculopapular eruption, red or purplish in color, the lesions frequently coalesce. Eruption of similar nature can be found in other disorders; these are referred to as morbilliform eruptions, e.g., morbilliform drug eruptions.

Complications include diarrhea, pneumonia, middle ear infection, and encephalitis. Encephalitis may lead to brain damage and mental retardation.

13.1.1.1 Treatment

The treatment is symptomatic. There have been reports that vitamin A and albumin have significantly reduced the intensity of eruption in the early stages of the disease. Treatment with vitamin A reduces the mortality and morbidity of measles. All children with severe measles should be given supplements of vitamin A.

- Below 6 months 50,000 IU
- 6 months–2 years 100,000 IU
- Above 2 years 200,000 IU

A repeated dose can be given on the following day.

13.1.1.2 Prophylaxis

On exposure to measles, human immunoglobulin is given to prevent or modify the disease in susceptible persons within 6 days of exposure. IgG 0.25 mL/kg of body weight is given by the I/M route.

13.1.1.3 Prevention

Children should be vaccinated soon after their first birthday.
> *The three C's of the prodromal stage of measles are coryza, cough, and conjunctivitis.*
> *In contrast to Rubella, lesions coalesce on the face and trunk; but often remain discrete on the extremities.*

13.1.2 Rubella (German Measles)

This is also a contagious viral infection. The most important complication of rubella is fetal abnormality (congenital rubella syndrome), which occurs if the infection takes place in the first trimester of pregnancy.

The incubation period is about 18 days. Mild symptoms of fever, malaise, and headache precede the rash by a few hours to a day. Lymphadenopathy especially of the posterior auricular and cervical glands may appear 4–7 days before the appearance of the rash. Petechiae occur in about 2% of cases on the soft palate in the early eruption phase.

The eruption begins on the face and neck; it then spreads to the trunk and extremities. The color is less livid than scarlet fever and lacks the violet tinge of measles. The lesions are usually discrete, but may coalesce on the trunk and face; the lesions are lentil-sized macules or faint papules (rubelliform). The rash fades in the same order in which it appeared, followed by a mild desquamation. In adults mild polyarthralgia and polyarthritis may occur.

Complications involving the CNS are likely to appear in adults and thrombocytopenia in children.

13.1.2.1 Congenital Rubella Syndrome

This syndrome includes sensory deafness, cataract, microphthalmia, glaucoma, chorioretinitis, patent ductus arteriosus, peripheral pulmonary artery stenosis, atrial ventricular septal defects, microcephaly, mental retardation, and postnatal growth retardation.

13.1.2.2 Treatment

Treatment is symptomatic.

The disease is also called "the 3 day measles."

13.1.3 Scarlet Fever

A streptococcal erythrogenic toxin (superantigen) causes this disease. The circulating toxin is responsible for the rash and systemic symptoms. The original infection may be in the skin or respiratory mucosa.

The incubation period is 2–4 days. There is a sudden onset of fever and pharyngitis, which is followed by nausea, vomiting, headache, and abdominal pain. The entire oral cavity is red; the tongue is covered with a yellowish white coat, through which the red papillae protrude. Diffuse lymphadenopathy may occur before the eruption of the rash.

The rash begins on the neck and face, it spreads within 48 h to the trunk and extremities; the palms and soles are not clinically involved. The face is flushed except for the circumoral pallor. All the other areas exhibit a vivid scarlet hue with innumerable pinpoint papules. Linear petechiae (Pastia's sign) are found in the skin folds, especially the antecubital area and the groin. The white coating of the tongue is then shed, leaving a red raw glazed surface with engorged papillae.

As the fever and rash subside, desquamation occurs. It begins on the face, progresses on the trunk and finally to the hands and feet. Large sheets of epidermis are later shed from the palms and soles in a glove-like cast. Beau's lines may be produced in the nails. Desquamation is complete in 4 weeks. Recurrences of scarlet fever are common.

Diagnosis of a recent infection can be confirmed by a rising antistreptolysin-O titre.

13.1.3.1 Treatment

Antibiotics such as penicillin, cephalosporin, erythromycin, ofloxacin, rifampicin, or the newer macrolides may be used.

Desquamation of the palms and soles and grooving of the nails are characteristic of scarlet fever.

The typical rash of scarlet fever may be found in other diseases such as some viral infections; it is known as a scarlatiniform eruption.

13.1.4 Hand, Foot and Mouth Disease

This is a contagious viral infection caused by an enterovirus. It occurs primarily in children. The orofecal or respiratory route spreads the disease.

The incubation period is 4 6 days. Fever, malaise, and sore throat are present for 1–2 days. Some patients develop submandibular and/or cervical lymphadenopathy. Oral lesions appear first. Apthous-like erosions appear anywhere in the oral cavity; they are small and asymptomatic. The cutaneous lesions appear 24 h after the enanthem. The lesions begin as red papules, which rapidly turn into vesicles, surrounded by a red halo. The lesions may be few or inconspicuous, or there may be many. The lesions are present on the hands, feet, palms, and soles. They heal in 7 days without scarring or pigmentation.

Beau's lines, and/or nail shedding may be followed in 3–8 weeks.

13.1.4.1 Complications

In severe cases especially in epidemics, cardiopulmonary complications such as pulmonary edema, and left ventricular dysfunction, resulting in cardiopulmonary arrest can occur. CNS complications such as meningitis, encephalitis, and flaccid paralysis may develop. MRI scans have shown evidence of brain stem damage.

13.1.4.2 Treatment

Treatment is symptomatic with analgesia as required.

13.2 Hypersensitivity Syndromes (Toxic Erythemas)

These syndromes are caused by "superantigens." Superantigens are those antigens that act directly on the T cells without being processed by the Langerhans cells. These antigens directly activate the T cells and cause the release of inflammatory mediators such as the cytokines. The cytokines, especially tumor necrotic factor-α, interleukin-1 and interleukin-2 are mainly responsible for the inflammatory reaction. The common hypersensitivity syndromes are:

- Group-A β-hemolytic streptococci produces an erythrogenic toxin; this is responsible for scarlet fever.
- Staphylococcal scarlatiniform eruption and Staphylococcal scalded skin syndrome (SSSS) are due to toxins produced by phage 11 Staphylococcus aureus.
- In toxic shock syndrome, several staphylococcal toxins are isolated, but the one most commonly implicated is an exoprotein designated toxic shock syndrome toxin-1. This toxin is different from that of SSSS. Streptococcal toxins are also responsible for producing toxic shock syndrome.
- The pathogenesis of Kawasaki's disease is unclear. An infectious origin is probably responsible; toxin-producing bacteria have been isolated in a few cases. The use of gamma globulin in the treatment may be helping in neutralizing the toxin.

13.2.1 Clinical Features

The clinical features of these erythemas are characteristic; the skin is generally red, the erythema is accentuated in the skin folds; it feels like sandpaper. Erythema of the hand, feet, palms, and soles is characteristic, followed by peeling and desquamation. Mucous membrane involvement is common, except in SSSS. The eyes, oral cavity, and lips are bright red in color. The skin is desquamated, once the inflammation is over. Most of the cases occur in childhood except toxic shock syndrome.

13.2.2 Treatment

All of the toxic erythemas are treated with appropriate antibiotics except Kawasaki's disease.

13.2.3 Kawasaki's Disease (Possibly Toxin-Mediated)

It has all the features described above; the differentiating points are:

- Fever is prolonged for more than 5 days.
- Cervical lymph nodes are enlarged.
- Dermatitis in the diaper area is common in children wearing diapers.
- Acquired heart disease is common in children, if the disease is not treated early. It is the most common cause of acquired cardiac disease in America. Cardiac disease is manifested by coronary aneurysm, arrhythmias, and cardiomegaly.
- The disease should be treated early with high doses of aspirin and I/V gamma globulin, to prevent heart disease.

13.2.4 Toxic Shock Syndrome

The differentiating points are:

- It occurs in adults (tampons were a common cause).
- It is due to the toxins of staphylococcus or streptococcus. Streptococcal toxic shock syndrome often has bacteremia and a focus of skin disease, not found in staphylococcal disease.
- High fever (above 38.9°C) and hypotension (systolic pressure of less than 90 mm) are characteristic.
- Loss of hair and nail may be seen after about 2 months of infection.

13.2.5 Staphylococcal Scalded Skin Syndrome (Ritter's Disease) (Fig. 13.1)

There are two hypotheses for this syndrome; it may be caused by an antigen antibody reaction to the toxin, or the staphylococcal toxin acts as a superantigen. The points in favor of the toxin being a superantigen are:

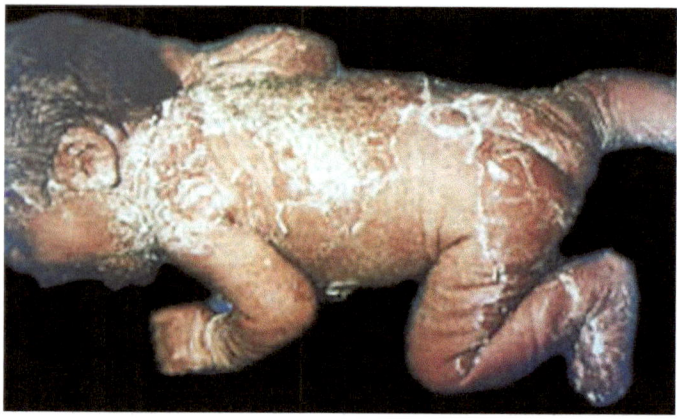

FIGURE 13.1. Staphylococcal scalded skin syndrome.

- The disease occurs in children.
- Erythema of the skin is followed by desquamation; erythema is accentuated in the flexures.

Points against the favor of superantigen:

- Mucous membranes not affected.
- Superficial blisters form after the generalized scarlatiniform erythema.
- Prodromal symptoms absent or mild.

> Scarlet fever is described with the exanthems.
> Toxic epidermal necrolysis (TEN) is not due to superantigens, but is described here as it resembles Staphylococcal scalded skin syndrome and it should be differentiated from it.

13.2.6 Toxic Epidermal Necrolysis (TEN)

In this condition there is complete detachment of the epidermis, through the dermo-epidermal junction; this leads to complications including death, from fluid loss and sepsis. Most cases of TEN follow a drug reaction, the common drugs being sulphamethoxazole/trimethoprim, sulphonamides, aminopenicillins, quinolone and cephalosporins. TEN may also follow Steven Johnson's syndrome; the etiology then is similar to erythema multiforme.

Fever, headache, and symptoms resembling an upper respiratory infection precede the skin rash by 1–2 weeks. Stomatitis and conjunctivitis appear 1–2 days before the onset of the rash.

13.2.6.1 Cutaneous signs

The skin becomes hot, painful, and erythematous. With slight pressure, the skin wrinkles and separates from the dermis (Nicolsky's sign). Small blisters and bullae appear and then the epidermis separates from the dermis. Nonerythematous skin remains intact; the scalp is often spared (Fig. 13.2).

13.2.6.2 Mucous membrane

Inflammation blisters and erosions are common in the oral mucosa; the rest of the GIT is not affected, except by sepsis if this occurs.

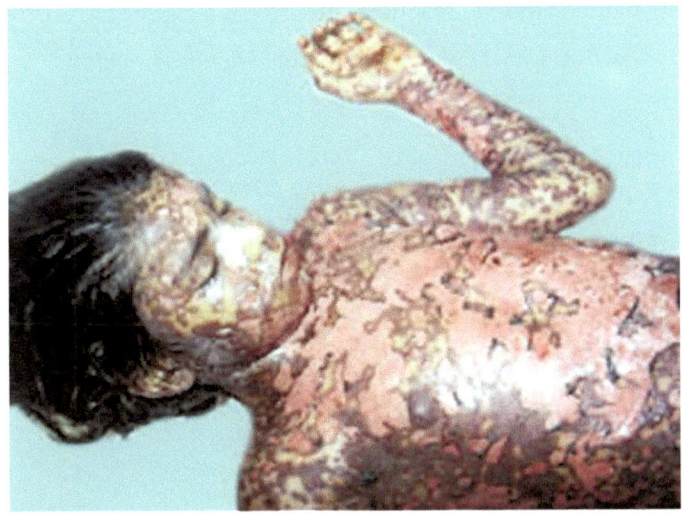

FIGURE 13.2. Toxic epidermal necrolysis.

Ocular complications are serious and include purulent conjunctivitis, conjunctival erosions, followed by fibrosis and adhesions. Corneal ulcerations and blindness may occur. Photophobia, increased mucinous discharge and decreased visual acuity may last for years.

Respiratory tract complications include dyspnea and bronchial hypersecretion which indicate respiratory involvement; bronchial injury indicates a poor prognosis. Septicemia and gram negative pneumonia are the most common causes of death.

13.2.6.3 Treatment

The offending drug should be removed. The use of corticosteroids is controversial; some authors do not indicate its use. All cases of TEN should be treated in a burns unit, where proper skin care is given, fluid and electrolyte balance and, above all, strict asepsis is maintained.

I/V IgG is safe and effective. Early treatment with a total dose of 3 g/kg over 3 consecutive days is recommended.

Cyclosporine or cyclophosphamide is used to inhibit cell-mediated cytotoxic reaction.

A patient with TEN should be treated in a burns unit.

Chapter 14
Urticaria

Urticaria, also known as hives or nettle rash, is a common skin disorder. It is characterized by the formation of a transient erythematous rash (wheal), often with a central pallor (Fig. 14.1). Urticaria is caused by temporary increase in capillary permeability leading to exudation of fluid in the dermis. The wheals do not last longer than 24 hours; new rashes develop at other sites. Urticaria may be acute or chronic. Urticaria that lasts for more than 6 weeks is regarded as chronic.

Urticaria is due to degranulation of mast cells (common variety) or it may be a manifestation of vasculitis (rarer form). Mast cells can be degranulated in response to immediate hypersensitivity (IgE mediated), immune complex disorders, complement activation, or there may be a direct release (non-immunological) of histamine from the mast cells. Mast cells when stimulated release histamine and other vasoactive mediators. Histamine causes the endothelial release of nitric oxide, a dilator of arteries and veins, leading to erythema and then edema.

The common antigens responsible for immunological cause of urticaria are food, food dyes and preservatives, drugs, parasitic infestation, insect bites, dust, and pollens. Urticaria can also be a manifestation of internal disease, malignancy, and serum injections. In a number of cases, the offending agent cannot be identified. Candida, which may be asymptomatic in the oral cavity or elsewhere, may be implicated in urticaria. A number of studies have shown that autoimmunity is the cause

Z. Zaidi, S. W. Lanigan, *Dermatology in Clinical Practice*, 281
DOI: 10.1007/978-1-84882-862-9_14,
© Springer-Verlag London Limited 2010

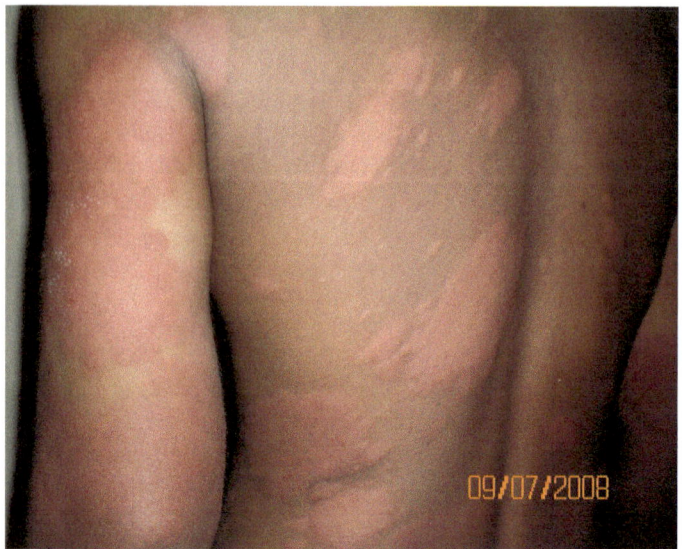

FIGURE 14.1. Urticaria.

of 30–50% cases of chronic urticaria. It may be associated with other autoimmune disorders; in particular autoimmune thyroid disease. Chronic urticaria may also be due to autoimmune IgG antibodies to IgE, or IgE receptors on mast cells. Clinically it is difficult to diagnose autoimmune urticaria, but can be supported by the Autologous Serum Skin Test (ASST). This test is not widely available at present.

Direct release of histamine from the mast cells may be due to drugs such as morphine, codeine, acetylcholine, polymyxin B, ethanol, aspirin; histamine containing foods such as fish of Scrombroidae family (tuna, mackerel) and some bacterial and plant toxins.

Physical urticaria is that produced by physical stimuli such as heat, sunlight, cold, water, and pressure. Pressure urticaria is caused by kinins or prostaglandins rather than histamine. It can occur on the buttocks after sitting, or on the feet after walking. It responds to nonsteroidal anti-inflammatory agents. Dermographism (skin writing) is the most common physical uticaria; wealing is produced by stroking the skin. Young patients are mostly affected. Dermographism may last for weeks, months or years. It is diagnosed by stroking the skin with a firm pressure (Darier's sign). Treatment is not necessary, unless the patients react continuously to minor trauma. Antihistamines are very effective; some patients may require continuous suppression.

Urticarial vasculitis lasts longer than 24 hours; it may be associated with fever, arthralgia, raised ESR, and immune-complexes in the blood. Urticarial vasculitis may be due to autoimmune diseases such as systemic lupus erythematosus, dermatitis herpetiformis, pemphigoid, and other similar disorders. The indurated wheals may contain purpuric foci, angiodema, livido reticularis; nodules and bullae may be associated. The urticarial lesions cause pain rather than itch. This type of urticaria responds better to corticosteroids than anti–histamines.

Angioedema (giant urticaria), is a variant of urticaria, affecting the subcutaneous tissue and deep dermis. The swellings are less demarcated and less red than the urticarial weal. Angioedema commonly occurs at the mucocutaneous junctions as perioral, periorbital, and genital regions. Involvement of the oral cavity and respiratory tract may occur. Laryngeal involvement may lead to asphyxia and death.

Hereditary angioedema is due to congenitally deficient C1 esterase levels. This should be suspected when there is a family history of wheals and angioedema, and sudden unexplained death. The condition often develops spontaneously and in response to minor trauma. Patients often have abdominal pain.

14.1 Investigations

The cause of acute urticaria can often be obtained from a detailed history rather than by investigations. In cases of chronic urticaria a full blood count, eosinophil count, erythrocyte sedimentation rate (ESR), urine examination, stool examination especially for parasites, ova and cysts, X-ray chest, liver function tests, and serum creatinine should be done to exclude systemic disease. If these fail to identify the cause of urticaria, then further tests may be required. Often after extensive evaluation and environmental change, the cause of chronic urticaria still cannot be found.

Challenge with relevant food, food additives, or physical stimulus may be done to find the possible cause of urticaria. An ice cube test is done for cold urticaria, phototesting for solar urticaria, and exercise challenge for cholinergic urticaria. Food sensitivity can be tested, by eliminating a certain food from the diet for a period and then seeing whether urticaria develops or not on reintroduction of the food.

14.2 Treatment

Any identifiable cause of urticaria should be removed, and avoided for the future such as drugs, food, food additives, etc. Reassure the patient, as itching can be exaggerated by psychological factors.

Acute urticaria is easy to manage; adequate doses of nonsedating anti-H_1 histamines e.g. cetirizine or loratidine are needed. If necessary, these can be supplemented by shorter acting antihistamines such as hydroxyzine 10–25 mg every 6 hours. Alternately a long-acting antihistamine such as chlorpheniramine maleate 1 mg sustained tablets taken every 12 hours. The idea is to block histamine activity during the day and night. If the rashes are still not controlled then the dose of hydroxyzine can be increased until tolerance occurs.

Cyproheptadine is useful in cold urticaria, hydroxyzine in cholinergic urticaria, diphenhydramine in solar urticaria. Hydroxyzine is also an anxiolytic and is often a very useful antihistamine for urticaria. Sedation usually occurs with hydroxyzine. Pressure urticaria is responsive to nonsteroidal anti-inflammatory agents as this urticaria is due to the action of prostaglandins.

Patients with chronic urticaria should avoid the use of colored foods, food additives, aspirin, and NSAIDS. In a number of cases urticaria resolves after the avoidance of the above substances.

In treating chronic urticaria long-acting, nonsedating antihistamines are preferred. If one H_1 antihistamine fails, then two antihistamines are given from two different groups. A combination of H_1 and H_2 antihistamines may be tried in some cases. Penicillinase has been successfully used in the treatment of patients with chronic urticaria who have a history of penicillin allergy. Sympathomimetic drugs can be tried, but the effect of adrenaline is short-lived. Pseudoephedrine 30–60 mg every 4 hours or terbutaline 2.5 mg every 8 hours can be helpful in some cases. Systemic steroids are best avoided in chronic urticaria.

In cases of recurrent urticaria, it is important to take the antihistamines regularly and prophylactically to control the disease, rather than taking them at the time of an attack. The antihistamines are continued until the disease has cleared and then tapered gradually. In some cases, admission to hospital may be helpful. It not only gives rest but also eliminates any antigenic factor present at home, which may be thought of and eliminated. Hospitalization also removes stress in some cases.

Systemic steroids are given in severe acute urticaria, and in serum sickness but these are not indicated for chronic urticaria. Adrenaline and tracheotomy may be life-saving in acute laryngeal edema.

Hereditary angioedema is treated by methyltestosterone, danazol, and tranexamic acid. Fresh plasma which contains C1 esterase inhibitor can be used during an attack. Respiratory obstruction is managed by intubation or tracheostomy as intubation may be difficult; and adrenaline 1/1000 0.5–1 mL subcutaneously or intramuscularly and hydrocortisone 200 mg intravenously.

> *History taking is important in managing urticaria; find the cause and eliminate it whenever possible.*
>
> *Antihistamines should be used in high doses.*
>
> *The patient should be warned about drowsiness while driving when taking antihistamines.*
>
> *Exclude systemic illness in chronic urticaria.*
>
> *Avoid the use of aspirin, food dyes, and food additives in chronic urticaria.*
>
> *In pregnancy avoid cetirizine and loratidine; chlorpheniramine or diphenhydramine are used.*

14.3 Mastocytosis

This is a disorder of proliferation of mast cells. The condition may be confined to the skin or it may also involve the internal organs; the central nervous is usually spared.

Cutaneous mastocytosis may be localized or generalized.

Localized mastocytosis. The disease occurs in infancy; it presents as reddish brown or yellowish brown nodules or plaques, and the disease evolves by the age of 2–3 years. The lesions urticate on rubbing (Darier's sign), as often seen on drying the skin after a bath. Solitary lesions (mastocytoma) can occur.

Generalized mastocytosis (urticaria pigmentosa). This form can occur in infancy or in adults. The lesions appear as reddish brown macules, which urticate on rubbing the skin. Some patients may exhibit dermographism. The internal organ involvement manifests as wheezing, dysnea, diarrhea, bone pains, or osteoporosis (bone is the most common organ involved after the skin), enlargement of the liver, spleen, and lymph nodes. Hematological abnormalities include anemia, leucopenia, and thrombocytopenia. Some cases manifest as mast cell leukemia.

Darier's sign is characteristic of mastocytosis. Injecting local anesthesia for biopsy directly into a lesion may degranulate the mast cells. If a biopsy is necessary the infiltration of local anesthetic should be around the lesion not directly into it. Histamine levels are raised in diffuse cutaneous mastocytosis.

14.3.1 Treatment

Itching can be treatment with antihistamines. The infantile variant resolves spontaneously. PUVA and mast cells stabilizers such as disodium cromoglycate may be used in resistant cases. Alcohol and other mast cell degranulators should be avoided. The treatment of malignant mastocytosis is unsatisfactory; death usually occurs in a couple of years.

> The classical diagnostic sign of cutaneous mastocytosis is Darier's sign.

Chapter 15
Pruritus

Pruritus is described as a sensation which produces the desire to scratch. It may be due to a cutaneous disease or as a manifestation of an internal disorder. These disorders may range from innocuous to malignant.

15.1 Etiology

15.1.1 Cutaneous

Almost any skin disease may itch. The common pruritic cutaneous diseases are scabies, lichen planus, dermatitis herpetiformis, eczema especially atopic dermatitis, prurigo, urticaria, insect bites, pediculosis, ichthyosis, and dryness of the skin from any cause. The changes caused by skin disease give a clue to their diagnosis.

In underdeveloped countries parasitic disorders such as scabies and diseases causing anemia should be excluded. Sometimes scratch marks give a clue to the diagnosis of pruritus. Different dermatoses react differently to scratching. Urticaria rarely produces scratch marks, scabies results in small excoriations, and atopic eczema produces large scratch marks. Patients with eczema use their nails to rub the skin; their nails then become highly polished. Neurotic patients often remove pieces of their skin.

Z. Zaidi, S. W. Lanigan, *Dermatology in Clinical Practice*,
DOI: 10.1007/978-1-84882-862-9_15,
© Springer-Verlag London Limited 2010

15.1.2 Systemic and Localized

The patients present with a history of itching often without a rash. The common causes are liver disorders, renal disease, thyroid disorders, diabetes mellitus, internal malignancy, iron deficiency anemia, and drugs (aspirin, morphine oral psoralens, etc.); carcinoid syndrome is a less common disorder. Candidiasis of the oral cavity or elsewhere may produce pruritus. Occasionally pruritus may be due to psychiatric causes. A diagnosis of psychogenic pruritus should not be made unless all the other causes are excluded.

PUO (pruritus of unknown origin), is defined as itching of more than 2 weeks duration, the cause of which remains unknown after 2 weeks of investigations and management. It is important to investigate the patient thoroughly as pruritus may be due to malignancy.

15.1.3 Localized Pruritus

15.1.3.1 Pruritus Ani

This can be due to localized dermatoses such as lichen simplex chronicus, psoriasis, seborrheic dermatitis, candidiasis, crab lice, tinea, erythrasma, and lichen planus.

Contact dermatitis in old age, which can be allergic or irritant, is often due to toilet paper, medicaments such as local anesthetics, diarrhea or discharge causing soiling of the perianal skin.

Rectal or anal diseases such as hemorrhoids or fissure in ano may also cause localized pruritus.

15.1.3.2 Pruritus Vulvae

Localized dermatoses such as candidiasis, trichomonal infestation, herpes simplex, warts, psoriasis, seborrheic dermatitis, tinea, lichen simplex chronicus, lichen sclerosis et atropicus, erythrasma, and crab lice can cause pruritus.

Threadworm infestation can cause both pruritus ani and vulvae.

15.2 Evaluation of the Itching Patient

It should be first determined whether the pruritus is due to a dermatological disease or whether it is a manifestation of an internal disorder. If a rash is present find out whether the itching occurred before the rash; this often points toward a systemic illness. If the itching occurred after the rash, this is often a pointer toward a cutaneous disorder.

First, exclude dermatological disorders such as scabies and other conditions by a thorough physical examination, especially in well-groomed individuals in whom signs of disease may be minimal. Scratch marks and excoriations indicate the degree of itching. Scratch marks of scabies are quite short; those of pediculosis corporis are often several centimeters long. Deep gouged-out excoriations may be present in delusional parasitosis and neurotic excoriations; subtle signs of persistent rubbing include the polished-nail sign.

Take a detailed history of the pruritus, e.g., specific time relationship (nocturnal, morning, monthly) etc., whether gradual or sudden, continuous or paroxysmal. Paroxysmal itching that wakes the patient from sleep may be of organic origin.

Signs of dermatological disease require no further investigations. More generalized itching without any cutaneous sign points to a systemic illness. Itching after a hot bath may point to polycythemia vera or aquagenic pruritus. Failure to obtain relief from symptomatic measures suggests severe disease. Itching from wool often points to atopy.

Information about pets should always be obtained in pruritus of unknown origin (PUO); fleas and mites of pets are often a cause of itching in household individuals. Unusual environmental causes include beetle-infested carpets, and fowl mites from air conditioners, where birds choose to build their nests.

A comprehensive drug history should always be obtained. The drugs that cause pruritus are opiates and its derivates, aspirin, quinidine, psoralen (PUVA), phenothiazine, oestrogens, progestins, testosterone, tolbutamide, and erythrocin estolate.

For practical purpose, itching may fall into one of the following groups:

- Cutaneous – due to recognizable dermatological disease, e.g., atopic dermatitis, lichen planus, etc.
- Systemic such as liver disease, kidney disease, hematological disorders, etc.
- Psychogenic

15.3 Investigations

A preliminary working diagnosis is required in systemic disorders causing pruritus. Tests usually include a complete blood count and differential, biochemical tests for thyroid, hepatic and renal function, and a chest X-ray examination. Stools should be examined for ova, cysts, and parasites. Urine should be tested for albumin and blood sugar.

Patients with PUO should be considered to have an internal disorder unless proved otherwise. Additional tests such as stool for occult blood, Papanicolaou smear, and further radiological examinations may be necessary. Radio contrast studies and CT scans are usually not indicated as a part of evaluation in every case, but in some cases, it may lead to the diagnosis of a treatable disorder. Electrophoresis of the blood and urine is required in some cases of pruritus.

15.4 Treatment

Symptomatic treatment falls into the following categories:

- Patient education and reduction of provocative factors
- Topical preparations

- Oral medications
- Physical modalities

15.4.1 Patient Education and Reduction of Provocative Factors

If the underlying cause of pruritus is known, treatment is straightforward. When the cause cannot be determined symptomatic treatment is required. Symptomatic treatment is also required when investigations are underway. Stimulants such as tea and coffee may aggravate itching; patients should be protected from external irritants such as wool. Soaps and detergents should not be used with dry skin. Baths containing small amounts of oil are helpful for dry skin. Nails should be kept short and clean. As pruritus is increased by an elevated temperature, wearing light clothes, maintaining a cool environment, and taking a tepid shower before sleep is helpful. Dryness of the skin produces itching; hence, simple emollients such as white soft paraffin, cold creams; moisturizers will help to reduce the itch.

The patient should also be taught to break the itch– scratch cycle. When the urge to scratch comes, distraction techniques using a cool washcloth, pressure, or will power may be helpful.

Fabrics that have been contaminated in the laundry, e.g., by fiberglass curtains, may have to be discarded. Drugs known to cause pruritus should be avoided.

15.4.2 Topical Preparations

Calamine lotion is one of the commonly used topical antipruritic agents. One percent menthol in ethanol relieves itching as it has a cooling sensation on the skin. Local anesthetics such as benzocaine and xylocaine are good antipruritics, but they cause contact dermatitis and therefore should be avoided. Liquor piscis carbonis 2–10% in alcohol, thymol, and tincture of benzoin are other topical antipruritics.

Phenol, menthol, and camphor may be added to a variety of vehicles such as calamine lotion. Camphor is used in 1–5%, menthol in 0.5–2%, and phenol in 0.5–2% concentrations. Phenol should not be prescribed to infants and pregnant women.

The following are some of the baths additives recommended for itching.

- Oatmeal baths; 1 lb of starch is added to a tubful of water, for generalized pruritus.
- Bath oils; 5–25 mL of olive oil is added to a tub of warm water, for dry and sensitive skin.
- Tar baths; 100 mL of coal tar solution is added to a tubful of water for pruritus due to psoriasis.
- Proprietary bath oils are available for purchase or on prescription.

15.4.3 Oral Medications

There are no effective specific antipruritic drugs. Antihistamines relieve itching by inhibiting the release of histamine and by causing sedation. Promethazine, diphenhydramine, cyproheptadine, and hydroxyzine are commonly used. Diazepam may provide useful sedation in an agitated or disturbed person. Opiod receptor antagonists including nalaxone are helpful in the management of intractable pruritus.

Cholestyramine may be effective in relieving the pruritus of renal and hepatic origin. It is also useful in relieving the itching of polycythemia rubra vera. It acts by removing the pruritogenic substances in the gut.

Activated charcoal is useful for the treatment of pruritus in patients undergoing renal dialysis.

Naloxone was used to treat pruritus of primary biliary cirrhosis. Enkephalin and endorphin blockage by naloxone is not used routinely for treatment of pruritus, but holds considerable promise. Because of the close relationship between pain and itch, aspirin is used for the treatment of itching in some patients. It is used in the treatment of polycythemia rubra vera. It blocks the release of prostaglandins and serotinin.

Thalidomide is used in the treatment of prurigo nodularis.

15.4.4 Other Modalities

Other suggested methods for the treatment of pruritus are transcutaneous nerve stimulation, phototherapy, and acupuncture. UVB therapy is especially useful in pruritus of renal failure and after dialysis. UVB radiation is administered two to three times a week starting with an initial dose of 75% of minimal erythema dose. Improvement is seen in 2–3 weeks; remission of several weeks or months may be obtained. PUVA is helpful in the treatment of atopic dermatitis. UVA alone has not been used in the treatment of pruritus as UVA itself may cause itching.

Stress can make anything worse; itching is no exception. Every effort should be made to reduce stress. Psychiatrists, social workers, and the dermatologist should all help the patient in coping with the problem of stress.

15.5 General Guidelines

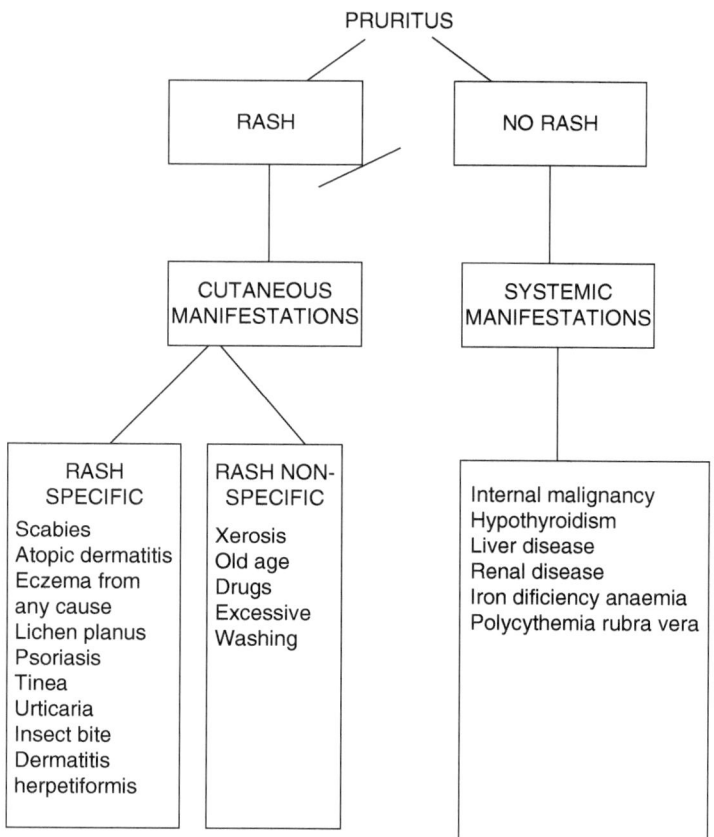

PRURITUS

RASH — NO RASH

CUTANEOUS MANIFESTATIONS — SYSTEMIC MANIFESTATIONS

RASH SPECIFIC
Scabies
Atopic dermatitis
Eczema from any cause
Lichen planus
Psoriasis
Tinea
Urticaria
Insect bite
Dermatitis herpetiformis

RASH NON-SPECIFIC
Xerosis
Old age
Drugs
Excessive Washing

Internal malignancy
Hypothyroidism
Liver disease
Renal disease
Iron dificiency anaemia
Polycythemia rubra vera

Chapter 16
Leg Ulcers

Ulcers on the leg may be due to venous or arterial disease, infections, infestations, neuropathy, trauma, diabetes, malignancy, burns, blood disease, vasculitis, immobility (decubitis ulcers), or due to psychosis (factitious ulcers). The most common ulcers on the leg are the venous, arterial, and neuropathic. In some tropical countries, ulcers due to leprosy are common; in Western countries venous ulcers predominate.

16.1 Venous Ulcers

These are due to increased pressure in the superficial veins of the legs. This may be due to deep venous thrombosis, incompetent valves in the deep and communicating veins, or tumors of the pelvis, which prevent the upward flow of blood. The blood flows back into the superficial veins, the valves of the perforating vessels between the superficial and deep vein are damaged, and the pressure of the superficial veins increases. The largest perforators are superior and posterior to the medial and lateral malleoli, the areas where the ulcers are most prevalent. Multiple tortuous veins are seen below and behind the malleoli due to localized venous incompetence; this is known as the "ankle flare." Superficial varicosities alone are very unlikely to produce venous insufficiency. Weakness of the calf muscles due to old age, immobility, or arthritis aggravates the problem.

Z. Zaidi, S. W. Lanigan, *Dermatology in Clinical Practice*,
DOI: 10.1007/978-1-84882-862-9_16,
© Springer-Verlag London Limited 2010

16.1.1 Etiology

The increased hydrostatic pressure in the superficial veins is transmitted to the capillaries. The single-cell capillary wall becomes stretched, leading to abnormal leakage of fluids into the tissues and skin. This results in pitting edema and leakage of RBC. The red blood cells release hemoglobin into the tissues where they disintegrate. The breakdown products of hemoglobin lead to irritation of the skin, discoloration, and eczema (not all patients develop eczema; this suggests that environmental and genetic factors also play a part). Fibrinogen from the leaked plasma is also deposited in the tissues as insoluble fibrin complex, which surrounds the capillaries; this "fibrin cuff" prevents the exchange of oxygen and nutrients leading to tissue death. Skin is thus depleted of oxygen and nutrients; it becomes ischemic and will eventually break down forming an ulcer. Ulcers may occur spontaneously or after slight trauma. The ulcer may remain small, or enlarge.

16.1.2 Clinical Features

Venous ulcers have a sharp or sloping border; they are superficial, becoming deep in long-standing cases. The base is granulomatous, healing is slow, and it may take weeks or months. After healing, the ulcer may rapidly recur. A constant dull pain is felt which improves on elevation of the leg (pain in an arterial ulcer is more intense and increases on elevation of the leg).

Chronic edema, trauma, infection, or inflammation of the skin, lead to fibrosis, giving the skin a firm, nonpitting edema. Fat necrosis is due to insufficient blood supply, or may follow thrombosis of the small veins. Loss of fat and fibrosis leads to decrease in the circumference of the lower leg (lipodermatosclerosis). The proximal part of the leg swells from chronic venous obstruction, giving rise to the "inverted bottle leg," appearance. Stasis papillomatous may develop in chronically congested legs due to lymphoedema. White atrophic scars (atrophic blanche) ultimately replace the ulcers (Fig. 16.1).

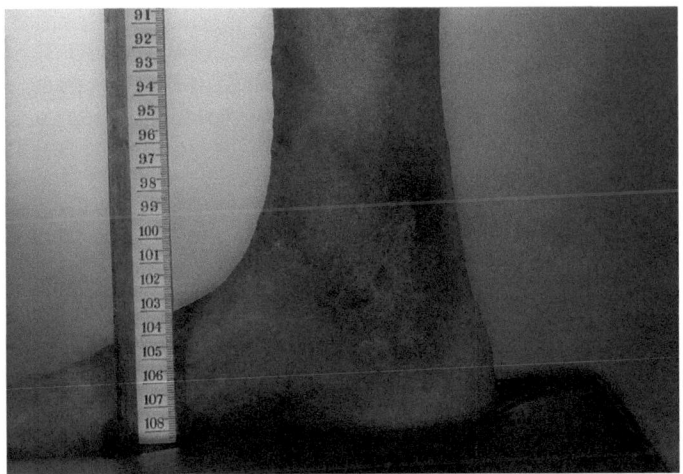

FIGURE 16.1. Venous ulcer.

16.1.3 Complications

These include infection, eczema, lymphangitis, osteomyelitis, septicaemia, lymphoedema, and malignancy.

Characteristics of venous ulcers are:

- Painless ulcers, on the medial or lateral surface of the legs above the ankle
- Pigmentation surrounding the ulcers
- Eczema
- Ankle flare
- Varicose veins
- Edema, pitting in early stages and nonpitting in the later stage
- Lipodermatosclerosis
- Atrophic scars

16.1.4 Treatment

Treatment of venous ulcers is a long-term process and the progress is usually slow. The initial examination includes testing for blood circulation by examination of the peripheral pulses; Doppler studies to exclude coexisting arterial disease are required if compression bandages are to be used. An evaluation of the contributing factors should be made such as anemia, obesity, cardiac failure, diabetes, and arthritis. These should be dealt with individually.

General measures:

- Stop smoking.
- Stop alcohol intake.
- Good nutrition, multivitamin supplements that contain Vitamin E, C, and zinc, iron, and folic acid if appropriate.
- Long-standing ulcers that do not heal, should have a biopsy for malignant change.
- Long-standing ulcers should have an X-ray of the leg to exclude osteomyelitis.
- Aspirin helps in the healing of ulcers.
- Short course of systemic antibiotics should be given in spreading infection.
- Pentoxifylline, in a dose of 400 mg given 2–3 times daily, increases the rate of healing of venous ulcer, by increasing the blood flow.
- Oxerutin 500 mg given twice daily relieves symptoms of edema associated with chronic venous insufficiency.
- Stanazol, an anabolic steroid, may not heal an existing ulcer, but it may prevent recurrences and ulceration in lipodermatosclerosis.

Local measures:

- Treat the ulcer. This includes measures that promote wound healing, such as medical or surgical debridement of the ulcer, occlusive dressings, treatment of infection, and good nutrition. Ulcers will not heal if there is infection, edema, eczema, and inflammation. These problems should be dealt with individually.
- *Compression* is the cornerstone of therapy in venous ulcers. Compression forces the fluid to pass from the interstitial spaces back into the vascular and lymphatic compartments. This is accomplished by the application

of external compression bandages during the healing phase, and graded compression stockings after healing, to prevent recurrence. Apply the bandage over the occlusive ulcer dressing.

(Always assess arterial blood flow to the legs before applying compression bandages. Occlusive dressings should be used when the infection and eczema have cleared.)

- Elevation of the legs 3–4 times a day, above the level of the heart for 30 minutes, helps the swelling to subside.
- Legs should be elevated at night, by raising the foot end of the bed by 15–20 cm.
- Measure the ulcer at each visit.
- Encourage periods of exercise and ambulation, to strengthen the calf muscles.
- Large ulcers may need skin grafting.
- Once the ulcer has healed, elastic compression stockings should be worn for the rest of the patient's life, otherwise there is a very high re-ulceration rate.

The goal of therapy is to normalize venous pathology.
In clean ulcers the dressings can be changed once or twice a week.
Infected ulcers should be cleaned and dressed more often, sometimes once or even twice daily.
Do not apply topical steroids on the ulcer.
Avoid compression bandage if the arterial supply is inadequate.
(Application of elastic bandages is explained in Appendix 1.)

16.2 Arterial Ulcers

These are less common compared to venous ulcers and are extremely painful. Varicose veins are usually absent but their presence does not exclude the diagnosis. Both sexes are involved more commonly after the age of 60 years.

16.2.1 Etiology

Arterial ulcers may be due to atherosclerosis in advanced age, vasculitis, diabetes, radiation damage, increased blood viscosity, and platelet adhesiveness. Patients with widespread arterial disease may have a history of stroke or coronary thrombosis.

16.2.2 Clinical Features

The ulcer appears on the area where the arterial supply is the poorest: on the tip of the toes, dorsum of the foot, the heel, and dorsum of the shin. The ulcers are sharply defined, punched out, and are deep. The ulcer may penetrate the deep fascia; at times even the tendons are exposed at the base (Fig. 16.2).

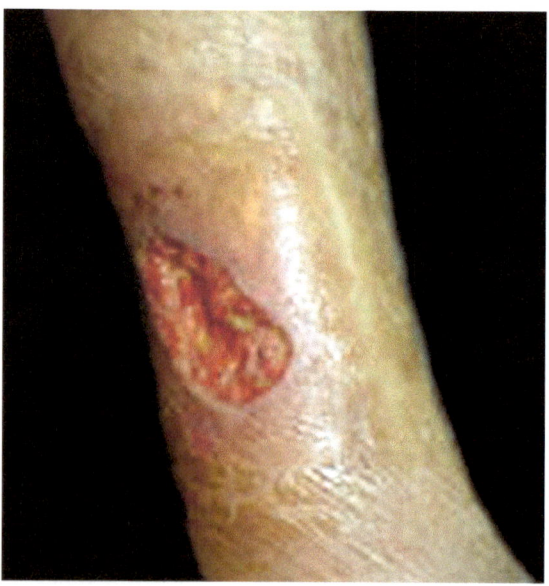

FIGURE 16.2. Arterial ulcer.

The pedal pulsations are absent, and the foot is cold. Doppler pressure indices are low. Intermittent claudication is usual; sometimes discoloration of the toes is present, indicating the onset of gangrene.

16.2.3 Treatment

- Treat the cause such as diabetes, vasculitis, and atherosclerosis.
- Increase the blood flow, by peripheral vasodilators such as nifedipine or pentoxifylline.
- Leg should be placed in a dependant position to help to reduce the pain and increase the arterial flow.
- If it is not possible to improve the vascular supply, the patient should be referred to a vascular surgeon.
- Treat the ulcer itself, remove the slough, and clean the ulcer. Once the ulcer is clean, it should be covered with a nonadherent dressing. The dressing is covered with a light bandage. A tight bandage will further impede the blood supply.

Differentiation between arterial and venous ulcer

Arterial ulcer	Venous ulcer
Site	
Shin, lateral malleoli toes	Medial side of the leg above and behind the medial malleolus
Clinical features	
Deep sharply defined, surrounding skin normal	Shallow, irregular edges, surrounding skin pigmented and oedematous
Painful	Not painful
Eczematization absent	Eczematization present
Foot cold, pedal pulsations absent	Foot warm, pedal pulsations present
Intermittent claudication present	Intermittent claudication absent

16.3 Decubitis Ulcers (Bedsore)

These ulcers commonly develop in a patient who is bedridden. Two most important factors in their development are pressure and loss of the trophic influence of nerves. Bedsores develop rapidly in anemic and malnourished patients. Moisture increases the rate of extension of a bedsore. The common sites for the development of bedsores are the sacrum, greater trochanters, and the heel.

16.3.1 Treatment

• The patient, who is bedridden, should be helped to change their position 3–4 times a day to avoid constant pressure on the ulcer site.
• The ulcer should be cleaned and debrided if required.
• Treat associated infection and edema if present. Local antibiotics should be avoided as they may cause sensitization.
• Urine and fecal contamination should be cleaned immediately.
• Occlusive dressings made of various polymers have made a significant contribution to ulcer therapy. These dressings keep the ulcer moist, a factor that helps in epidermal repair, through migration of epithelial cells over the ulcer. Initially large amounts of exudates form under the dressings (crust and necrotic debris). These dressings are changed every day: as the ulcer heals, they can be changed at 2–3 day intervals.

16.4 Neuropathic Ulcers

These ulcers are due to the lack of sensation of the skin, as seen in diabetic and leprosy patients. The sole of the foot is a common site. The trauma goes unnoticed, until an ulcer appears. The ulcers are common over the head of the metatarsal bones.

16.4.1 Treatment

- To get the ulcers to heal, further injury must be avoided. The simplest way of achieving this is by the patient resting in bed. An alternative is to apply a below-the-knee walking plaster for 2 months at a time.
- The aim of treatment is to remove the pressure over the ulcer. Special bandages or shoes that elevate the foot above the floor, so that the area of the ulcer does not rest on the floor can be used.
- The ulcer is treated in a similar way to other ulcers described above; remove the slough, clean the ulcer, and apply nonadherent dressings.

> *Long-standing ulcers should have a biopsy to exclude malignancy.*
>
> *Patients with nonhealing ulcers should be investigated for diabetes, hypertension, peripheral vascular disease, pyoderma gangrenosum, obesity, and malnutrition.*
>
> *Avoid local medicaments while treating leg ulcers due to sensitization.*

Common leg ulcers
Venous
Arterial
Neuropathic
Traumatic
Vasculitis
Diabetes
Immune bullous disorders
Pyoderma gangrenosum
Malignancy
Tuberculosis
Tropical ulcer
Leishmaniasis

Chapter 17
Disorders of Pigmentation

The color of the skin is due to a number of factors. Melanin is responsible for the shades of brown, eumelanin for brown and black, and pheomelanin for red pigmentation as seen in red heads; the pink color of untanned Caucasoid skin is due to oxyhemoglobin. Other substances responsible for skin color are the carotenes, found in the subcutaneous fat and stratum corneum. The blue color of blue naevus is due to an optical effect from melanin transmission through the skin. Optical effects are also responsible for other colors such as purple in lichen planus. There are a number of endogenous and exogenous substances responsible for skin color. Excess bilirubin in jaundice is an endogenous pigment and, skin tattooing and henna are some of the exogenous pigments.

The number of melanocytes is the same in all races; the difference in color is due to the production, distribution, and degeneration of melanosomes. Abnormalities of skin color can cause considerable psychological stress in many people; for example, vitiligo in dark skin, and pigmented naevi in a lighter skin population.

17.1 Albinism

This is a congenital abnormality of autosomal recessive inheritance. Melanocytes are present in the skin, but they are unable to produce melanin or produce very little

Z. Zaidi, S. W. Lanigan, *Dermatology in Clinical Practice*,
DOI: 10.1007/978-1-84882-862-9_17,
© Springer-Verlag London Limited 2010

melanin, due to a defect in the enzyme tyrosinase. Accordingly patients can be tyrosinase positive or tyosinase negative. The tyrosinase positive patients have a waxen yellow complexion, freckles may develop with age, and they slightly tan on exposure to light. Tyrosinase negative patients have white hair, their skin is pink, and their pupils are red in color (Fig. 17.1).

Patients with albinism have poor vision, rotatory nystagmus, and photophobia. There is extreme photosensitivity due to loss of melanin and there is an increased tendency to the formation of skin tumors. The patients have melanocytes so they can develop nonpigmented melanocytic naevi and amelanotic malignant melanomas.

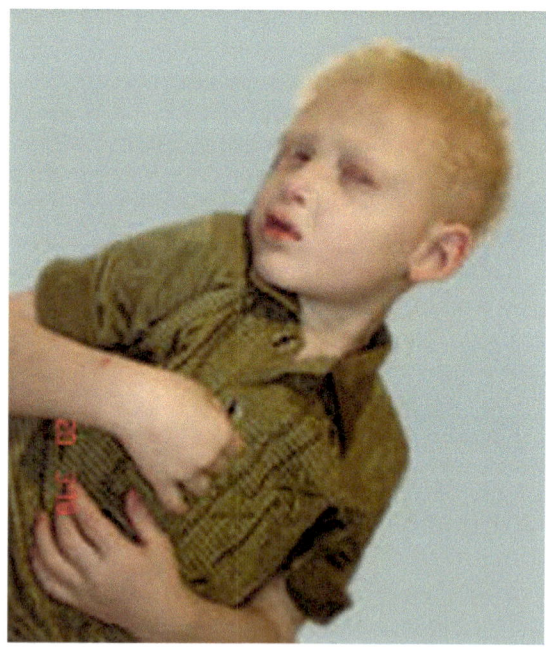

FIGURE 17.1. Albinism.

17.1.1 Treatment

Avoid sun exposure, use sunscreens, wear broad brimmed hats, and opaque clothing. Patients should have regular checkups for the early diagnosis and treatment of skin tumors. Eyes should be examined periodically by an ophthalmologist, and protected by the wearing of UV protective sunglasses.

17.2 Vitiligo

The word vitiligo comes from the Latin – vitellus, meaning veal, for pale or light pink flesh. It is an acquired disorder of pigmentation, in which the melanocytes are absent from the skin. There is a family history in about 30% of patients; an autoimmune pathogenesis is thought to play a role in its etiology. Vitiligo is often associated with diabetes, pernicious anemia, and thyroid disorders.

17.2.1 Etiology

The exact cause of vitiligo is not known, the following are some of the hypotheses proposed:

- Autoimmune.
- Neurogenic – some neurotoxic agent is liberated near the melanocytes, which causes their destruction. This may also explain some cases of dermatomal vitiligo.
- Self-destruction of melanin – melanin production produces a toxin that destroys the melanocytes.
- Exogenous chemicals such as thiols, phenols catechols, etc.

17.2.2 Clinical Features

Vitiligo often begins before the age of 20 years; both men and women are equally affected. The patches of vitilgo are found on the face, hands, flexures, genitals, front of the knees, and elbows. These are the sites often subjected to trauma and/or ultraviolet light. The patches are chalky white and surrounded by a hyperpigmented halo in dark-skinned people. As the condition progresses the hair in the patches also depigments. The lesions are often bilateral and symmetrical. Spontaneous repigmentation is seen in 10–20% of patients, most frequently in the sun-exposed areas. The pigmentation is at first perifollicular (lesions around the lips and fingertips have a bad prognosis due to lack of hair follicles) (Figs. 17.2–17.4).

In some patients, the distribution of vitiligo is segmental; lesions may or may not follow a dermatome. The segmental variety is seen at an earlier age, it is not associated with autoimmune diseases, and spontaneous repigmentation occurs more often in this type of vitiligo.

Mode of presentation in the west is different from people with dark complexions. Fair-skinned people often complain that areas of skin did not tan on exposure to sunlight, rather than patches of depigmentation.

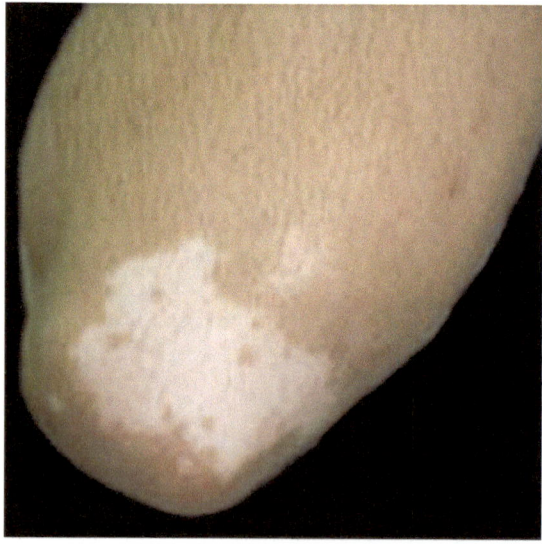

FIGURE 17.2. Vitiligo.

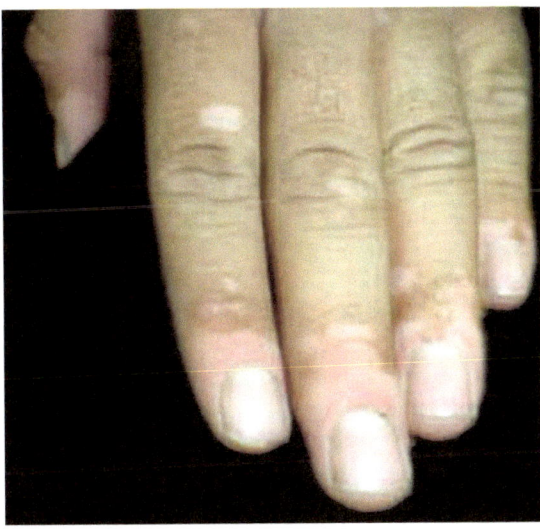

FIGURE 17.3. Vitiligo – finger tip vitiligo has a bad prognosis due to lack of hair follicles.

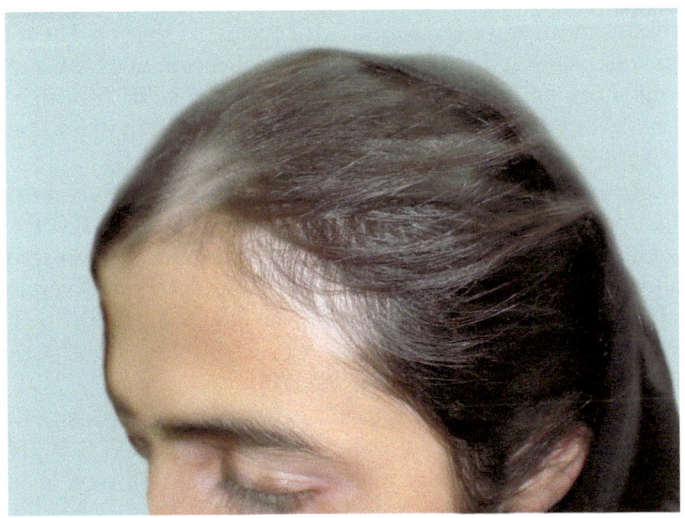

FIGURE 17.4. Vitiligo scalp – the patch with black hair has a better prognosis that the one with white hair.

17.2.3 Treatment

The treatment is unsatisfactory in most cases; an effective cosmetic camouflage for lesions on the exposed skin is required. Cosmetic covers up with vitadye and dyoderm stains are used. These cosmetics are mixed to match the skin hues to mask the white skin. In sunny climates, sunscreens are necessary.

A small percentage (recent onset) respond to topical potent steroid therapy. Topical steroids may be used with careful monitoring of cutaneous side effects. These are especially effective on the face of dark-skinned patients.

A more effective treatment is psoralens and ultraviolet light (PUVA). The best results are obtained with oral rather than topical psoralens. The treatment is time consuming and may have to be continued for up to 2 years. Asians and Negroes respond better to treatment than Caucasoids. If follicular pigmentation has not occurred in 3 months, it should be considered as a therapeutic failure and treatment should be stopped.

Psoralens can be applied topically or taken orally. Topical treatment is more appropriate for localized lesions. The local psoralen should be diluted before application or else the skin will show marked irritation. Oral psoralens (tri-psoralen or 8-methoxy psoralen) are given in a dose of 0.6 mg/kg of body weight, 2 h before exposure to sunlight. Starting with a 15-min exposure and then increasing to 5 min per exposure until a faint persistent erythema is obtained. About 30–100 treatments may be required to elicit repigmentation. A sunscreen should be used in the non-vitiliginous area to avoid sun tanning and thereby increasing the color contrast. UV protective glasses should be worn to protect eyes and the patient should avoid sunlight for the rest of the day.

Tacrolimus and narrow band UVB therapy are also effective in the treatment of vitiligo. Narrow band UVB is given two to three times weekly for at least 6 months; new lesions respond the best.

Khellin, a furanochromone, is being investigated for the treatment of vitiligo. Furanochromone is a photosensitizer in combination with ultraviolet light. It does not produce photo-toxic erythema.

Patients with vitiligo involving more than two-thirds of the body may prefer to have the normal skin bleached with hydroquinone preparation. Twenty percent monobenzoylether cream or 20% hydroxyquinone cream is applied to the skin in qd or bid dose. Depigmentation of the normal skin takes 2–3 months to show initial lightening and may take 1–3 years to complete. Bleaching is permanent.

Minigrafting – grafts of pigmented skin are transplanted to nonpigmented areas. Melanocyte and stem cell transplants, in which single cell suspensions are made from unaffected skin and applied to the dermabraded-affected skin, are also being tried for the treatment of vitiligo.

Micropigmentation (tattooing) involves injecting colored pigments, mostly iron oxide into the dermis. This may be most useful in the lip area, particularly those with dark skin. Unfortunately, many patients experience significant pigment loss within the first several weeks after the procedure. It is difficult to obtain a perfect match of the color of the surrounding skin.

Treatment of vitiligo in white-skinned patients is disappointing.

Do not promise a cure for vitiligo.

Lip and finger tip vitiligo, and patches of vitiligo with white hair have a bad prognosis.

17.3 Melasma (Chloasma)

This is a very common condition seen in pigmented skin. Dark brown irregular patches of pigmentation occur on the cheeks, nose, and forehead mainly in women. The highest incidence is in the reproductive years of life. The exact etiology is unknown; it may be due to ovarian disorders, oral contraceptives, pregnancy, or perhaps associated with high estrogen levels. The condition is less common in males, but

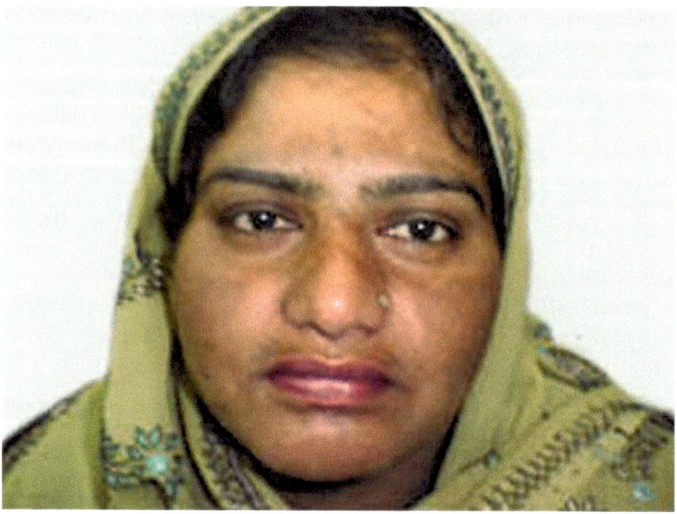

FIGURE 17.5. Melasma.

when it does occur, it is more difficult to treat. Sunlight and genetic factors are also implicated. Melasma also occurs after hydantoin therapy and in AIDS (Fig. 17.5).

Most of the extra melanin lies in the epidermis, but some pigment is also dermal. If the area is viewed with a Wood's lamp, an increase in contrast of the pigment indicates epidermal pigmentation; loss of contrast would suggest dermal pigmentation.

17.3.1 Treatment

Treatment is difficult; a combination of hydroquinone, tretinoin, and dexamethasone is often used. Five percent hydroquinone is used initially for about 4–6 weeks, later a 2% concentration is used for maintenance. Sunlight should be avoided; sunscreens are helpful. Use of oral contraceptives with high estrogen content should be avoided. Chemical peels may induce temporary improvement if the pigmentation is epidermal; the area first turns red and then black, the black eschar peels off within a week. Postinflammatory hyperpigmentation is a complication.

17.4 Freckles

Freckles are probably of autosomal dominant inheritance. They appear by the age of 5 years as small brown macules on the sun-exposed skin. The macules are less than 5 mm in diameter. They are common in fair complexions and red-haired people. Freckles multiply and become darker in summer with sun exposure. The number of melanocytes is unaltered, but the melanosomes are longer and more active. People with freckles tend to sunburn easily and are more prone to the development of cutaneous malignancy (Fig. 17.6).

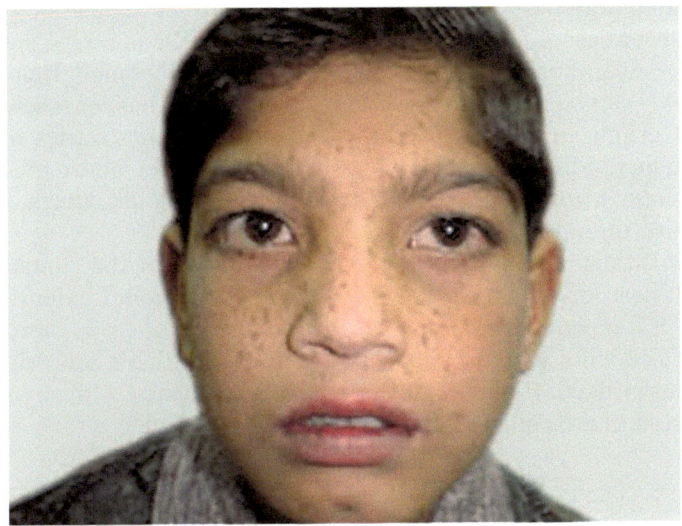

FIGURE 17.6. Freckles.

17.4.1 Treatment

Avoidance of sunlight and the use of sunscreens are advised. A depigmenting cream may lighten freckles. If the patient wants treatment for cosmetic reasons then solid carbon dioxide, phenol, or lasers may help.

17.5 Acanthosis Nigricans (AN)

As with the terminology of so many dermatoses, this is also a misnomer. Histologically there is no acanthosis, but papillomatosis, with or without thickening of the stratum malpighian, associated with hyperkeratosis and increased pigmentation. AN is often associated with insulin resistance. Prolonged hypersecretion of insulin can lead to pancreatic impairment, glucose intolerance, and type 2 diabetes mellitus.

AN affects the flexures such as the axillae, neck, and groin. The skin is thickened and pigmented. It later becomes papillomatous and ridged, giving the skin a velvety appearance. In severe cases, it may become warty (Fig. 17.7).

Acanthosis nigricans can be malignant or benign. Benign AN can be hereditary, due to hormonal disturbances (such as Cushing's disease, Addison's disease, polycystic ovaries, and hyperandrogenic states), obesity (pseudo AN), and medications (nicotinic acid, fuscidic acid, glucocorticoids, contraceptive therapy).

Malignant AN is associated with tumors of the stomach, breast, or lungs. The disease is more severe, and extensive. Oral mucous membrane is involved in 50% of cases, there is thickening of the palms (tripe palms), and nails are brittle and ridged. Removal of the tumor is associated with regression of the clinical signs. Relapses are frequent.

17.5.1 Treatment

Removal of the cause results in moderate improvement of AN. Pseudo AN may improve with weight loss. Etretinate has been used in the treatment of hereditary benign AN.

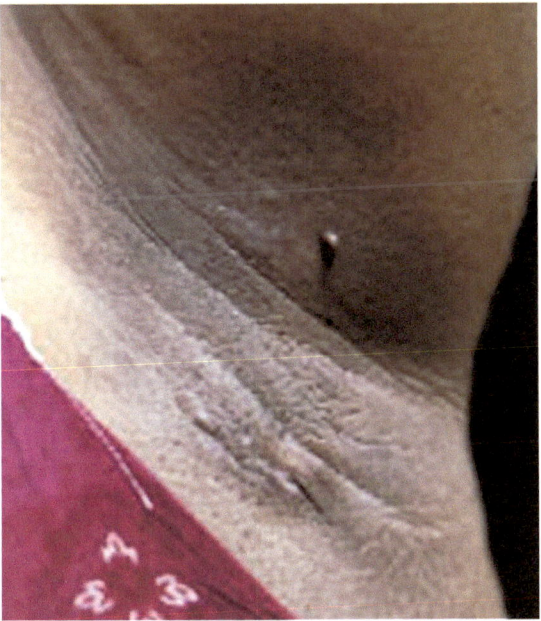

FIGURE 17.7. Acanthosis nigricans.

17.6 Periocular Hyperpigmentataion

The pigmentation may be genetic with an autosomal dominant inheritance. Genetic factors are more frequent in people with dark skin. The pigmentation may extend to involve the eyebrows and the cheeks. The pigmentation is melanin. There is an increase in basal melanocytes with upper and mid-dermal melanophages.

Periorbital pigmentation may be due to cosmetics or it may be a part of generalized pigmentation such as Addison's disease; it is seen in AIDS, and chronic diseases such as renal or liver failure (Fig. 17.8).

Treatment is unsatisfactory; treat any chronic illness when present.

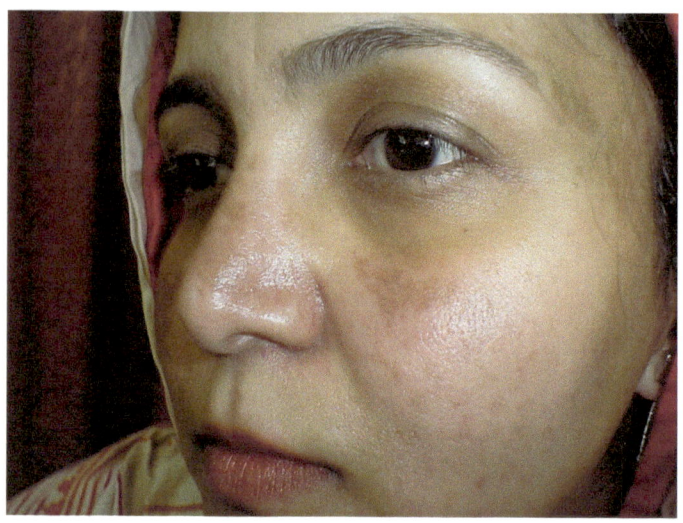

FIGURE 17.8. Periocular pigmentation.

Chapter 18
Disorders of Ultraviolet Radiation and Injuries Due to Cold

Skin is protected against the harmful effects of ultraviolet radiation by a number of factors, melanin being the main protective barrier for ultraviolet light (UVL). Exposure of the skin to UVL results in tanning of the skin and sunburn. Cumulative effects of UVL on the skin over the years can give rise to skin malignancy. Different types of skin react differently; type I suffer the most damage and type VI the least. The different skin phototypes are:

- *Type I*: always burns and never tans.
- *Type II*: burns easily, tans minimally.
- *Type III*: burns minimally, tans gradually and uniformly.
- *Type IV*: burns minimally, tans easily.
- *Type V*: rarely burns but tans darkly; genetically brown skin, e.g., Mongoloids and Indians
- *Type VI*: never burns, tans darkly as genetically black skin of Negroid.

The sun emits a continuous spectrum of light, ranging from the short cosmic rays to long radio waves (Fig. 18.1). Ultraviolet spectrum comprises UVC, UVB and UVA. UVC wavelength ranges from 200 to 290 nm, UVB from 290 to 320 nm, and UVA from 320 to 400 nm (Fig. 18.2). The most harmful effect on the skin is by UVB. UVC is prevented from reaching the earth's surface by the ozone layer; it is therefore currently irrelevant to skin disease; but it is of concern if the injurious effects of the changes in the environment disrupt the ozone

Z. Zaidi, S. W. Lanigan, *Dermatology in Clinical Practice*,
DOI: 10.1007/978-1-84882-862-9_18,
© Springer-Verlag London Limited 2010

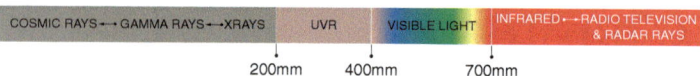

FIGURE 18.1 Spectrum of sunlight.

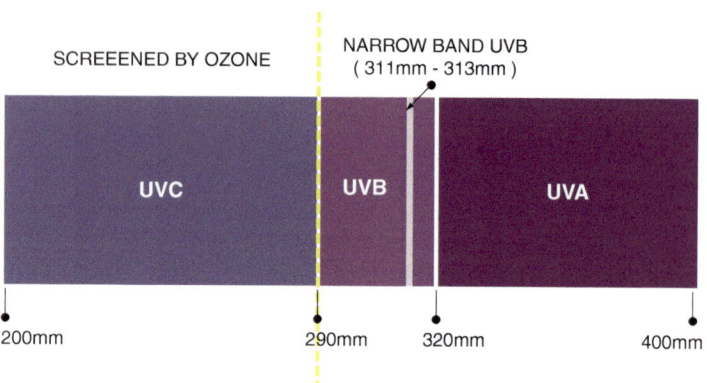

FIGURE 18.2. Ultraviolet radiation (UVR).

layer. UVA has little short-term effects on normal skin; it is invisible to man, and is called the "black light".

18.1 Sites of Photosensitive Eruption

These are the areas exposed to sunlight such as the forehead, nose, cheeks, rim of the ears, sides and back of the neck, V area of the chest, extensor surfaces of the forearm, dorsum of the hands, shins, and feet when exposed.

Sparing of the shielded areas is characteristic of photosensitive eruptions; these are the retroauricular folds, submental region, upper eyelids which are protected by the supraorbital ridge, nasolabial folds, and flexor aspect of the forearm (Figs. 18.3 and 18.4).

The effects of ultraviolet radiation on the skin can be studied under the following headings:

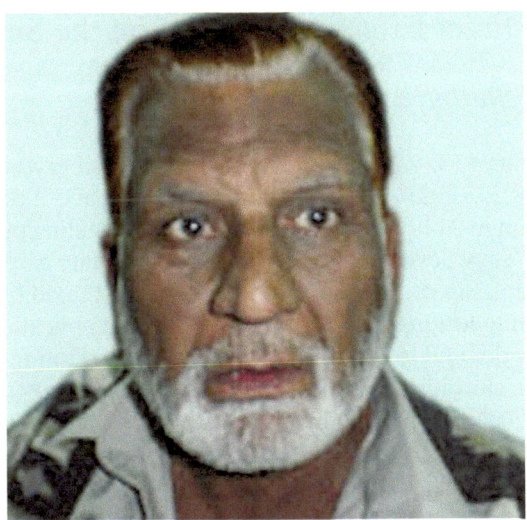

FIGURE 18.3. Sunburn.

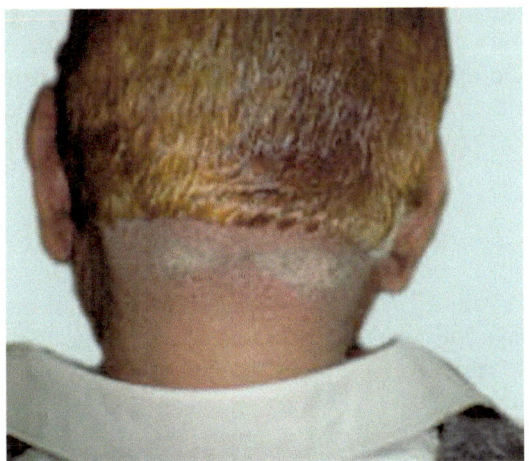

FIGURE 18.4. Sunburn – neck.

- Direct effect of sunlight on the skin
- Effect on the skin due to photosensitivity
- Diseases affected by ultraviolet light

18.2 Direct Effect of Sunlight on the Skin

18.2.1 Sunburn

This is due to UVB, it is manifested by painful erythema that develops 2–3 hours after exposure to the sun, and it reaches its maximum in 24 hours. It is then followed by peeling of the skin in a few days. Severe blistering can occur in some cases. Use of sunscreens can prevent sunburn. Sunburn is treated by the use of soothing lotions such as calamine; liberal application of talcum powder and in some cases a topical steroid lotion or spray. Systemic steroids are indicated in severe cases. Prostaglandins are produced in the skin in sunburn; indomethacin inhibits the enzyme prostaglandin synthetase, and can therefore decrease the severity of sunburn due to UVB.

Sunburn is best treated with wet cool compresses such as calamine lotion, and staying indoors in a cool environment. Lidocaine may provide some relief, but it is a cutaneous sensitizer. When sunburn is severe topical steroids should be used.

Sunburn can be prevented by the use of sunscreens; these should be applied half an hour before going out in the sun and limiting sun exposure appropriately. They need reapplication at regular intervals.

18.2.2 Tanning

Both UVA and UVB stimulate the formation of melanin for some days following exposure to the sun. The new melanin forms a "cap" over the keratinocyte nuclei to protect DNA from further damage.

18.2.3 Epidervmal Thickening

The epidermis may double its thickness following UV radiation, it is important in providing protection against further damage by UVL.

18.2.4 Vitamin D Production

Vitamin D3 (calciferol) is formed in the skin from dehydrocholesterol with the help of UVR. Exposure to sunlight is thus helpful in preventing rickets and osteomalacia in those persons who have a deficient dietary intake of these vitamins.

18.2.5 Immunological Effects

It is now well-established that PUVA therapy causes a temporary suppression of type IV or delayed hypersensitivity reactions in the skin. This is associated with a depletion of epidermal Langerhans cells. The success of PUVA therapy in treating T cell lymphomas suggests that this irradiation also affect lymphocytes. Recent work suggests that ordinary sunburn can also produce immunosuppression. In previous generations patients with tuberculosis were advised to avoid sunbathing as it was supposed to exacerbate the infection probably due to immnuosuppression.

18.2.6 Chronic Effects of Ultraviolet Radiation

Many of the changes associated with ageing of the skin such as wrinkling, solar keratosis, lentigenes, dryness, inelasticity and thinning of the skin are due to chronic exposure of the skin to the ultraviolet radiation of the sun. Chronic exposure of the sun can cause precancerous lesions and can lead to malignancy. The following are the changes due to prolonged exposure to the sun.

18.2.6.1 Actinic Keratosis

These are premalignant scaly lesions, which develop on skin exposed to UVB; common sites are the backs of the hands, forehead, and the ears. Clinically they appear as scaly hyperpigmented plaques that may ulcerate (Fig. 18.5). There is usually a

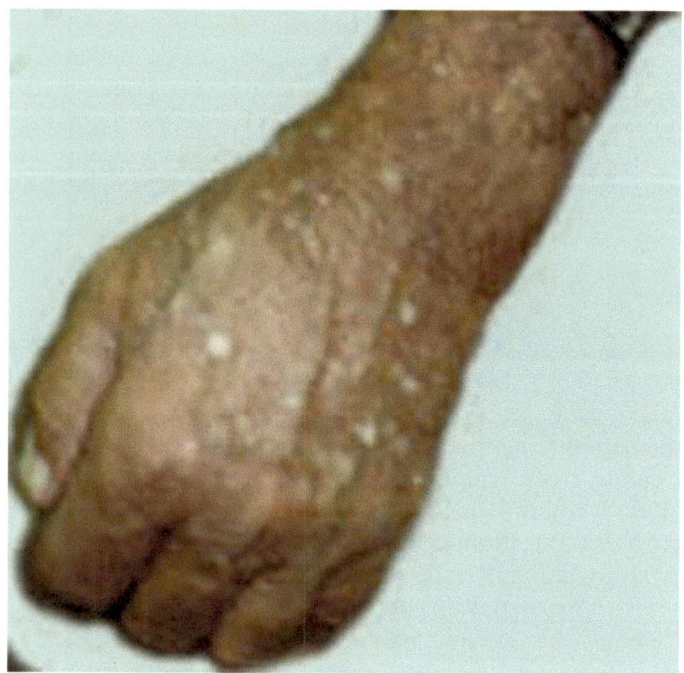

FIGURE 18.5. Actinic keratosis.

period of several years between the development of solar keratosis and its transformation to squamous cell carcinoma.

18.2.6.2 Actinic Elastosis

Small yellowish papules and plaques develop on the face or
back of the hands. The skin assumes a dull yellowish color
with deep furrows and wrinkles.

18.2.6.3 Nodular Elastoidosis
(Favre-Racouchot Syndrome)

This is seen mainly around the eyes and extends on the cheeks,
seen in the elderly particularly in men. The lesions consist of

comedones, follicular cysts, and large folds of furrowed and yellowish skin. Treatment consists of removal of comedones and the cysts. Retinoic acid cream is often helpful.

18.2.6.4 Cutis Rhomboidalis Nuchae

The skin over the back of the neck becomes thickened, rough, and leathery, the normal skin markings become exaggerated. The condition is often seen in farmers, sailors, or those people who are exposed to excessive sunlight.

18.2.6.5 Actinic Cheilitis

This occurs on the lower lips, excessive sunlight produces dryness, scaling, atrophy, and telangiectasia. Fissures, keratosis, leukoplakia, and carcinoma may develop (Fig. 18.6). It responds well to cryotherapy and 5% flourouracil.

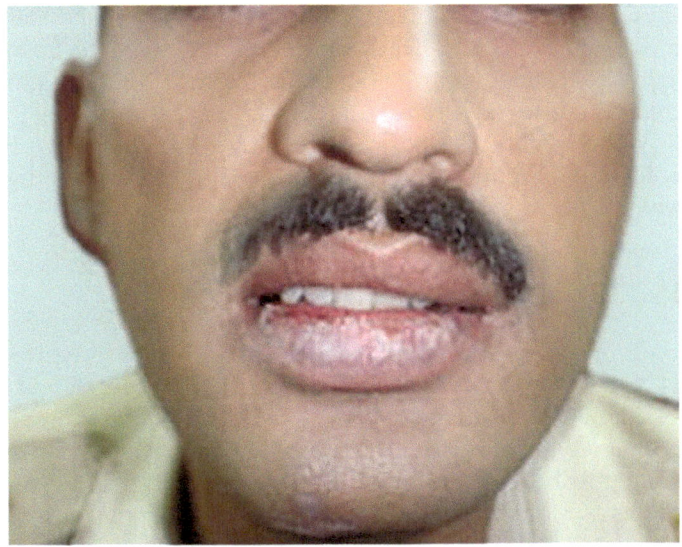

FIGURE 18.6. Actinic cheilitis.

18.2.6.6 Poikilodermic Changes

Characterized by telangiectasia, hyperpigmentation, hypopigmentation, and atrophy are often seen on the sides of the neck, and V of the chest.

18.2.6.7 Skin Cancer

Squamous cell cancer, basal cell carcinoma, and malignant melanoma are enhanced by the total hours of exposure to UVB and perhaps UVA. These are more common in fairskinned people. The more sensitive skin types (skin type I-III) should take care to avoid excessive exposure to the sun and should use sunscreens.

18.2.7 Protection Against Ultraviolet Radiation

18.2.7.1 Clothing

Protective clothing should be worn such as long-sleeve shirts, broad-brim hats, etc. Dark-colored clothes tend to absorb light and heat and these should therefore be avoided. Lighter colored fabrics are preferred.

Weave tightness, fabric type, and color determine the potential for photoprotection. Loose clothing with a tight weave is most appropriate.

18.2.7.2 Time of the Day

UVB reaching the earth's surface is most intense between 11.30 am and 4 pm; exposure to the sun at this time should be avoided. Window glass prevents UVB but it does not prevent UVA. Clouds absorb only 70% of the sunrays and so it is quite possible to sunburn on a cloudy day. Snow reflects 85% of the rays of sun, sand 17–25%, and water vapor up to 5%. Therefore people can easily burn on a snowy day.

18.2.7.3 Sunscreens

These are of two types; those that absorb ultraviolet radiation and those that reflect it. Para-amino benzoic acid (PABA) absorbs ultraviolet radiation; sunscreens containing this are cosmetically acceptable. Some also permit tanning, which may be useful for skin types I and II.

Other sunscreens containing cinnamates and benzaphenones are also efficient and cosmetically acceptable; sensitization may occur rarely.

The opaque sunscreens such as zinc oxide and titanium dioxide are very effective; they reflect the ultraviolet radiation, but are cosmetically less acceptable.

Sun protecting factor (SPF) is the ratio of the dose of ultraviolet light to produce minimal erythema of the skin to which a sunscreen has been applied, compared to the dose of ultraviolet light to produce minimal erythema of the skin without the use of a sunscreen. SPF of 10 means that when applied to the skin, exposure to UVB could be ten times longer than if the sunscreen was not applied to the skin to achieve the same effect.

18.2.7.4 Chemical Photoprotective Agents

Antimalarial drugs such as chloroquine 250 mg a day help to protect the skin against UVL. They probably absorb the UVL, and through the anti-inflammatory properties protect the skin against UVR. Chloroquine causes reversible skin pigmentation but irreversible eye damage. Ocular function should be carefully monitored. β carotene absorbs visible light. Psoralens are used to increase skin pigment production and thereby help in tanning.

Vitamin C, vitamin E, and carotenoids. In some studies the daily use of vitamin C 2 gm, and vitamin E 1000 IU has been shown to reduce sunburn reactions. Carotenoids and vitamin E also prevent the erythema of sunburn.

18.3 Photosensitive Skin Reactions

Photosensitivity may be due to chemicals such as tar, coal, pitch, dyes, drugs such as calcium channel blockers, NSAIDS, sulphonamides, tetracycline, phenothiazine, nalidixic acid, frusemide, plants such as psoralens, some perfumes and cosmetics.

Some people are sensitive to ultraviolet radiation without any cause (idiopathic), on exposure to the sun; they develop rashes on the exposed parts of the body. The condition is more common in Caucasians, but it is also seen in pigmented skin. It presents in different morphological forms such as polymorphic light eruption (the eruptions are polymorphic including macules, papules, vesicles, and urticarial lesions), Hutchinson's summer prurigo (excoriated papules), and hydroa vacciniforme (umbilicated vesicles). Actinic reticuloid is the name given to extreme photosensitivity, in which the patient is even sensitive to visible light. These patients have a miserable existence; they lead a secluded life in the dark. The lesions begin in the sun-exposed areas; these later extend to the whole body. Actinic reticuloid presents as persistent eczema, lichenification, and poikilodermic changes. The condition occasionally progresses to lymphoma.

18.4 Skin Diseases Affected by Sunlight

Some skin diseases are aggravated by sunlight such as herpes simplex, lupus erythematosus, rosacea, pellagra, lichen planus, carcinoid syndrome, and congenital disorders such as Darier's disease, porphyria, and xeroderma pigmentosa. Diseases helped by sunlight are psoriasis, vitiligo, some cases of acne, etc. PUVA and narrow band UVB are important methods of treatment in cutaneous disorders. Venous leg ulcers appear to be helped by UVR, perhaps due to decreased secondary infection and promotion of healing. Acne vulgaris and eczema usually benefit from UVR, but some cases deteriorate. Sunlight has been used for thousands of years as a therapeutic modality, but its precise mode of action is unknown.

18.5 Congenital Disorders Leading to Increased Photosensitivity

18.5.1 Porphyrias

These are a group of diseases in which there is a deficiency of enzymes, required for the formation of heam. Excessive quantities of porphyrins or their precursors are produced. The biochemical defect is either in the liver or RBC depending upon the site of porphyrin production. Porphyrias are thus erythropoetic, hepatic, or erythrohepatic. The different types of porphyria can be differentiated by the biochemical analysis of the blood, urine, and feces for porphyrins. Most of these diseases cause photosensitivity at 400 ± 10 nm (Soret band). This wavelength is able to penetrate through glass, which makes the patient suffer even indoors.

18.5.1.1 Congenital Erythropoetic Porphyria

Patients have photosensitivity soon after birth, which is severe with the formation of blisters leading to scarring. This may lead to mutilation of the ears, nose, and fingertips. There is sclerosis of the skin and hypertrichosis, the urine is pink in color and the teeth are brown due to deposition of porphyrins (Figs. 18.7 and 18.8). Hemolytic anemia is present. Because of the hairy appearance, tendency to avoid sunlight, and discolored teeth, patients with this form of porphyria were often referred to as werewolves.

18.5.1.2 Erythrohepatic Porphyria

Photosensitivity is less severe and it develops in childhood, the child often not wanting to play outside. A burning sensation occurs on exposure to the sun; plunging the affected part in cold water can relieve this. The skin becomes swollen and crusted and characteristic linear scars develop on the sun-exposed skin. Liver disease and gallstones occur.

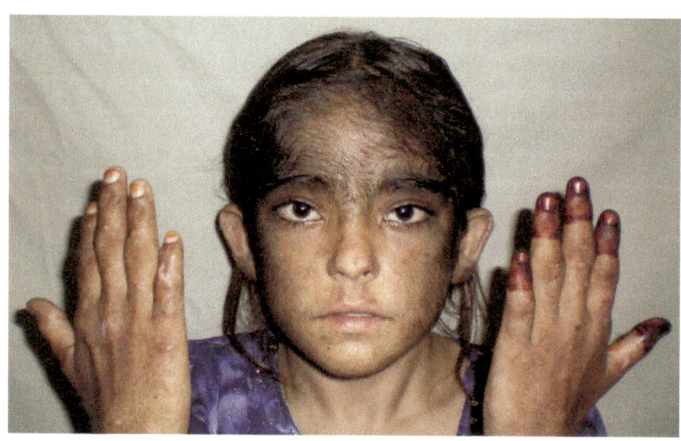

FIGURE 18.7. Porphyria – note the hypertrichosis.

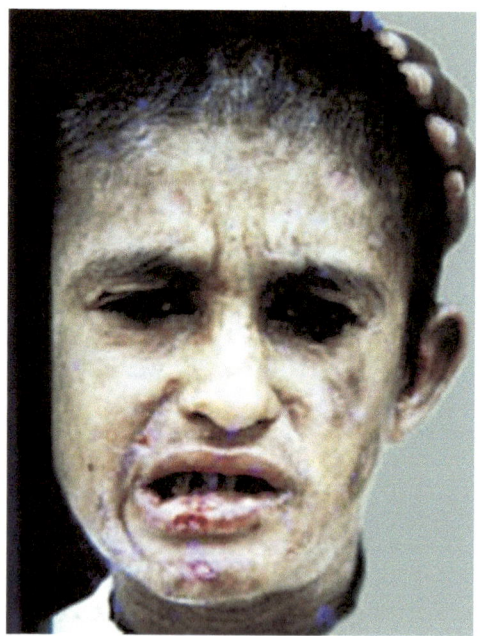

FIGURE 18.8. Porphyria – scarring prominent.

18.5.1.3 Hepatic Porphyrias

There are a number of hepatic porphyrias. *Porphyria cutanea tarda* (PCT) is the most common. There is a defect in uroporphyrin decarboxylase. In 80% of cases, it is sporadic; hepatic disease, secondary to alcohol intake is the most common cause. Twenty percent are hereditary. Some cases are caused by hepatitis C virus. Plasma iron is increased in 50% of cases; the cause is unknown, possibly due to increase absorption of iron from the gut. There are no systemic signs in PCT.

18.5.1.4 Acute Intermittent Porphyria (AIP)

It has no cutaneous signs. It is associated with acute attacks of abdominal pain and GIT disturbances, paralysis, and psychiatric disorders, often precipitated by medication. AIP is characterized by the patient's urine turning dark on standing.

In Africa variegate porphyria is relatively common; it has the features of both AIP and PCT.

18.5.1.5 Pseudoporphyria

Is a term used when the cutaneous changes are like prophyria but there is no abnormality of porphyrin metabolism. It can occur after intake of drugs such as NSAIDS, frusemide, and with hemodialysis. Sometimes use of sun beds can produce pseudoporphyria.

18.5.1.6 Treatment

Protection from sunlight is important in all forms of porphyrias. β carotene 150 mg/day is an active oxygen quencher and can be used in most cases of porphyrias. Low dose of chloroquine 125 mg twice a week is helpful in a number of cases. How chloroquine works is not fully understood, it seems to form a complex with porphyrins deposited in the liver, to form water soluble compounds that are excreted in the urine. Chloroquine also absorbs melanin. Chloroquine must be given with care as higher doses may exacerbate the symptoms, or produce ocular changes and hepatic toxicity.

Phlebotomy at 10–15 days interval will decrease the hemoglobin level to 10–12 g/100 mL, and is helpful in decreasing the iron overload seen in porphyria cutanea tarda. Iron chelation therapy; with cholestyramine, plasmaphoresis, or activated charcoal has been used to decrease the iron levels.

> *Glucose loading to decrease levels of aminolaevulinic acid (ALA) synthetase in a dose of 300–500 mg daily is used in porphyrias that have increased ALA levels.*
> *Alkalization of the urine also increases porphyrin excretion.*

18.5.2 Xeroderma Pigmentosum

This is an autosomal recessive disorder; the disease is characterized by a deficiency of the enzyme endonuclease, which repairs the damage done in the DNA of keratinocytes by UVL. As a result of this deficiency there is excessive photosensitivity. The face has all the markers of photoageing including dryness of the skin, freckles, telangiectasias, angiomas, solar keratosis, wrinkles, and development of cutaneous malignancy at an early age. The skin is normal at birth; symptoms develop from about 6 months of age and progress, by about 2 years when freckles, roughness, and solar keratosis are seen. In severe cases blisters, followed by ulcers and scarring add to the disfigurement of the face. Eye problems are common such as conjunctivitis, photophobia, and ectropion. The disease is often fatal by the age of 10 years (Figs. 18.9 and 18.10).

When xeroderma pigmentosum is associated with CNS abnormalities such as microcephaly, mental retardation, stunted growth, deafness, and ataxia, it is known as De Sanctis-Cacchione syndrome.

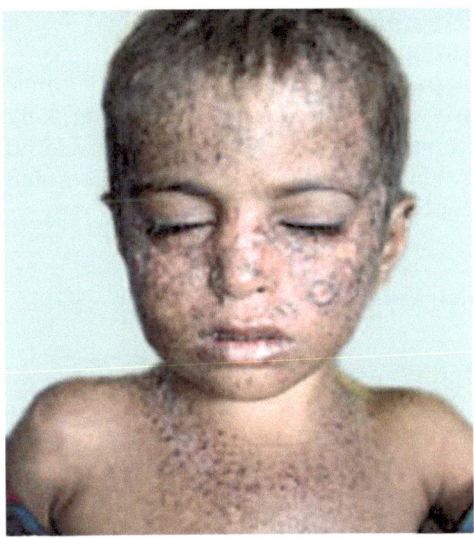

FIGURE 18.9. Xeroderma pigmentosum.

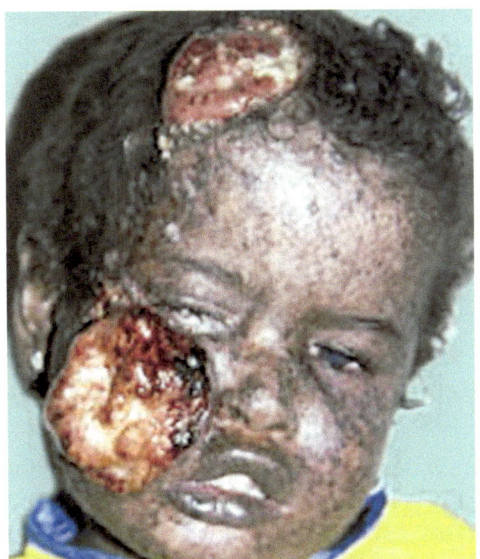

FIGURE 18.10. Xeroderma pigmentosum with squamous cell carcinoma.

18.5.2.1 Treatment

Protect the patient from sunlight. Actinic keratosis should be treated early. Oral retinoids help in reducing skin cancers, and a trial of prophylactic therapy should be considered. Protection is only present while the retinoid is taken, and there is a relapse on stopping the treatment.

18.6 Injuries Due to Cold

18.6.1 Asteotosis (Eczema Craquele)

This is a common skin problem in winter; cold and dryness lowers the extensibility of the stratum corneum. It affects the lower limb in all age groups, and the trunk and extremities in the elderly, and those with severe asteotosis. The skin becomes dry and scaly, and shows the accentuation of the skin lines. As the condition advances long horizontal fissure lines appear, then a cracked porcelain or crazy paving pattern of fissuring develops. The term "eczema craquele" is given to this condition. In severe cases the fissures become deep and wide, they may become purulent and ooze.

18.6.1.1 Treatment

Moisturizers are the mainstay of treatment; topical steroids are used for severe cases. Antibiotics are required if the condition becomes infected.

18.6.2 Chilblain (Perniosis)

This occurs in susceptible individuals when exposed to cold. The blood vessels produce an exaggerated vasoconstriction, leading to tissue anoxia. The parts of the body exposed to cold; fingers, toes, ears, and nose, first become pale, accompanied by burning and itching. The lesions then become purplish, in severe cases blistering and ulceration may occur (Fig. 18.11).

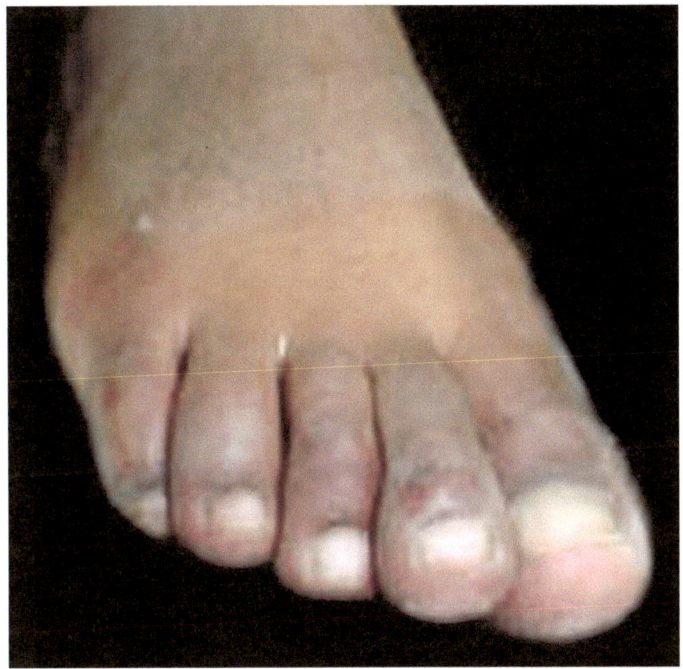

FIGURE 18.11. Chilblains.

18.6.2.1 Treatment

Warming of the exposed parts of the body is the best way to prevent chilblains. Wearing of warm thermal gloves, socks, hats covering the ears help to keep the body warm. Smoking should be prohibited. Nicotinamide and nifedipine help to improve peripheral circulation in persistent cases.

18.6.3 Frostbite

This follows exposure to extreme cold. Many factors influence its occurrence such as wind velocity and length of exposure to cold. The injury is due to the freezing of tissues marked by the formation of ice crystals; the area is deprived of its blood supply. The ears, nose, fingers, and toes become pale and waxy; there is hardly any pain or discomfort. Clinical features vary from erythema, soreness, blistering, to necrosis and gangrene.

18.6.3.1 Treatment

Rapid rewarming is recommended. Slow thawing results in tissue damage. Analgesics are given if pain is experienced during thawing. When the skin flushes then the thawing should stop.

Symptomatic treatment is advised with bed rest, wound care, and avoidance of trauma; antibiotics are given to prevent infection. Nicotinic acid is used to treat vasoconstriction. Recovery may take several weeks.

18.6.4 Raynaud's Phenomenon

This is caused by intermittent contraction of small digital arteries and arterioles. The disease is characterized by pain, and color changes of the digits on exposure to cold. The classic color changes are in sequence – white, purple, and red. White color is characteristic of vasoconstriction. If the condition persists then the fingers and toes are persistently cyanotic, painful, and gangrene may even occur.

Raynaud's phenomenon when primary is called Raynaud's disease, and when secondary to some underlying disease is known as Raynaud's phenomenon. It may be secondary to collagen disorders especially systemic sclerosis, vascular occlusion, drugs such as ergot and bleomycin, poliomyelitis, syringomyelia, neoplastic disorders, etc.

18.6.4.1 Treatment

In Raynaud's phenomenon the underlying disease should be treated. Symptomatic treatment consists of warm clothing, vasodilators such as nifedipine 10–20 mg three times daily oxpentifylline 400 mg three times daily, nicotinamide 30–60 mg a day. In severe cases sympathectomy may be required.

Raynaud's disease is generally benign, and it can be managed without vasodilators. The patient should avoid cold, wear warm clothing, and protect the hands and feet with thermal gloves and socks. Smoking should be prohibited.

Chapter 19
Diseases of the Sebaceous, Sweat, and Apocrine Glands

19.1 Acne Vulgaris

Acne is a very common disorder of the pilosebaceous unit; it affects about 80–90% of adolescents. Acne is characterized by the formation of comedones, papules, pustules, and in some cases cysts and nodules. The face, chest, and back are the common sites affected; at these sites, the density of the sebaceous glands is high; these glands are under the influence of androgens. At puberty, the glands become activated under androgenic influence and give rise to acne. The disease gradually subsides by the late twenties in the majority.

19.1.1 Etiology

The precise mechanism for the formation of acne is unknown. There are four major etiological factors involved:

- Increased production of sebum
- Ductal hyperkeratosis
- Colonization of the duct with Propionibacterium acnes (P acnes)
- Production of inflammation

At puberty the androgen receptors in the skin convert testosterone into dehydrotesterone (DHT), by the enzyme: 5-α reductase. DHT is a more potent androgen, it stimulates the

Z. Zaidi, S. W. Lanigan, *Dermatology in Clinical Practice*, 337
DOI: 10.1007/978-1-84882-862-9_19,
© Springer-Verlag London Limited 2010

sebaceous glands, increasing sebum production, and follicular hyperkeratinization follows.

Comedones are the first lesions of acne, these are due to follicular hyperkeratinization; this results from increased sebum production and decreased levels of linoleic acid in the sebum. The inflammatory lesions of acne are the papules, pustules, cysts, and nodules; these are due to increased proliferation of Propionibacterium acnes (P acnes) following the formation of comedones and the release of cytokines into the dermis initiating inflammation. The source of these inflammatory mediators could be P acnes or their extracellular products. The inflammatory reaction is maintained by a type IV immune reaction to one or more antigens in the follicle.

19.1.2 Clinical Features

Lesions of acne are confined to the face, shoulders, upper chest, and back. Seborrhea is always present. Comedones are the noninflammatory lesions of acne, the rest of the lesions; papules, pustules, nodules, and cysts are the inflammatory lesions of acne.

Closed comedones or "whiteheads" appear as flesh-colored or yellowish dome-shaped papules; these are the first lesions of acne. The open comedone or "blackhead" appears as a dilated pore filled with black keratinous material and sebum. The black color is due to the oxidation of keratin rather than dirt as was once commonly thought (Fig. 19.1).

Inflammatory lesions of acne are papules, pustules, and in severe cases nodules and cysts. Scarring occurs on healing of nodules and cysts. The scars may be depressed or hypertrophic (Figs. 19.2).

19.1.3 Variants of Acne

Other causes of acneform lesions are: drugs (isoniazid, halogens such as iodides and bromides, steroids, lithium, and anticonvulsants); occupations (people working with halogenated

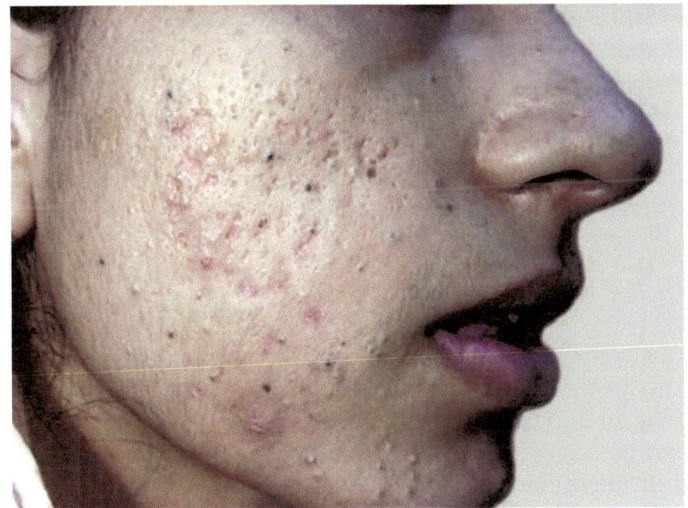

FIGURE 19.1. Acne vulgaris – note the comedones.

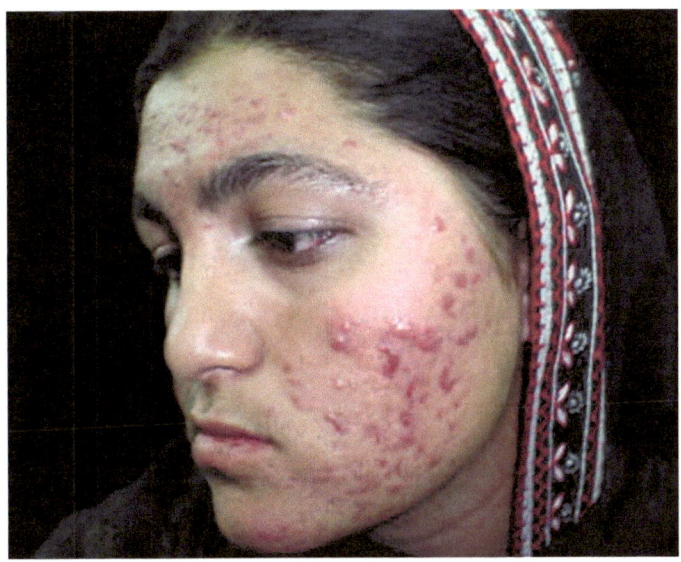

FIGURE 19.2. Acne vulgaris – note the papules and pustules.

hydrocarbons, electrical insulators, tar, oils); cosmetics (greasy creams and cheap pomades); and occlusion (headbands, rucksack straps). These conditions should always be excluded while treating acne.

Rarely endocrine disorders such as polycystic ovaries, Cushing's syndrome, virilizing neoplasms, or exogenous corticosteroids/androgens, may underlie the acne.

19.1.4 Complications of Acne

Acne conglobata (gathered into balls, globus is Latin for ball). This form of acne consists of abscesses or nodules and cysts with intercommunicating sinuses. Multiple fused comedones and extensive scarring are characteristic features. Therapy is difficult; oral isotretinoin is the treatment of choice.

Acne fulminans. A severe form of nodulocystic acne, with systemic signs and symptoms of fever, malaise, joint pains, and swelling, is called acne fulminans.

Pyoderma faciale. In this condition, the acne suddenly develops purulent nodulocystic lesions; there are no systemic symptoms.

Gram-negative folliculitis. This is seen when the patient has been on antibiotic treatment for a long time for their acne. A sudden eruption of small monomorphic follicular pustules occurs; some patients have nodulocystic lesions. Gram-negative organisms such as Klebsiella. E coli, Proteus, or Pseudomonas, are responsible for the condition.

Scars. On the chest the scars are usually hypertrophic or keloidal, and on the face the scars are atrophic due to the loss of collagen resulting in "ice pick" and other forms of atrophic scars.

Calcification occurring in the scarred areas is an unusual complication of acne.

Pyogenic granuloma. This is a rare complication of healing nodular lesions; it occurs more frequently with isotretinoin therapy.

Solid facial edema. This may be symmetrical or asymmetrical; it is due to abnormal lymphatic drainage. The condition is slowly progressive and it should be treated aggressively.

19.1.5 Assessment of Acne

For proper management of acne, accurate assessment of the disease is necessary. There are a number of ways of assessing acne. The two common methods used are lesion count and grading of acne. The lesion count is usually used for clinical trials, and grading of acne is done in routine clinical practice. Acne is treated according to the type and severity of acne. General guideline for assessment is as follows:

- 0 – Normal skin, with no evidence of acne vulgaris.
- 1 – Few noninflammatory and few inflammatory lesions present.
- 2 – Multiple noninflammatory and inflammatory lesions; noninflammatory lesions predominate.
- 3 – Multiple noninflammatory and inflammatory lesions; inflammatory lesions predominate. Few nodules/cysts may be found.
- 4 – Severe acne with nodules and cysts.

(Note – always palpate the skin while examining acne patients; as sometimes papules and nodules can only be felt and not seen, because they are deep in the skin.)

19.1.6 Management of Acne

Acne is treated according to its severity, type of lesions present: noninflammatory or inflammatory, duration, psychological impact on the patient, socioeconomic condition of the patient, compliance of the patient, and response to previous treatment.

The treatment is aimed at targeting the abnormal pathology present:

- Reduce abnormal sebum production
- Reduce the number of P acnes bacteria
- Normalize the abnormal keratin

The other factors to be considered before initiating the treatment of acne are the duration of acne, previous treatments, presence of scarring, and socioeconomic status of the patient.

There are numerous antiacne drugs available in the market. Mild acne can be treated by topical medications; systemic treatment is required in the following cases:

- Severe acne
- Acne not responding to local treatment
- Prolonged duration
- Acne excoriee
- Patients with gram negative folliculitis
- Active acne, causing postinflammatory hyperpigmentation and scarring

19.1.7 Topical Treatment

The noninflammatory lesions respond to keratolytic agents and the inflammatory lesions to antibiotics. There are a number of topical preparations available in the market most of these act on both the lesions.

- Those that are mainly comedolytic are: the vitamin A derivatives, azeliac acid, salicylic acid, benzoyl peroxide.
- Those that are predominantly antimicrobial are: clindamycin, erythromycin, tetracycline, benzoyl peroxide, azelaic acid.
- The predominantly antiinflammatory drugs are: antibiotics, adapalene and tazarotene (third generation retinoid).

Keratolytic agents often irritate the skin and can cause dryness. This side effect has to be explained to the patient before initiation of therapy; the use of moisturizers and adjusting the application schedule can minimize this side effect. Patients often avoid the use of antikeratolytics leading to therapeutic failure.

It is important that while applying the topical therapy that it should be applied to the whole area prone to acne and not just to the acne spots, the reason being that the apparent normal skin adjacent to the acne lesion is likely to have microscopic lesions not seen by the naked eye. In most cases, it is appropriate to use an anti inflammatory agent in the morning and a comedolytic in the evening.

19.1.8 Systemic Treatment

Oral medications for acne include tetracycline and erythromycin antibiotics, hormones, and the retinoids. Other drugs, which may be used, are dapsone, trimethoprin, clofazamine, zinc sulphate, and clindamycin. Oral medication has to be taken for a minimum of 6 months. Only 20% improvement is to be expected at the end of 2 months, 60% improvement by the end of 4 months, and about 80% at 6 months. Most of the patients expect a dramatic improvement as soon as the treatment is started; it is important to explain the duration of treatment on the first visit and likely outcome.

Oral antibiotics are used worldwide in the treatment of acne. The tetracyclines are the treatment of choice. These include tetracycline, oxytetracycline, lymecycline, minocycline, and doxycycline. Both tetracycline and erythromycin should be given in a dose of 1 g a day. Tetracyclines should be given half an hour before meals and should be taken with water not milk, the latter interferes with their absorption due to chelation with calcium-containing foods. Minocycline and doxycycline are given in a dose of 100 mg/day.

Tetracyclines should be avoided in pregnant women and children.

Hormonal therapy can be used in females when antibiotics fail or when they are poorly tolerated. These can be used alone or in combination with antibiotics. The hormones commonly used are estrogens and antiandrogens. Cyproterone is often used in combination with estrogen. This treatment is given to selected female patients. A standard screening work-up of androgens should be done before prescribing hormonal therapy. Patients taking hormonal therapy require regular breast and pelvic examination because of the risks of certain types of cancer. Topical cyproterone is not very effective, but trials are ongoing to find a suitable vehicle for this antiandrogen.

Hormonal therapy is not used in men, as it decreases libido, produces gynecomastia and azoospermia.

Retinoids have revolutionized the treatment of acne; isotretinoin (roaccutane) is the drug of choice. It acts on all the areas of pathogenesis, i.e., reduces sebum production, reduces the number of P. acnes and inflammation; it also corrects abnormal keratinization. The drug has to be monitored very carefully due to its side effects, and it is also teratogenic. It should not be given in pregnancy, and pregnancy should be excluded before starting treatment and during the course of treatment. There are concerns that this drug may precipitate or aggravate depression.

Only dermatologists currently should prescribe oral retinoids.

19.1.9 Other Modalities

Intralesional steroids are used for large inflamed cysts; if injected deeply, skin atrophy may occur, so care should be taken in ensuring accurate placement. The injection should be in the appropriate dilution and at the correct site in the skin.

Dermabrasion, laser resurfacing, and collagen injections can be used in some cases of superficial scarring. Deep scars do not respond to dermabrasion, and those on the trunk respond poorly to both dermabrasion and laser. Persistent noninflamed cysts can be excised.

For resistant comedones, superficial peeling and electrodessication are effective. Peeling can lead to numerous side effects; and should only be performed by experienced practitioners.

Regardless of the treatment, the patient should observe the following guidelines:

- Do not squeeze the pimples.
- Use noncomedogenic cosmetics.
- Gently wash the face two to three times a day, depending upon the greasiness of the skin, too much washing may worsen acne.

- Avoid aggravating factors that block the pilosebaceous ducts, e.g., oil, airborne grease, clothing, or occlusive sporting equipment.
- Avoid drugs that aggravate acne; oral contraceptives that contain progestogens, halogens, phenobarbitone, isoniazid, androgens, and lithium.
- Avoid humid conditions.

Acne is a very common disorder and so are the myths associated with it. Much folklore exists regarding diet and acne. There is very little scientific proof to implicate that diet plays a significant role in acne, but studies are ongoing.

> *Antibiotics and other drugs in acne have to be taken for 4–6 months.*
>
> *Do not prescribe short courses of different antibiotics. This encourages bacterial resistance.*
>
> *Tetracyclines should not be given to pregnant women and children.*
>
> *A dermatologist should only prescribe retinoids.*
>
> *If depression occurs in a patient on retinoids, stop the treatment immediately.*

19.2 Rosacea

Rosacea characteristically affects middle-aged females of fair complexion. The disease is characterized by the appearance of flushing in association with erythema, papules and pustules. Pustules can be seen sitting on erythematous papules. Close examination shows a number of telangiectasia. Alcohol, hot drinks, and sunlight exacerbate the flushing. As the disease progresses the flushing is replaced by permanent erythema. Uncommonly significant lymphoedema can develop. The cause is unknown; sunlight plays an important role in its pathogenesis. There has been an interest in the role of demodex mites and H pylori bacteria in the pathogenesis of the disorder. About one-third of the patients have conjunctivitis. Rhinophyma is characterized by hypertrophy of the lower third of the nose, due to sebaceous gland hypertrophy, associated with marked erythema and telangiectasia (Fig. 19.3).

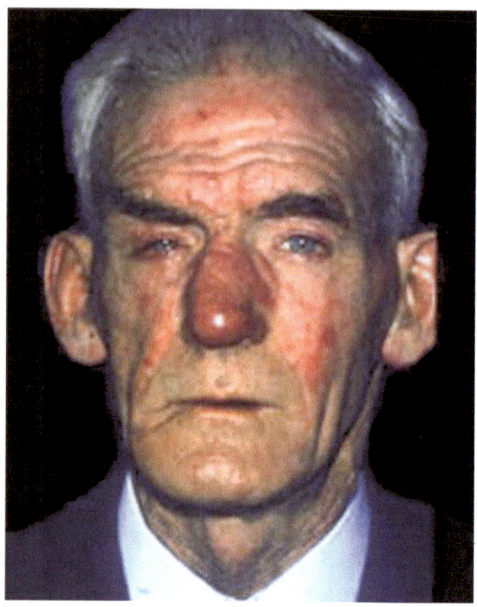

FIGURE 19.3. Rosacea.

19.2.1 Differential Diagnosis

Rosacea should be differentiated from acne, seborrheic dermatitis, and other photosensitive disorders such as systemic lupus erythematosus. In rosacea comedones are absent, the lesions are only found on the face, and the rash has an erythematous background with telangiectasia.

19.2.2 Treatment

Hot drinks, spices, alcohol, and exposure to sunlight should be avoided. Fluorinated corticosteroids are contraindicated as they significantly aggravate the erythema and telangiectasia.

Systemic tetracycline is the most effective form of treatment. The dose is similar to acne, initially 1 g daily, reducing to 250 or 500 mg daily after a few weeks, and the treatment is continued for 2–3 months. If there is no recurrence, the tetracycline should be stopped. Tetracycline also improves the eye lesion but has no effect on rhinophyma.

Metronidazole 200 mg twice daily is also effective. The duration of the treatment is the same as that for tetracycline.

Isotretinoin should be reserved for patients with severe involvement. The dose is 0.5–2.0 mg/kg/day for 16–20 weeks.

Topical metronidazole (0.75–1%), azaleic acid and 1–2% sulphur ointment, are effective. Most topical agents are applied twice a day on the affected areas. Patients require 3 months of therapy for optimal diminution in erythema, papules, and pustules

Topical corticosteroids may temporarily suppress inflammation, but usually make rosacea worse over long-term use. These should be avoided.

Flushing and telangiectasia do not respond to the above treatment. Oral clonidine 50 μg twice a day may be effective in reducing flushing. β blockers such as propranolol twice daily may also be effective. The pulsed dye laser is also helpful in reducing redness.

Mild ocular lesions respond to oral tetracycline and steroid eye drops, but keratitis needs the care of an ophthalmologist.

Rhinophyma does not respond to medical treatment, surgical treatment gives good results as does laser resurfacing.

Potent topical steroids should never be used in rosacea.

19.3 Perioral Dermatitis

Perioral dermatitis has become more common since the introduction of potent corticosteroids. It tends to affect young women; papules and pustules occur around the mouth and the nasolabial folds, sparing the lip margin. It is probably a variant of rosacea and responds to the same treatment. Facial flushing and telangiectasia are not seen in perioral dermatitis (Fig. 19.4).

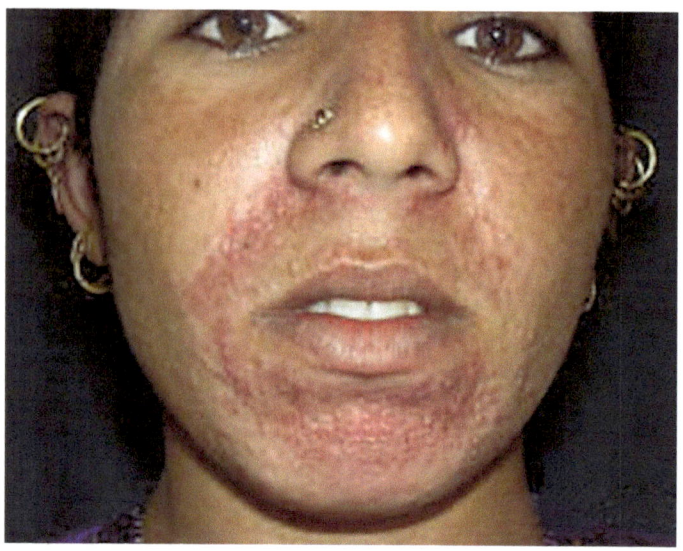

FIGURE 19.4. Perioral dermatitis.

19.3.1 Treatment

The condition can be eradicated if the patient stops applying potent topical steroids on the face. In chronic cases there may be a rebound. A 4-week course of oral tetracycline clears the eruption. Topical tetracycline and 1% metronidazole cream are also effective.

> The topical steroid that the patient was using should not be stopped suddenly; otherwise, there will be a rebound and worsening of the reaction. The strength of steroid should be gradually reduced.

19.4 Hyperhidrosis of the Hands, Feet, and Axilla

Excessive sweating of the hands impairs the performance of many tasks such as typing, writing, sewing, knitting, etc.

Hyperhidrosis of the feet can result in malodor; it may lead to infections with dermatophytes and candida and it may predispose to eczema. Axillary hyperhidrosis stains the underclothing leaving visible marks causing embarrassment. The disease is common in young adults, often precipitated by anxiety. In these cases, the sweating is precipitated by emotional stimuli and stops during sleep. An organic cause is seldom found, but thyrotoxicosis, acromegaly, tuberculosis, and Hodgkin's disease should be excluded.

19.4.1 Treatment

Treatment is not satisfactory. Topical drugs are generally used to treat hyperhidrosis.

For hyperhidrosis of the axillae, 20% aluminium chloride in absolute ethanol is applied at night initially daily and then at weekly intervals. It should be applied after washing and then drying the axillae with or without a polythene occlusion. Mild irritation of the skin by this therapy can be treated with topical steroids.

For the palms and soles aluminium chloride is not very successful, 1% formalin solution or 10% glutaraldehyde in a buffered solution of pH 7.5 swabbed into the feet three times weekly has helped some persons. Staining may occur.

Iontophoresis is another method of treating hyperhidrosis of the hands and feet, using either tap water or anticholinergic drugs. A direct current of low voltage can be used to introduce ionized drugs into the skin. The electric current selectively damages and blocks the sweat duct.

Botulinum toxin inhibits the release of acetylcholine; it is used to treat severe cases of hyperhidrosis. It is more popular in the treatment of hyperhidrosis of the axillae and feet. On the hands, there is the disadvantage of paralyzing the intrinsic muscles of the hand and multiple injections are painful. Subdermal injections are given to the whole area in a single session. Sweating is abolished after 2–3 days. Repeat injections (after 6–8 months) are necessary as the effect wears off with new nerve connections developing.

Systemic drugs such as propanthelene in a dose of 15 mg three times a day may be used; the dose is increased gradually to 150 mg daily if tolerated. However, the side effects of the drug such as dryness of the mouth, glaucoma, hyperthermia, and convulsions limit its use.

19.4.1.1 Surgical Treatment

Axillary hyperhidrosis can also be cured by excision and undercutting of the affected skin. The area of the densest sweat glands is first identified, by staining with iodine and starch, which is then removed.

Cervical and lumber sympathectomy which can be performed endoscopically will reduce hyperhidrosis of the hands, feet, and axillae, but the operation is not free from risks, most patients develop compensatory hyperhidrosis of the trunk.

19.5 Miliaria (Prickly Heat)

This is a condition common in the tropics due to excessive sweating causing overhydration of keratin, which results in blocking of the ducts of the sweat glands. The clinical picture depends upon the site of obstruction. The patient presents with vesicles (blockage of duct in the stratum corneum), itchy erythematous papules (blockage of duct in the stratum malpighian), or skin-colored elevations resulting from deep vesicles; this gives the skin a goose flesh appearance. The common sites involved are the flexures and the trunk. Patients may become susceptible to heat stroke. The condition is also seen in overclothed infants, in hot nurseries (Fig. 19.5).

Prevention and treatment by fans, coolers, etc. help in sweat evaporation and thereby preventing the hydration of keratin. In hot weather, cotton clothes are preferred as they help in the evaporation of sweat.

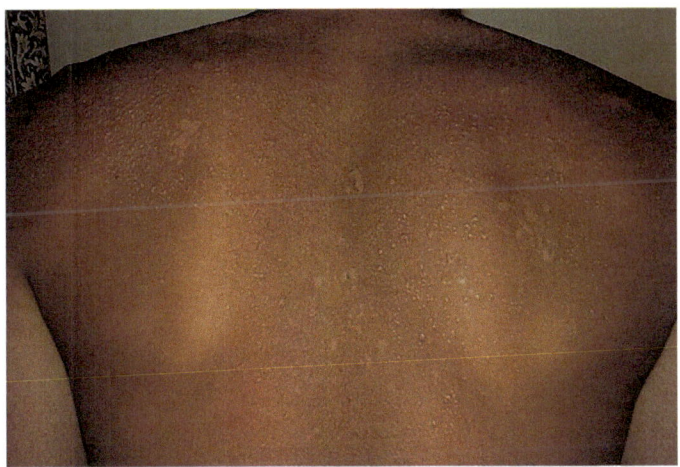

FIGURE 19.5. Miliaria crystalline.

19.5.1 Treatment

It is essential to cool the patient. This can be achieved by cooling lotions such as calamine, baths, liberal application of dusting powders, the use of electric fans or if possible air conditioning. Removal of the keratin plug can be attempted by salicylic acid lotion. Vitamin C 1 g daily may be helpful. Topical and systemic antibiotics should control any secondary bacterial infections.

19.6 Congenital Disorders of the Sweat Glands

19.6.1 Anhidrotic Ectodermal Dysplasia

The classical triad of this disorder consists of hypotrichosis, anodontia, and anhidrosis. The inheritance is X linked recessive; males are commonly affected.

These patients have a typical facies. The nasal bridge is depressed forming a saddle shaped nose. The supraorbital

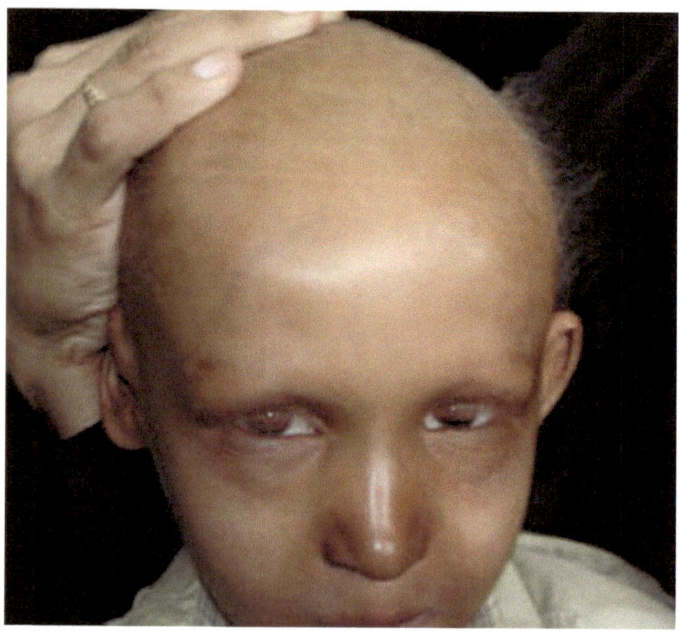

FIGURE 19.6. Anhidrotic ectodermal dysplasia.

ridge is prominent, cheekbones are high and wide, the eyebrows are scanty, there are radiating furrows at the buccal commisures, and lips are thickened. There is partial or complete anodontia. The incisors and/or canines if present are conical and pointed. Nails may be thin and brittle. Hypotrichosis is generalized. The alopecia is not complete, the hair are thin sparse and dry. Mental retardation is present in some cases. The patients are unable to tolerate heat, fever-induced sweating is absent or slight. Seizures may occur (Fig. 19.6).

Anhidrotic ectodermal dysplasia – note the conical incisors.

The patients should be advised against physical exertion; choice of a suitable occupation; avoidance of warm climate. Regular dental supervision is essential. Genetic counseling should be advised; the condition could be diagnosed on prenatal examination.

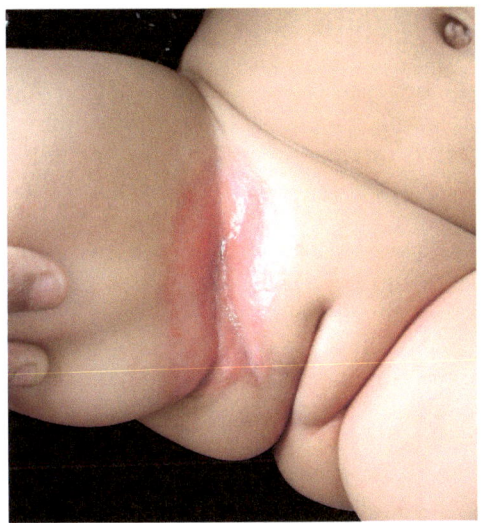

FIGURE 19.7. Intertrigo.

19.7 Intertrigo

This is a superficial, inflammatory dermatitis occurring when two skin surfaces are in apposition. It is due to heat, friction, and moisture. It is common in obese individuals, on areas of excessive sweating such as axillae, groins, and intergluteal folds, beneath pendulous breasts, and between the toes. The skin folds are red, tender, and itchy, fissures may develop. Maceration, leads to secondary infection with pyogenic bacteria and candida, infective eczema may result (Fig. 19.7).

19.7.1 Treatment

This is similar to that of superficial dermatitis. Appropriate antibiotics or fungicides are applied locally. The opposing skin surfaces may be separated with gauze or appropriate dressings. Castellani's paint and liberal use of dusting powder is helpful.

19.8 Hidradenitis Suppurativa (HS)

This is now believed to be a disease of hair follicles rather than of apocrine glands as thought previously. The initial lesion of HS is due to the blockage of hair follicles. HS is a part of the follicular occlusion triad – acne, dissecting cellulitis of the scalp, and hidradenitis suppurativa. The disease has its onset after puberty; it affects the flexures in particular the axillae, groin, and natal clefts; areas rich in apocrine glands. Androgens, heat and moisture play a part in blocking the ducts of the hair follicles, but the exact mechanism is unknown. The disease is more common in obese patients.

The hallmark of HS is the double comedone; this is a black head with two or more surface openings that communicate under the skin. These may be present before the other signs appear. Later the duct dilates, ruptures and gets infected, with the formation of nodules and abscess. This progresses to the formation of cysts and sinuses. The disease is chronic; the chronic state represents secondary bacterial infection. All patients with HS should have any discharge tested for culture and sensitivity especially for tetracycline and erythromycin (Fig. 19.8).

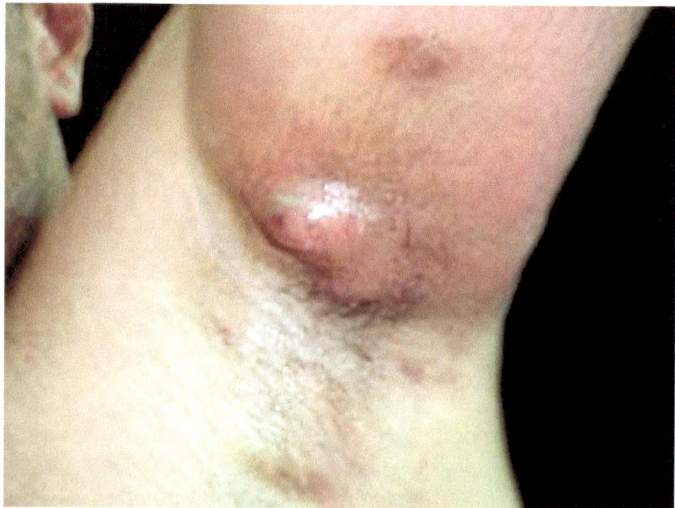

FIGURE 19.8. Hidradenitis suppurativa.

19.8.1 Treatment

The treatment is difficult and similar to acne and it also requires long-term treatment. If antibiotics, fail to bring about a response then oral retinoids and dianette in women may be tried. An acute episode can be helped by oral or intralesional steroids. Recalcitrant cases require wide excisional surgery and skin grafting.

The infected area should be kept dry, obesity should be treated, and smoking avoided.

19.9 Bromhidrosis (Fetid Sweat)

Bromhidrosis is commonly encountered in the axillae; it is due to the bacterial decomposition of apocrine sweat, producing fatty acids with distinctive offensive odors. Various ingested substances such as garlic may also affect the odor of the sweat.

19.9.1 Treatment

Antibacterial soaps and many commercial deodorants are quite effective in controlling the odor. Frequent bathing and changing of underclothes are helpful. Sweating can be reduced by the use of aluminium chloride.

Plantar bromidrosis may be treated, by washing with anti bacterial soaps, and use of dusting powders on the feet. Soaking the feet in 1:5,000 potassium permanganate for 30 min daily may help in reducing the fetid odor. Plantar hyperhidrosis should be treated as mentioned earlier.

19.10 Tumors of the Sweat Glands

19.10.1 Syringomas

Syringomas are benign neoplasms with differentiation toward eccrine acrosyringium. They are most common in women

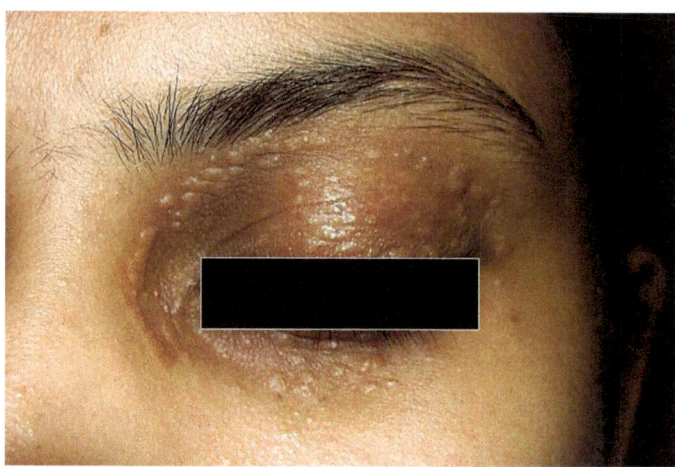

FIGURE 19.9. Syringoma.

starting at puberty. The lesions appear as multiple, yellowish or skin-colored small, firm papules, most commonly located around the periorbital region (Fig. 19.9). The lesions are bilateral, but syringomas can also occur at other sites such as the axillae, umbilicus, and genital areas. Eruptive syringomas have a sudden onset; the tumors are multiple, and are most commonly found on the trunk.

Syringomas should be differentiated from plane warts, trichoepitheliomas, adenoma sebaceum, xanthelasma, and other xanthomas. Syringomas on the trunk should be differentiated from disseminated granuloma annulare.

The tumors are benign and are best left alone as there is a tendency for recurrence after treatment.

19.10.2 Cylindroma (Turban Tumor)

Cylindroma is a sweat gland tumor differentiating toward either an eccrine or apocrine line. The tumors can be solitary or multiple.

The solitary tumor begins at middle age or later, men and women are equally affected. It is a slow growing rubbery

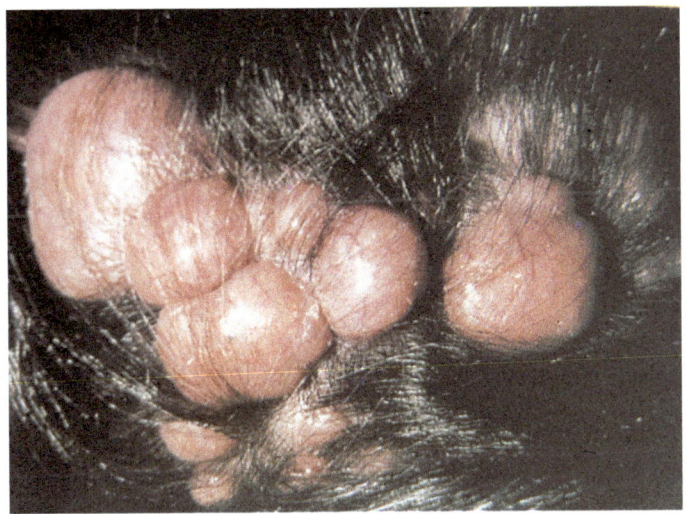

FIGURE 19.10. Cylindroma.

symptomless nodule. The dominantly inherited multiple variety begins shortly after puberty, with numerous rounded nodules of various sizes. The tumors are most commonly found on the scalp. The surface is smooth with multiple telangiectasias (Fig. 19.10).

19.10.2.1 Treatment

Single tumors can be excised. The treatment of multiple tumors is difficult, extensive laser ablation, or wide excision of the scalp followed by skin grafting may help.

> When treating hyperhidrosis, always dry the skin, before applying antiperspirants.
> Oral anti-cholinergic drugs are seldom used because of their side effects.
> Exclude organic causes for hyperhidrosis such as thyrotoxicosis, acromegaly, tuberculosis and Hodgkin's disease.

Chapter 20
Hair Disorders

Hair plays a very important role in the psychological buildup of man. No one would like to have too much or too little hair; we want the right amount of hair in the right place. Hair is not only important for psychological reasons; it also serves many useful purposes. Vellus hair protects us against cold, by piloerection. Eyelashes and eyebrows give protection to the eye, axillary and pubic hair help in the dissemination of body odor. Hair also helps to protect against foreign material by entrapment, e.g., nasal cilia.

Hair disorders can be studied under the following headings:

- Excessive hair (hirsutism and hypertrichosis)
- Loss of hair (alopecia)
- Disorders of colur and texture
- Miscellaneous

Hair loss can be localized or generalized. It may be scarring (cicatricial) or nonscarring (noncicatricial).
Causes of localized noncicatricial hair loss:

- Fungal infections such as tinea capitis
- Bacterial infections such as folliculitis
- Alopecia areata
- Androgenetic alopecia
- Trichotillomania
- Traction alopecia

Z. Zaidi, S. W. Lanigan, *Dermatology in Clinical Practice*,
DOI: 10.1007/978-1-84882-862-9_20,
© Springer-Verlag London Limited 2010

Causes of localized cicatricial hair loss:

- Fungal infections such as kerion, favus
- Bacterial infections such as furuncle, carbuncle
- Chronic discoid lupus erythematosus
- Burns
- Radiation
- Malignancy
- Follicular lichen planus (lichen planopilaris)
- Naevus sebaceous
- Necrobiosis lipoidica
- Sarcoidosis

Causes of generalized hair loss – noncicatricial:

- Alopecia areata universalis
- Telogen effluvium
- Anangen effluvium
- Hypothyroidism and hyperthyroidism
- Hypopituitarism
- Chronic iron deficiency
- Malnutrition
- Congenital disorders such as anhidrotic ectodermal dysplasia

20.1 Excessive Hair

Hirsutism – growth of terminal hair in females in a male pattern, due to increased circulating androgens or sensitivity of the hair follicles to androgens.

Hypertrichosis – growth of terminal hair in males or females, that is not due to increased sensitivity to androgens, e.g., racial, anorexia nervosa, porphyria, drugs such as minoxidil and ciclosporin, Beckers naevus, and hair overlying spina bifida.

Hypertrichosis lanuginosa – excessive growth of lanugo hair, e.g., secondary to internal malignancy. It may also be congenital as in congenital hypertrichosis lanuginosa.

20.1.1 Hirsutism

Hirsutism is defined as excess hair growth in women from increased androgenic production or skin sensitivity. The hair growth follows a male pattern, being predominantly facial (moustache or beard) thoracic and abdominal (Fig. 20.1). The pubic hair also has a male pattern, the triangle pointing towards the umbilicus. Minor degrees of hirsutism are common after the menopause.

Hirsutism is due to increased response of the hair follicle to circulating androgens, or due to the over production of androgens, by the ovaries or the adrenal cortex.

20.1.1.1 Etiology

Hirsutism may be due to obesity, polycystic ovarian syndrome, familial or idiopathic, drugs such as androgenic steroids, Cushing's syndrome, congenital adrenal hyperplasia, and androgenic secreting tumors in the adrenals or ovary. In cases of malignant tumors the onset of hirsutism is rapid. Most cases of hirsutism are familial or idiopathic.

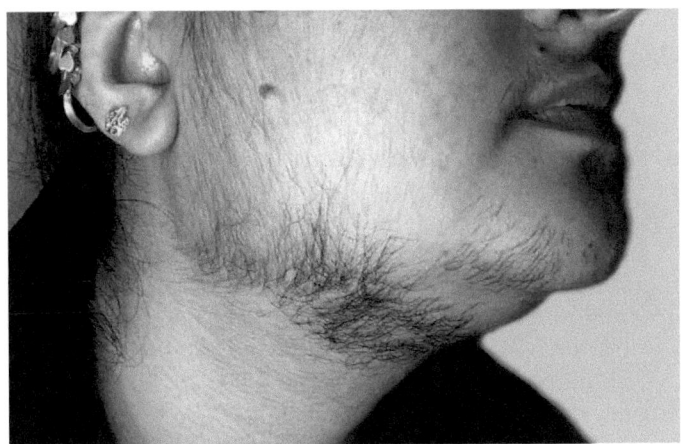

FIGURE 20.1. Hirsutism.

20.1.1.2 Assessment of Hirsutism

- Quantitative assessment of hirsutism.
  This is graded according to the extent of area involved.

  On the beard region

  Grade I: Circumscribed area of hair growth on one side of the chin
  Grade II: Involvement of both sides of the chin
  Grade III: Fusion in the midline, Grade I and II
  Grade IV: Complete cover of the chin

  On the chest

  Grade I: Circumaerola hair
  Grade II: Circumaerola hair and midline chest hair
  Grade III: Fusion in the midline, Grade I and II
  Grade IV: Complete cover of the chest

- Clinical and laboratory assessment

A careful history and physical examination is essential in all cases of hirsutism. Significant hormonal abnormalities are not found in patients with a normal menstrual history. The history should focus on the age, acuteness of onset, progression, virilization, menstrual history, family and racial background.

Physical examination may reveal signs of Cushing's disease, acromegaly, and other endocrinal disorders. Other signs to be evaluated are distribution of muscle mass, body fat, size of clitoris, voice depth, and galactorrhoea. Sudden onset of virulism points towards malignancy.

Investigations are required if hirsutism occurs in childhood, there is a sudden onset of hirsutism, when signs of virilization are present, if the patient has menstrual irregularities, infertility or if the patient has premature cessation of menstruation.

Laboratory evaluation should include levels of free testosterone, dehydroepiandrosterone (DHEA), leutinizing hormone (LH), follicular stimulating hormone (FSH), 17-hydroxy progesterone level, and prolactin.

A pelvic ultrasound should be done, if an ovarian abnormality is suspected.

20.1.1.3 Treatment

These may be:

- Cosmetic
- Suppressive
- Antiandrogenic

Cosmetic

Cosmetic methods are the cheapest and easiest for therapy of hirsutism. These include shaving, waxing, chemical depilation, bleaching of the hair, and electrolysis. Chemical depilatories previously contained barium sulphide; these corrode the projecting hair shaft, and they have no action on the intrafollicular growing portion of the hair. They also irritate the skin and are therefore not used. Currently depilatories contain sodium thioglycolate; this acts by reducing the disulphide bond of the hair follicles. These are nonirritating. Lasers are now a popular method of hair removal.

Reduction of weight in obese women may help in reduction of hirsutism.

Suppressive Therapy

These include oral contraceptives and glucocorticoids. These suppress hirsutism due to ovarian and adrenal causes. Ovarian suppression can be achieved by a combination of ethinylestradiol 35 mg and norethindrone 0.5 mg. Birth control pills are helpful in 75% of hirsute women.

Antiandrogens

Combination of cyproterone acetate and ethinylestradiol has been widely used to treat hirsutism. Cyproterone acetate 100 mg a day, from days 5 to 14 of the menstrual cycle, and ethinyestradiol from 5 to 25 days of the cycle. Strict contraception is indicated during its use.

Spironolactone is a stronger antiandrogen. It is used in a dose of 75 –200 mg/day. A combination of spironolactone and oral contraceptives is also used to treat hirsutism. It limits menstrual irregularities and prevents contraception.

Other Drugs

5-α reductase inhibitors. Finasteride, a 5-α reductase inhibitor has been used with promising results, its effects are seen after 6 months of therapy. It may feminize a male fetus; therefore it should not be used in women of childbearing potential. A recently described treatment of hirsutism is eflornithine cream, an ornithine decarboxylase inhibitor. Studies have indicated a reduction of hirsutism by 20%. Metformin is also used to treat hirsutism in polycystic ovarian syndrome.

> Hormonal abnormalities are rarely found, if the patient has a normal menstrual cycle.
>
> Sudden development of hirsutism should be investigated for malignancy.

20.2 Loss of Hair (Alopecia)

20.2.1 Nonscarring Alopecia

20.2.1.1 Androgenetic Alopecia (AGA)

This is the most common pattern of alopecia. It is familial, but the mode of inheritance is not clear; it is probably autosomal dominant with reduced penetrance.

In males, it follows a particular pattern. Hair is first lost from the temporal region, and then a patch of baldness appears at the vertex. Later these two areas merge, with loss of hair from the surface of the scalp. The terminal hair first becomes vellus, and these are then lost. Parietal and occipital areas are not affected, as these are not dependent on androgens for growth (Figs. 20.2 and 20.3). Scalp devoid of hair is prone to actinic damage.

The process begins at any age after puberty; temporal recession is noticed between the age of 20 and 30 years.

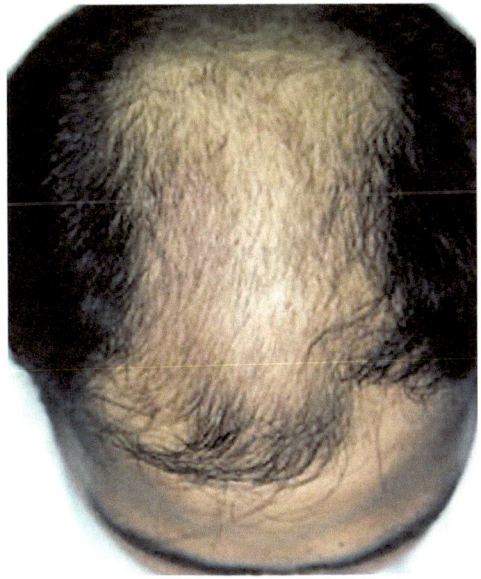

FIGURE 20.2. Androgenetic alopecia.

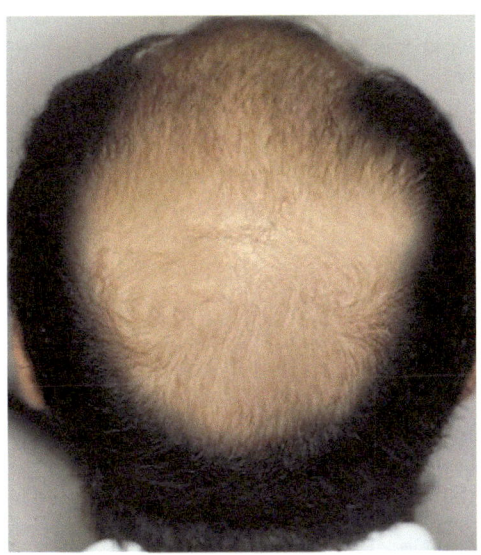

FIGURE 20.3. Androgenetic alopecia – does not affect the occipital and parietal hair.

The onset and progression are gradual.

In females, the loss of hair is generalized and tends to progress slowly. There is no loss of frontal hairline.

Hamilton's classification:

Type I. Normal prepubertal scalp pattern

Type II. Slight recession of the frontotemporal region

Type III. Deeper recession of the frontotemporal region

Type IV. Associated patch of baldness at the vertex

Type V. Patch at the vertex enlarges

Type VI. Joining of the frontotemporal patch and that of the vertex by a narrow path

Type VII. Widening of the joining patch, both frontotemporal patch and that of the vertex appear as a single patch

Type VIII. Only a narrow rim of hair remains at the occipital and parietal region

Treatment

Treatment of baldness dates back over 5,000 years ago, record of its treatment is found in Egyptian papyri. Hippocrates prescribed opium mixed with an essence of roses or lilies and oil of vinegar, olive oil, or acacia juice.

In men. Most medical treatment is ineffective. Topical application of minoxidil is said to increase blood flow but how it produces hair growth is not established. Two percent solution of minoxidil is applied locally; clinical improvement is seen after 3–4 months of treatment. If this has no effect then a 5%, solution is applied. This treatment has to be continued for life; for baldness reappears once, minoxidil has stopped.

Minoxidil is most effective if the patient is less than 30 years and has alopecia for less than 5 years. It should be applied on a dry scalp twice a day.

More recently, 0.5% minoxidil has been studied in combination with topical tretinoin for AGA.

Finastride 1 mg, a 5α-reductase inhibitor, given once daily, it may increase hair growth in a number of patients. Finasteride is less effective in men over the age of 60, due to decrease in the amount of 5α-reductase. Finasteride is contraindicated in women of childbearing age, because of a teratogenic effect on male offsprings.

Supplementary zinc therapy 60 mg/day has been used to inhibit 5-∝-reductase activity, but the role of zinc in AGA remains uncertain.

Surgical Treatment of AGA. AGA can be treated with full-thickness hair-bearing punch autografts obtained from AGA resistant occipital hair. In their new position, the transplanted follicles continue to produce hair of the same texture and color, at the same rate as they did in the occipital area.

Scalp reduction techniques can reduce the area requiring hair transplants.

In women. Antiandrogens given in a cyclical form may be of benefit. This may increase the thickness of the hair.

Surgery is difficult, as the hair loss is diffuse. A wig can conceal such hair loss effectively.

20.2.1.2 Alopecia Areata (AA)

This is a localized patch of hair loss, without any signs of inflammation. It is common in young adults. It is commonly seen on the scalp, or the beard region. Patches may be single or multiple. Spontaneous recovery occurs in the majority of cases. The hair that grows is often white in color, which repigments later (Figs. 20.4 and 20.5).

Alopecia totalis occurs when the entire scalp is involved and alopecia universalis when the whole body hair is affected. A less common diffuse type of alopecia areata, affects the whole body in patches, this preferentially affects the black hair, these fall out leaving the white hair intact. This diffuse pattern can lead to alopecia universalis.

The pathognomonic feature of AA is the presence of "exclamation hair" at the periphery of the patch of hair loss. This hair has an expanded club at the distal end with the constriction above. Some patients may show fine pitting of the nails, pitting of the nails signifies a poor prognosis.

An immunological basis is suspected for the etiology of AA. It may be associated with vitiligo, autoimmune thyroid disorders, diabetes mellitus, atopy, etc. Histologically T lymphocytes are present as a cluster around the hair bulbs.

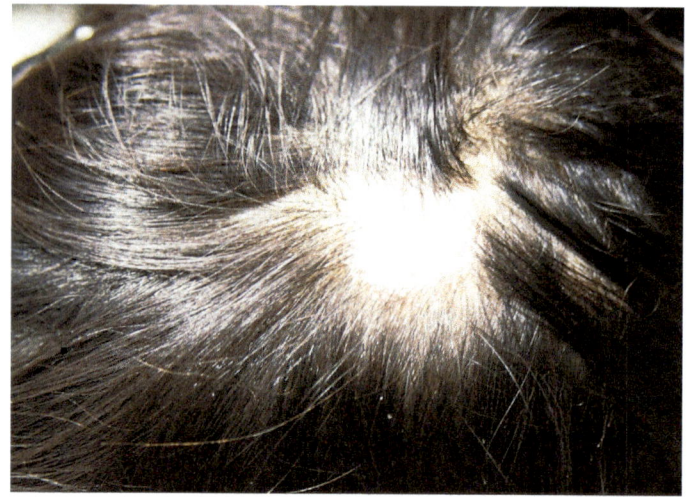

FIGURE 20.4. Alopecia areata.

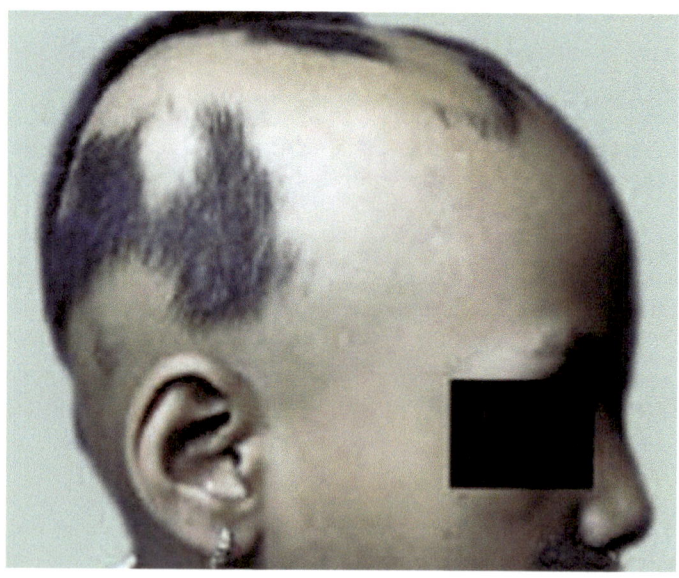

FIGURE 20.5. Alopecia areata – extensive.

Spontaneous regrowth is seen in most cases after the first episode. The new hair is fine and light-colored or white. It slowly regains the normal color and thickness. Subsequent episodes tend to be more extensive and the regrowth is slower.

Bad Prognostic Signs
Early onset – before puberty
Associated with atopy
Diffuse widespread alopecia
Involvement of the scalp margin
Pitting of the nails
Long history

Treatment

- Recent patches respond to I/L injection of triamcinolone (5 mg/mL).
- Topical minoxidil.
- Contact sensitizers such as diphencyprone, anthralin.
- Topical immunomodulators such as tacrolimus.
- PUVA.
- Generalized AA responds to systemic steroids, oral cyclosporine.
- Wigs may be required for extensive cases.

  The hair of Marie Antoinette is said to have turned white overnight, after hearing her death sentence – this was due to alopecia areata. Alopecia areata preferentially affects the black hair.

  My hair is gray, but not with years,
  Nor grew it white,
  In a single night.
  As men's have grown with sudden fear.

                                                              Byron

20.2.1.3 Trichotillomania (Hair Pulling)

Trichotillomania is defined as recurrent pulling of hair that leads to a patch of hair loss. It is seen mostly in young children, adolescents, and women. The patch of hair loss is irregular; it is present at areas most susceptible to removal of the hair, such as the

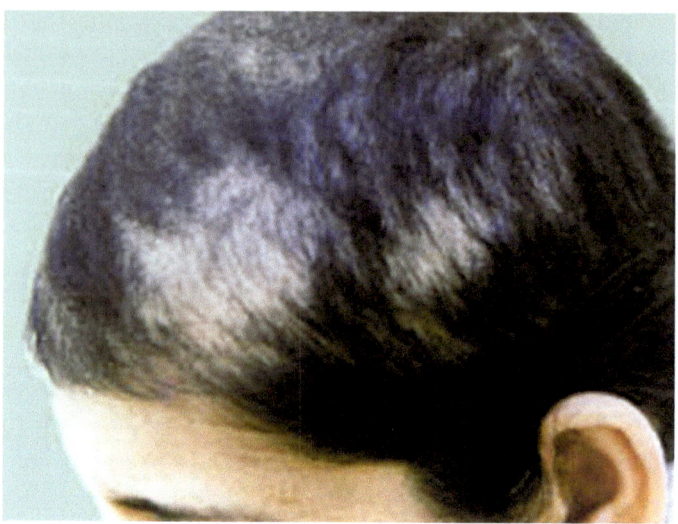

FIGURE 20.6. Trichotillomania.

frontoparietal region, but any area of the scalp may be affected. The hair tends not to be lost but is short, as the child can no longer pull the shortened hair. The eyebrows and eyelashes may even be involved. Several short broken hairs are found in the patch of alopecia (Fig. 20.6). In children, there is a tendency for the disorder to grow out by itself, but in some cases, it may persist. Stress is documented to be a factor, for the pathogenesis of trichotillomania. In adults, the disease shows the similarities to obsessive-compulsive disorders, predominantly in females. The condition may become worse during pregnancy.

The disorder is easy to diagnose, the personality of the person often points to the disease. The patch of alopecia can be occluded, and then examined after a week, if the hair grows in the patch, it confirms the diagnosis.

Treatment

Children usually grow out of the disorder. Many patients are psychologically stable, and require only a discussion of the problem. There should be a good patient-physician relationship.

Adults may need support with behavioral treatment and pharmacotherapy. Pimozide, haloperidoal, paroxotine, and vanlatidine, have been found useful for the treatment of trichotillomania. It is better to refer the patient to a psychiatrist if the habit persists

Differences between tinea capitis, alopecia areata, androgenetic alopecia, and trichotillomania

Characteristics	Tinea Capitis	Alopecia Areata	Androgenetic alopecia	Trichotilo-mania
Age of Onset	Children	Children and young adults	Young adults	Children and women
Area of baldness	Inflamed, scaly, and irregular	Not inflamed, round or oval	Particular pattern in males, generalized in females	Not inflamed, may show mild folliculitis. Irregular
Hair in bald patch	Broken hair near scalp	No hair in bald patch	Complete hair loss in males, diffuse hair loss in females	Small irregular hair in bald patch
Effect of occlusion	No effect	No effect	No effect	Hair re-grows in bald patch
Scraping	Positive for hyphae	Negative	Negative	Negative
Exclamation marked hair	Absent	Present	Absent	Absent
Other immune disorders	Absent	Present	Absent	Absent

Table showing differentiation of hair loss in common forms of localized non-scarring alopecia.

20.2.1.4 Generalized Hair Loss

This includes systemic illness such as tuberculosis, chronic renal failure, internal malignancy, thyroid disorders, iron deficiency anemia, drugs such as cytotoxic medication, lithium, and malnutrition. In females, androgentic alopecia is generalized.

Telogen Effluvium

In a number of disorders, the anagen phase prematurely terminates and causes a number of hairs to enter the telogen phase together, these hair are shed synchronously. There is no inflammation or scarring. Telogen effluvium may be due to fever, severe infections, post partum, stress, hypothyroidism, excessive dieting, and drugs such as retinoids, lithium, antithyroid medication, anticonvulsants, and indomethacin. There is no specific therapy; in most cases, the hair loss stops spontaneously within a few weeks and the hair regrows again.

Anagen Effluvium

This is an abrupt loss of hair from follicles that are in their growing phase. Anagen effluvium is commonly seen after the use of chemotherapy and radiation; mitotic inhibition stops the reproduction of matrix cells, but does not destroy the follicle. A pressure cap applied to the scalp during chemotherapy may prevent such an arrest; scalp hypothermia is also used for the same reason.

> *Plucked telogen hair have small, unpigmented ovoid hair bulb, they do not contain an internal root sheath.*
>
> *Plucked anagen hair have larger elongated pigmented hair bulb, surrounded by a gelatinous internal root sheath. The plucked root may show an angle of 20° or more with the shaft; this is probably artifactual.*

20.2.2 Scarring Alopecia

It is important to differentiate the scarring from the nonscarring alopecias. The hair will not grow back in scarring alopecia, as the hair follicles are replaced by fibrous tissue. The skin in scarring alopecia is devoid of hair and there are no skin markings. It may be thick and hypopigmented or hyperpigmented, or thin from epidermal atrophy (Fig. 20.7). A careful history and examinination of the skin will help to diagnose cases of

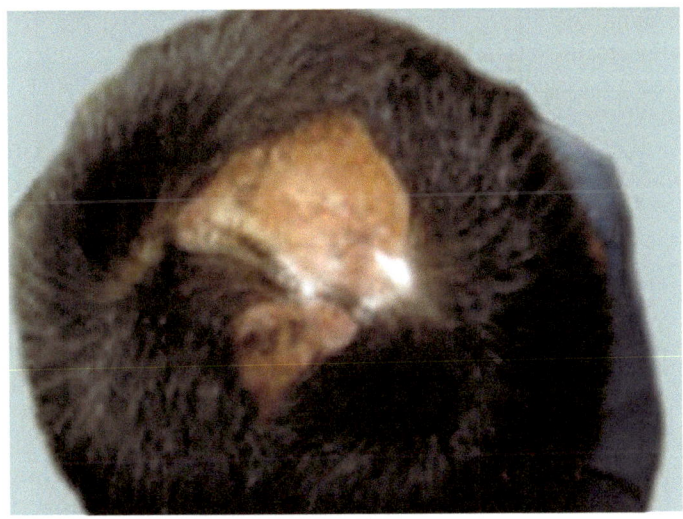

FIGURE 20.7. Scarring alopecia.

scarring alopecia. Many cases will have associated skin disease; such as lichen planopilaris will have signs of lichen planus in other parts of the body. The common diseases giving rise to scarring alopecia are discoid lupus erythematosus, lichen planus, scarring secondary to severe bacterial, fungal and viral infection, dissecting cellulitis, acne keloidalis, trauma, follicular mucinosis, tumors, or surgical scars.

Diagnosis and treatment must be prompt to minimize further hair loss. Treat the underlying disorder.

Alopecia due to fungal disease is discussed in the Chapter 5

20.3 Disorders of Color and Texture

A number of congenital disorders can cause changes in texture and color, many of which are rare. These include disorders of the hair shaft such as monolithrix, pili torti, bamboo hair, trichorrhexis nodosa, etc. The hair in these disorders is short and brittle, and there is change of texture. There is increased susceptibility to trauma and injury. These hair shaft defects may be due to an abnormality of amino acids. Examination of the hair under the microscope helps in diagnosis, and a urinary screening for abnormalities of amino acids is advisable.

When a mother brings a child with short, unruly hair, that fails to grow, think of hair shaft defects.

20.3.1 Premature Graying of the Hair

Graying is a normal process in ageing; however, in some patients graying occurs at an early age. Premature graying of the hair may be hereditary, associated with pernicious anemia, deficiency of iron, protein deficiency (kwashiorkor), drugs such as triparanol and fluorobutyrophenone, and the premature ageing syndromes such as progeria, acrogeria, and pangeria.

20.3.2 Dryness of the Hair

This is associated with a dry environment, malnutrition, or damage to the hair by chemicals and heat. Hair is often subject to different procedures and application of chemicals in hair dressing salons such as bleaching, perming, styling, back combing, etc., which can damage the hair and cause dryness.

20.4 Tumor of the Hair Follicles

20.4.1 Pilomatricoma

This is the most common tumor of the hair follicles. It is a benign tumor, which arises from the matrix cells. Calcification is very common in these tumors.

The tumor can occur at any age, it is more common in children, females are more often affected than males. The tumor is often found on the face, neck, or arms. It is a symptomless, deep nodule, skin or pinkish in color. The tumor has a firm to stony hard consistency, due to calcification. Stretching the skin over the tumor shows the "tent sign," with multiple facets and angles. It may be subject to periods of inflammation. Malignancy has been recorded.

20.4.1.1 Treatment

Surgical removal.

20.4.2 Trichoepithelioma

These hair follicle tumors are usually multiple and are inherited as an autosomal dominant trait. The onset is at puberty, lesions are commonly seen on the head and neck, mainly on the face. On the face, the tumors are distributed in the perinasal and midfacial regions. The tumors are flesh-colored; and appear as papules or nodules, which may be solid or cystic (Fig. 20.8). A malignant change can rarely occur. Solitary trichoepithelioma is not inherited; lesions occur on the scalp, neck, or trunk.

Multiple trichoepitheliomas should be differentiated from adenoma sebaceum, multiple basal cell carcinomas and syringomas.

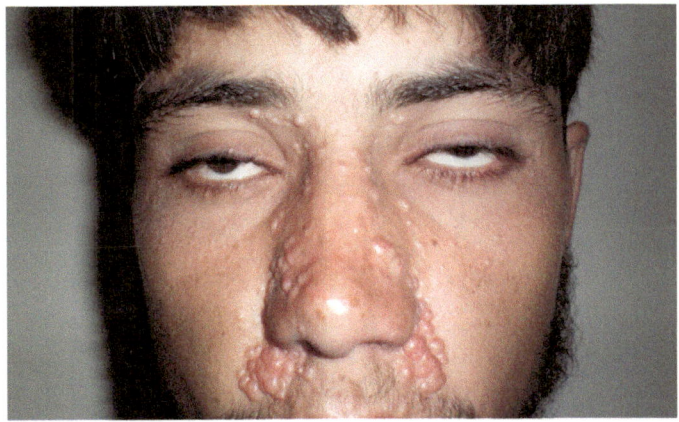

FIGURE 20.8. Trichlorepithelioma.

20.4.2.1 Treatment

A single tumor may be excised. Multiple tumors may be treated for cosmetic reasons by laser ablation but recurrences are common.

20.5 Miscellaneous Disorders

20.5.1 Pityriasis Amiantacea

The disease is characterized by thick, asbestos-like (amiantaceous-like), shiny scales on the scalp. This is localized to one or more areas of the scalp; in some cases it may be generalized. The tuft of hair is matted together by laminated crusts (Fig. 20.9). The cause is unknown; it may be secondary to seborrheic dermatitis, psoriasis, pediculosis, and neurodermatitis. Secondary bacterial infection can occur.

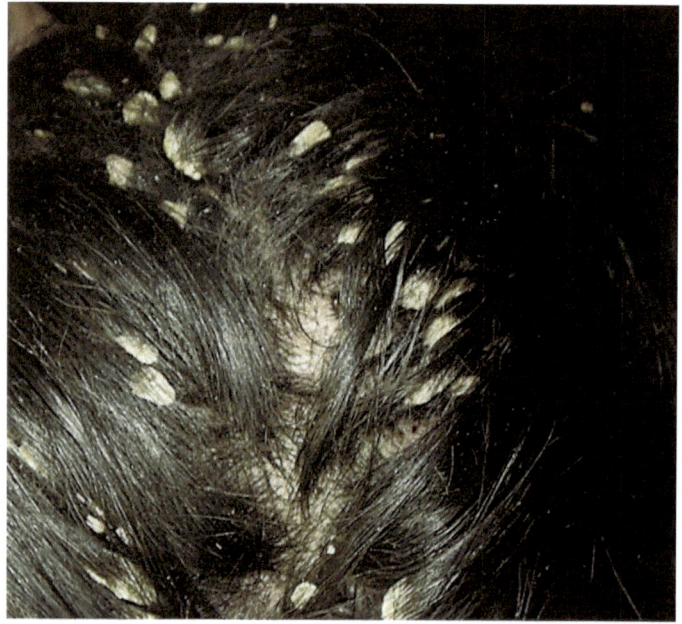

FIGURE 20.9. Pityriasis amiantacea.

20.5.1.1 Treatment

The underlying cutaneous disorder should be treated. The thick crusts are removed by salicylic acid preparations. Appropriate antibiotics are required to treat any secondary infection.

20.5.2 Pseudofolliculitis Barbae

The condition is produced due to tightly curved hair re-entering the skin after coming out of the hair follicle. The condition is common in Afro-Caribbean patients. The hair on reentering the skin excites an inflammatory reaction, with the formation of papules and pustules (Fig. 20.10). Normal bacterial flora may eventually be replaced by pathogenic organisms if the condition becomes chronic.

Pseudofolliculitis barbae can also occur in the axillae, pubic area, and legs.

20.5.2.1 Treatment

Definitive treatment is by laser hair removal.

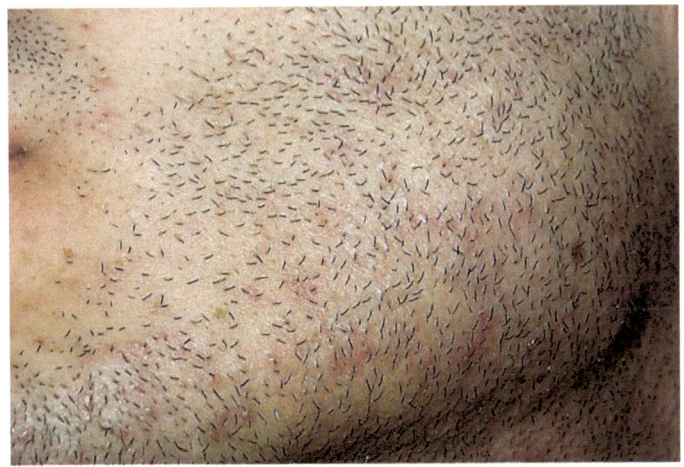

FIGURE 20.10. Pseudofolliculitis barbae.

20.5.2.2 Shaving Techniques

Patients should not shave close to the skin. A special razor with a single-edged blade should be used. Shaving with electric clippers to leave a minimum of 1 mm of hair length can also be tried.

Some hair releasing techniques, such as washing the beard with a toothbrush using a circular movement may help to dislodge the ingrown hair.

A short course of antibiotics may hasten resolution.

20.5.3 Acne Keloidalis

The condition occurs on the nape of neck, in young male adults after puberty, mostly confined to black people. Acne keloidalis is due to the penetration of hair back into the skin, similar to pseudofolliculitis barbae. The problem is more severe in the neck area, where the hair follicles are more likely to be oriented at low angles to the skin surface, making repenetration of the skin more likely. There is a tendency to scar formation, which is hypertrophic and keloidal (Fig. 20.11).

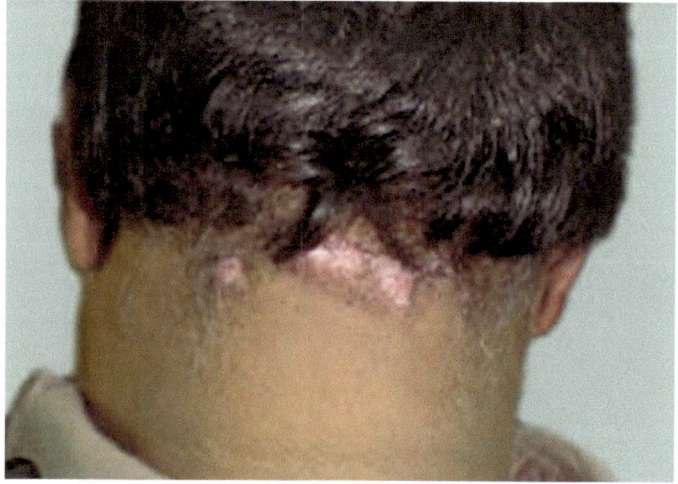

FIGURE 20.11. Acne keloidalis.

20.5.3.1 Treatment

The treatment of acne keloidalis is generally difficult.

Avoid close shaving on the back of the scalp. Intralesional injection of steroids may help in reducing scarring and keloid formation. Surgical excision and grafting is reserved for severe cases. Carbon dioxide laser can also be used to excise the affected skin, healing occurs by secondary intention. A short or long course of antibiotics may help in resolution.

20.5.4 Dissecting Cellulitis of the Scalp (Perifolliculitis Capitis Abscedens et Suffodiens)

This is a suppurative disease of the scalp of unknown etiology. The condition is associated with acne conglobata, hidradenitis suppurativa, and pilonidal sinus disease. These grouped disorders form the follicular tetrad. Follicular blockage is the proposed etiological factor for these diseases. Blockage of the duct leads to dilatation of the hair follicle and subsequent rupture, resulting in inflammation.

The disease begins as simple folliculitis on the occiput or vertex of the scalp; as the disease progresses papules, nodules, abscess and sinus formation occurs. The hairs over the nodules are shed, and the follicular openings discharge pus. The nodules heal with scarring and the scars may become keloidal. There are no systemic symptoms but there is a tendency to recurrences.

20.5.4.1 Treatment

Treatment is difficult. Oral isotretinoin is the treatment of choice. External beam radiation has been used in some cases. Intralesional steroids may be used to reduce inflammation; it should not be used as a monotherapy. Surgical excision of the affected scalp may be required in severe cases, followed by skin grafting.

Practical points
Treat all hair disorders with a sympathetic and supportive approach, as these disorders may be associated with significant anxiety and distress.

Chapter 21
Nail Disorders

Nails are specialized epidermal appendages, found on the dorsum of each finger and toe. Nails protect the phalanx against trauma; they are also used for performing fine movements such as grasping and scratching. Nails also have aesthetic value. Nail disorders are difficult to diagnose, as the same pathology e.g. subungal hyperkeratosis is found in a number of skin diseases, and a single disease can present with many different nail changes. Nail changes can be due to cutaneous or systemic disorders, or due to injury. The common nail disorders seen by a general practitioner will be discussed here.

21.1 Paronychial Disorders

21.1.1 Acute Paronychia

This is an acute inflammation of the nail fold, this can be the proximal and/or the lateral nail fold. The causative organism is usually Staphylococcus aureus. The nail fold is red, swollen, and tender. Pus is often seen coming through the cuticle (Fig. 21.1).

21.1.1.1 Treatment

Pus if present should be evacuated, by incision and drainage. An appropriate antibiotic such as cefalexin 500 mg twice

Z. Zaidi, S. W. Lanigan, *Dermatology in Clinical Practice*,
DOI 10.1007/978-1-84882-862-9_21,
© Springer-Verlag London Limited 2010

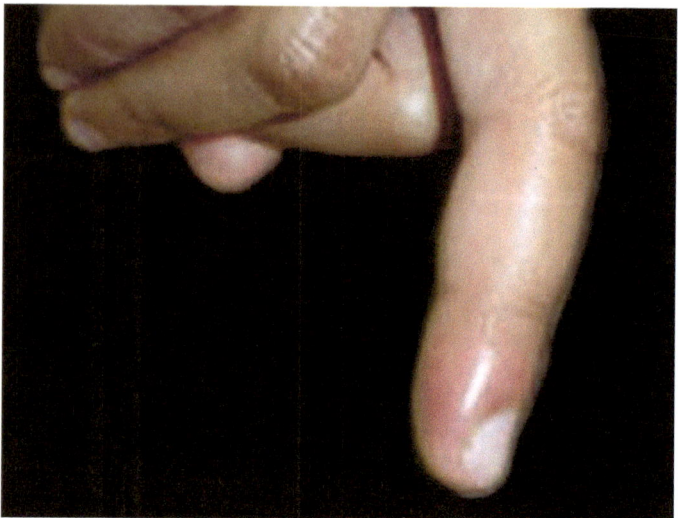

FIGURE 21.1. Acute paronychia.

daily, erythromycin 500 mg twice daily, or dicloxcillin 500 mg twice daily is prescribed.

21.1.2 Chronic Paronychia

The condition is common in housewives, bartenders, nurses, cooks, and other people who do wet work. Interruption of the cuticle and wetness creates an environment for the growth of yeast and bacteria. Predisposing factors include diabetes mellitus, poor peripheral circulation, vaginal candidiasis, and overzealous pushing back of the cuticle. Candida is the most common pathogen, often associated with bacterial infection. The nail folds are swollen; there is slight tenderness and erythema. Loss of cuticle is a characteristic finding of chronic paronychia. The nail plate is discolored and ridged. Acute exacerbations are common due to secondary invasion of bacteria. Pus is discharged at intervals (Fig. 21.2).

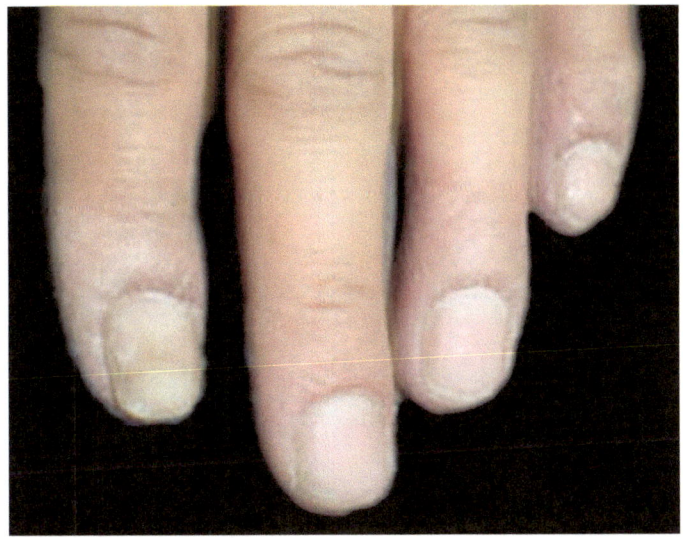

FIGURE 21.2. Chronic paronychia.

21.1.2.1 Treatment

The most important factor for treatment is to keep the hands dry, and use of gloves while doing wet work. Manicuring should be avoided. An antifungal cream for the day and topical antibiotic at night should be used. If Candida is positive on culture then oral itraconazole 100 mg orally for 4–6 weeks, should be instituted. Oral antibiotic may be needed for acute exacerbations.

21.1.3 Ingrowing ToeNail

This is often caused by nail spicules, which when separated from the nail plate, penetrate the lateral nail fold. The nail spicules result from compression of the nail by ill-fitted shoes. The nail pierces the lateral nail fold and enters the dermis, where it acts as a foreign body. This causes pain and swelling. The area of penetration later becomes infected with the formation of granulation tissue.

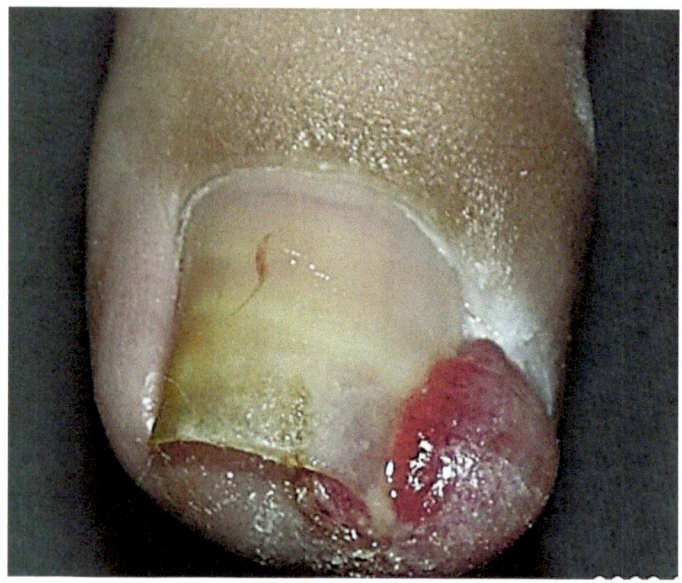

FIGURE 21.3. Ingrown toenail.

The great toenail is most commonly affected as this is the nail which is compressed by the shoes. If the nails are improperly cut, i.e., in a semicircle rather than straight, the chances of getting an ingrowing nail become much higher (Fig. 21.3).

21.1.3.1 Prevention

Wear fitted shoes that do not compress the toes. Nails should be cut when they extend beyond the hyponychium; the nails should be cut straight rather than in a semicircle.

21.1.3.2 Treatment

Treat the infection when present, locally with antiseptics if the infection is mild, or by systemic antibiotics when the infection is severe. Separate the toenail gently from the nail fold with a wisp of absorbent cotton coated with collodion.

Pain is relieved immediately. The collodion fixes the cotton in place and waterproofs the area. The cotton insert may need replacement after 3–4 weeks. If granulation tissue is present, this should be removed chemically by silver nitrate or surgically.

Recurrent Ingrown Nail

This may require permanent destruction of the lateral portion of the nail matrix by liquid phenol. In some cases, nail avulsion may be required.

> *The nails should neither exceed nor come short of*
> *the fingernails – Hippocrates*

21.1.4 Trauma and Haemorrhage

Damage to the nail matrix results in splits and ridges. Splinter hemorrhages in a linear manner, are seen under the nails of manual workers caused by minor trauma. This is also a feature of psoriasis and subacute bacterial endocarditis.

Damage to the proximal nail fold often occurs while playing a sport, unnoticed at the time of injury; the patient becomes aware of the injury when the nail plate emerges from the nail fold, dark in color. If this is not producing any discomfort then it should be left as such, until the nail grows out and a new nail takes its place. The dark color of the nail should not be confused with dark nails from pseudomonas, proteus, and some fungal infections.

Large subungal hematomas are due to trauma to the nail bed. If pain is obvious at the time of injury then the blood should be removed to decrease the tension. The traditional method of puncturing the nail with a red-hot paper clip or pin remains the quickest and effective way of removing the blood. A carbon dioxide laser can be used to perforate the nail and decompress the hematoma. Drilling the nail to remove the blood requires local anesthesia.

21.2 Common Nail Dystrophies

21.2.1 Lamellar Dystrophy (Distal Plate Splitting)

A condition found in about 20% of the adult population, it is analogous to the scaling of dry skin. The brittleness of the nails is determined by its hydration. It is important to protect such nails from detergents, cleaning agents, and trauma. Regular use of emollients and protection of the nails with rubber gloves over cotton gloves while doing wet work is advisable.

21.2.2 Onychogryphosis

In this condition the nail, usually the toenail, thickens in both the vertical and longitudinal plane with excessive curvature; it commonly occurs in old age. The nail is thickened, yellowish in color and hard (horn-like). The nail is very difficult to cut. The exact cause is unknown, the following factors may contribute to its formation – trauma, an inadequate matrix as seen in old age, the bulk of the nail being formed by the nail bed, failure to trim the nails as seen in the elderly. The nails then increase in length and later become curved. Nail infections such as onychomycosis may be a contributing factor.

21.2.2.1 Treatment

Trimming is difficult; it may be facilitated by the use of a 20% urea preparation to soften the nail. A chiropodist may trim thickened nails; special clippers are also available. When the condition occurs in young patients, the nail should be avulsed, so that a new nail grows.

21.2.3 Clubbing (Hippocratic Nail)

This is a feature of a number of diseases, or may occur as a normal variant. The digital phalanges of the fingers and toes are enlarged to a rounded, bulbous shape. The nail enlarges and becomes curved, hard, and thickened. Clubbing may be seen in diseases of the lungs such as bronchiectasis, tuberculosis, and bronchogenic carcinoma. It can occur in GIT disorders such as Crohn's disease and ulcerative colitis. It is also seen in congenital heart disease, hyperthyroidism, and biliary cirrhosis.

Treatment is directed at the underlying disease.

21.2.4 Koilonychia (Spoon-Shaped Nails)

Koilonychia may be familial, or it may be associated with a local nail dystrophy. It is often secondary to poor peripheral circulation; or iron deficiency anemia, or with dermatoses such as psoriasis and lichen simplex.

21.2.5 Beau's Line

These are transverse depression on the nail plate due to temporary interference with nail formation. These lines are commonly seen during convalescence from severe diseases, such as pneumonia, measles, mumps, coronary thrombosis, and other conditions causing prolonged fever. The line appears first at the cuticle and then moves forwards with the nail growth. It is a self-limiting condition and requires no treatment.

21.2.6 Onycholysis

This means separation of the nail plate from the nail bed. Because of the separation from the nail bed, the nail appears whitish. The nails separate due to a number of causes such as increased hyperkeratosis of the nail bed in psoriasis, subungal tumors, trauma, thyroid disorders, extreme photosensitivity, drugs, etc.

21.2.7 Pitting

Pitting is defined as ice-pick-like depressions on the nail plate. The distribution, pattern, and diameter vary in different diseases. The pits reflect the persistence of parakeratotic cells. The parakeratotic cells of the nail plate are shed in much the same way as skin scales are shed, leaving tiny punched-out depressions on the nail surface. Many diseases produce pitting of the nail such as psoriasis, eczema, fungal infections, and alopecia areata; it may also occur as an isolated finding in normal individuals (Fig. 21.4).

21.2.8 Pterygium

The condition typically develops in lichen planus, and following trauma. A fibrous band fuses the proximal nail fold with the nail

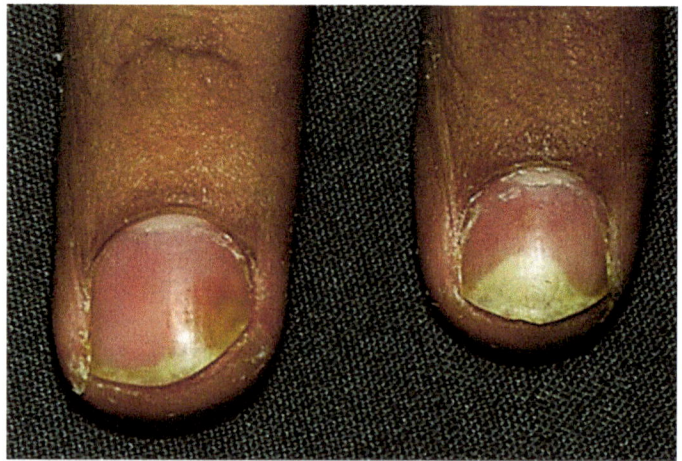

FIGURE 21.4. Psoriasis – note the pitting and onycholysis.

bed; this obstructs the normal nail growth. An inflammatory destructive process precedes pterygium formation.

21.3 Discoloration

21.3.1 White Spots

Patients are often worried about the white spots they see on their nails, and think it is due to calcium deficiency. Calcium has nothing to do with it. The white spots are often incidental and can be due to trauma, they are also seen in superficial fungal infections, in arsenic poisoning, and renal disease. White nails are also indicative of liver and renal failure. Any discoloration on the nail plate will grow out with it; a discoloration due to lesion of the nail bed will remain at its site, until treated (Fig. 21.5).

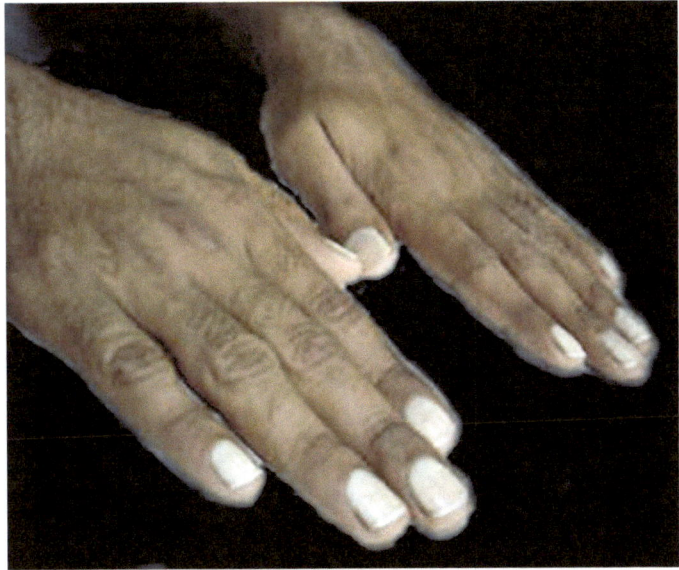

FIGURE 21.5. Leukonychia.

21.3.2 Yellow Nail Syndrome

The syndrome occurs spontaneously in association with certain respiratory diseases such as bronchiectasis and chronic respiratory infections, and diseases associated with lymphoedema including edema of the lower extremities, pleural effusion, and facial edema. The syndrome is thus a combination of lymphoedema, chronic respiratory disease, and yellow nails. The condition is also reported in AIDS. The growth of the nails is extremely slow; the surface of the nail usually remains smooth. It is a disease usually seen in adults. There is no treatment; yellow nail syndrome may at times spontaneously improve with treatment of the associated disorder.

21.3.3 Nail Discoloration

White discoloration (leukonychia)	Yellow discoloration	Blue discoloration	Black discoloration
Cirrhosis of the liver	Jaundice	Cyanosis	Junctional naevus
Hypoalbuminemia	Dyes – saffron, turmeric, varnish	Drugs – gold, mepacrine	Drugs – chloroquin, cytotoxics, adriamycin
Nephrotic syndrome	Psoriasis	Fixed drug eruption	Trauma – deep
Trauma – superficial	Fungal infection – dermatophytes.	Blue lunula in Wilson's disease	Fungal infection – scytalidium, aspergillosis, scopulariopsis
Chronic arsenic poisoning	AIDS		Addison's disease
Superficial fungal infection	Pulmonary diseases and malignancy Smoker's nail		Normal in Negroid Malignancy – melanoma

21.4 Tumors Adjacent to and Under the Nails

21.4.1 Mucoid Cyst

These are dome-shaped, translucent to skin colored, firm to fluctuant nodules found on the dorsal surface of the distal phalanx. The cysts are found on the proximal nail fold, or on the dorsolateral surface of the distal phalanx. Etiology is uncertain, but thought to be due to the mucoid degeneration of connective tissue of the distal phalanx. The cysts do not have an epithelial lining, they are thus pseudocysts. Compression on the nail matrix leads to a longitudinal depression on the nail plate. The underlying bone may show changes of osteoarthritis. The disease is more common on the dominant hand and in females. The condition is often symptomless. Treatment if required can be done by injection of triamcinolone into the cyst, multiple punctures and expression of the cysts contents, or surgical removal. Recurrences are common.

21.4.2 Glomus Tumor

These are the most characteristic of the vascular nail bed tumors. Pain may be spontaneous or evoked by mild trauma or temperature changes. Nail plate changes depend upon the site of the tumor. Matrix tumors cause splitting, and distortion of the nail plate. Nail bed tumors appear as reddish or blue lesions beneath the nail. MRI scan reveals the exact site of the tumor. Histology confirms the diagnosis. The tumor is treated by excision.

21.4.3 Malignant Tumors

These may be squamous cell carcinoma or malignant melanoma. They present as chronic paronychia, ingrown nail, pyogenic granuloma, onycholysis or as a nail dystrophy. Subungal melanoma may also simulate onychomycosis or subungal hematoma. Pigmented macules or nodules in the periungal region should be referred for diagnostic biopsy, to rule out malignant melanoma. Symptoms such as pain, itching, and throbbing may occur, metastasis is rare but local spread may occur; X-ray of the underlying bone should be done to see the extent of the disease. Moh's surgery or amputation of the digit is the treatment of choice.

ABCDEF of malignant melanoma in a nail:

1. Age of the patient (peak incidence between fifth and seventh decade)
2. Breadth of the pigmentation (3 mm or more)
3. Change in nail morphology
4. Digit involved
5. Extension beyond the nail folds
6. Family history, of dysplastic naevi or melanoma

21.5 Differential Diagnosis of Common Nail Disorders

Nail changes	Psoriasis	Eczema	Onychomycosis (dermatophytes)	Chronic paronychia
Color	Yellow or normal	Normal	Yellow	Normal, edges maybe brown
Onycholysis	Present	Absent	Present	Absent
Pitting	Present	May be present	May be present	Absent
Ridging	Absent	Present	Absent	Present
Subungal hyperkeratosis	Present	Absent	Present	Absent
Proximal nail fold	Normal	Normal	Normal	Swollen and inflamed
Lesions in other parts of body	Present-knees, elbows, lumbosacral, scalp	Present – hand	Present – feet	Absent

Before treating any nail disorder, first establish whether the disorder is due to an underlying systemic disease, or if there is a local cause for the nail dystrophy.

Nail disorders often require systemic medication, due to the hard keratin that makes local medicines difficult to penetrate.

Nail therapy is often of a long duration, due to time taken for the growth of the nail from the proximal to the distal end.

Dystrophic nail is a misshapen disorganized nail.

Nail clippings for onychomycosis should be taken from the proximal end of involvement in the affected nail.
Fungal nail infections (onychomycosis) discussed in Chap. 5
Periungal warts discussed in Chap. 6
Dystrophy of nails in psoriasis, lichen planus are discussed in Chap. 9
Removal of nail by urea in Appendix 3.

Chapter 22
Diseases of the Subcutaneous Tissue

The subcutaneous tissue is an important metabolic organ; it functions as a thermal and mechanical insulator. The three major components of the subcutaneous tissue are lipocytes present in the fat lobules, fibrous septa, and blood vessels.

22.1 Panniculitis

Panniculitis represents an inflammation of the adipose tissue involving cutaneous or extracutaneous sites. Cutaneous panniculitis usually appears as erythematous to violaceous deep-seated nodules, these are usually painful and may be accompanied by systemic symptoms. The inflammation may be primary, e.g., erythema nodosum (septal panniculitis), erythema induratum (lobular panniculitis), cold injury (cold panniculitis), idiopathic (Weber Christian disease), or it may be secondary to other diseases such as systemic lupus erythematosus (lupus profundus), erythema induratum (Bazin's disease-associated with tuberculosis) and pancreatic disorders. The diagnosis of panniculitis requires a deep skin biopsy to include an adequate amount of subcutaneous fat. A fully evolved lesion should be biopsied and not a new or resolving one.

Microscopically, panniculitis may be categorized according to the dominant location of the inflammatory infiltrate (lobular or septate) and the presence or absence of vascular injury such as polyarteritis nodosa (septal panniculitis with vasculitis).

Z. Zaidi, S. W. Lanigan, *Dermatology in Clinical Practice*, DOI 10.1007/978-1-84882-862-9_22, © Springer-Verlag London Limited 2010

The cutaneous manifestations are tender nodules or plaques that appear on the trunk or extremities, chiefly on the thighs and lower legs. The skin over the nodules may be erythematous, mottled, or pigmented. The nodules regress slowly leading to localized depressed atrophic scars. Sometimes the nodules may undergo liquifaction and discharge an oily liquid.

Systemic panniculitis may be due to pancreatic disorders, immune disorders such as systemic lupus erythematosus, sarcoidosis, etc. These diseases are usually accompanied by fever, arthralgia, arthritis, abdominal pain, and hepatosplenomegaly.

22.1.1 Evaluation of Panniculitis

An excisional biopsy, is preferred to a punch biopsy, the latter often does not include the subcutaneous fat. The biopsy should be taken from an active lesion rather than from a lesion in the late stage.

Laboratory investigations are done to exclude systemic disorders such as connective tissue diseases; serological tests for syphilis should be performed as appropriate. Blood levels of calcium, phosphorus, serum amylase, lipase, α anti trypsin levels will help to detect the presence of pancreatic disorders.

For isolated lesions consider a drug reaction, exposure to cold, malignancy, and psychiatric disorders.

22.1.2 Treatment

This depends upon the cause of panniculitis. In idiopathic panniculitis such as Weber Christian Disease therapeutic responses to sulphapyridine, dapsone, azathioprine, thalidomide, cyclophosphamide, and tetracycline have been reported. The use of corticosteroids in the acute inflammatory phase is sometimes beneficial.

Ernest Bazin (1807–1878)

Ernest Bazin studied scabies thoroughly, and revolutionized its treatment at the Hospital St Louis. He used epilation in addition to parasiticides for the treatment of ringworm of the scalp and favus. He described acne keloidalis and eythema induratum.

22.2 Fat Dystrophies

Fat dystrophies are due to atrophy of subcutaneous fat; this can be congenital or acquired, it may be partial or generalized. The cause is often unknown; the patient has a characteristic appearance. On the face many wrinkles are present and the patient appears prematurely aged. The chin and cheeks are prominent. On the limbs due to the loss of fat the muscles and veins appear prominent. The overlying skin is of normal color, texture, and elasticity. Some cases are associated with acanthosis nigricans and hepatosplenomegaly.

In partial lipodystrophy the loss of fat usually starts from the face and gradually spreads down; it may stop at any level above and middle of the thigh. Simultaneously fat hypertrophy occurs in the lower limbs.

Treatment is unsatisfactory.

22.3 Dercums Disease (Adiposis Dolorosa)

The disease affects obese menopausal women. Multiple areas of the body are affected. The disease begins gradually; it is characterized by overgrowth of fat with formation of tender subcutaneous plaques and ecchymosis. The pain is characteristically unresponsive to analgesics.

22.3.1 Treatment

Fat reduction or surgical excision. Intralesional lidocaine may be effective.

22.4 Sclerema Neonatorum

This condition is seen in seriously ill premature or full-term infants. It affects debilitated infants with serious underlying illness such as congenital heart disease or respiratory distress syndrome. Hypothermia, shock, and sepsis are identified as predisposing factors.

The lobules of adipose tissue are poorly formed, and the fat is replaced by cystic cavities. The skin is bound to the underlying structures. A diffuse rapidly spreading hardening of the skin is noticed within the first few weeks of life. The skin appears waxy and cold. The infants become immobilized with fixed mask-like faces. Most of the patients succumb to intercurrent illness; in those who survive the condition resolve without complications.

Treatment is supportive and directed to the underlying disease.

22.5 Subcutaneous Fat Necrosis of the Newborn

This condition is a self-limiting disease of healthy full-term infants. The specific cause is not known; it is associated with hypothermia, asphyxia, maternal diabetes mellitus, traumatic deliveries, etc. Infants are predisposed to this condition because of the increased ratio of unsaturated to saturated fat in the newborn.

Subcutaneous indurated nodules appear in the first 2 weeks of life, some nodules may coalesce to form plaques. The cheeks, buttocks, arms, and thighs are commonly affected. As the lesions resolve they become fluctuant. The nodules resolve spontaneously within a period of 6 months. Significant hypercalcemia may occur as the lesions disappear. Hypercalcemia is associated with symptoms such as irritability, vomiting, and weight loss.

No treatment is required. During the resolving period: calcium levels should be monitored and treated accordingly.

22.6 Cellulite

This is an altered topography of the skin that occurs mainly in women in the pelvic region. It is due to structural changes in the dermal microcirculation and in the adipocytes. The exact etiology is not known, oestrogens is said to play a role in its production as the condition is predominant in females, where it is a common occurrence. It is found in young women who perform physical activity, or in inactive women who suddenly reduce weight. The surface of the skin looks dimpled. Fat deposits that push and distort the connective tissue contribute to the lumpiness.

Cellulite is graded according to its clinical appearance and histology.

Grade I. No symptoms, no clinical changes, there is increase thickness of areola tissue and increase in capillary permeability.

Grade II. No skin changes at rest, but on muscular contraction several clumps appear. There is local pallor, decrease in temperature and decrease in elasticity of the skin.

Grade III. The skin is orangish pink in appearance; pain may or may not be present. On histology there is fatty tissue destruction.

Grade IV. Skin surface appears wavy; there are visible painful purple nodules. The lobular structure of adipose tissue has disappeared, and the nodules are encapsulated by dermal connective tissue.

22.6.1 Treatment

Weight reduction should be gradual, performing regular exercises improve circulation, and the use of nonhormonal contraceptives may help in preventing cellulite. The condition is difficult to treat; ultrasound, mesotherapy and thermotherapy may be helpful.

Erythema nodosum described in Chapter 12
Lupus profundus described in Chapter 10

Chapter 23
Tumors of the Skin

Tumors of the skin may be benign, premalignant or malignant.

23.1 Benign Tumors

23.1.1 Skin Tags

These are small polypoid growths, often multiple, present on the neck and axillae of the elderly, and especially in obese people. They are symptomless, unless they catch on jewelry or clothing of patients. They can occur in large numbers in diabetes and in patients with hyperlipidemias. These growths are also called fibroepithelial polyps as they consist of an outer core of normal epidermis with a connective tissue core. The lesions are skin-colored or pigmented (Fig. 23.1).

23.1.1.1 Treatment

Skin tags can easily be removed by cautery, liquid nitrogen, or they can be snipped off with fine scissors. After treatment new ones can occur.

Z. Zaidi, S. W. Lanigan, *Dermatology in Clinical Practice*,
DOI 10.1007/978-1-84882-862-9_23,
© Springer-Verlag London Limited 2010

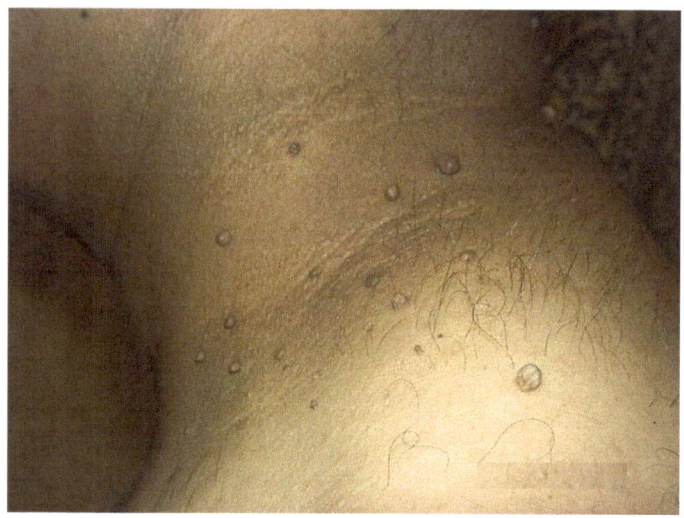

FIGURE 23.1. Skin tags.

23.1.2 Pyogenic Granuloma (Acquired Hemangioma)

This is a reddish growth that bleeds easily; it is due to proliferation of new blood vessels. This often develops after minor trauma. Pyogenic granulomas are seen most commonly in children and young adults, particularly during pregnancy they are also seen as a side effect of isotretinoin therapy (Fig. 23.2).

23.1.2.1 Treatment

Curettage and cauterization of the growth.

23.1.3 Milia

These are keratin cysts; these may be primary or secondary. They occur at all ages, from infancy onwards. Primary milia occur spontaneously and are found on the face near the eyelids and cheeks. These are due to the involvement of the most

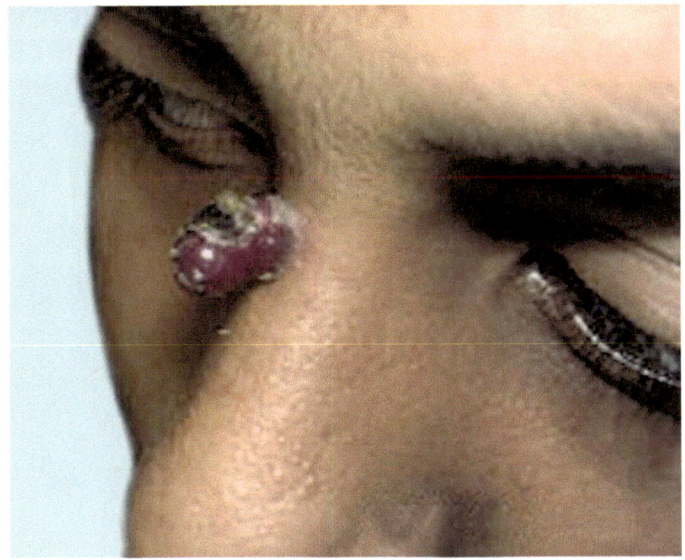

FIGURE 23.2. Pyogenic granuloma.

distal part of the infundibulum of the hair follicle. They appear as small whitish papules. Secondary milia are found secondary to disease; the most common being blistering disorders such as acquired epidermolysis bullosa, porphyria cutanea tarda, also after dermabrasion, laser surgery, burns, sunbathing, etc. Secondary milia are similar to primary milia in morphology and histology (Fig. 23.3).

23.1.3.1 Treatment

Milia are easily expressed after incision. They can also be treated by electrodessication.

23.1.4 *Dermatosa Papulosa Nigra*

These are small multiple brownish black papules on the face, especially the cheeks, of dark-skinned people. They occur at puberty, and are probably genetically determined (Fig. 23.4).

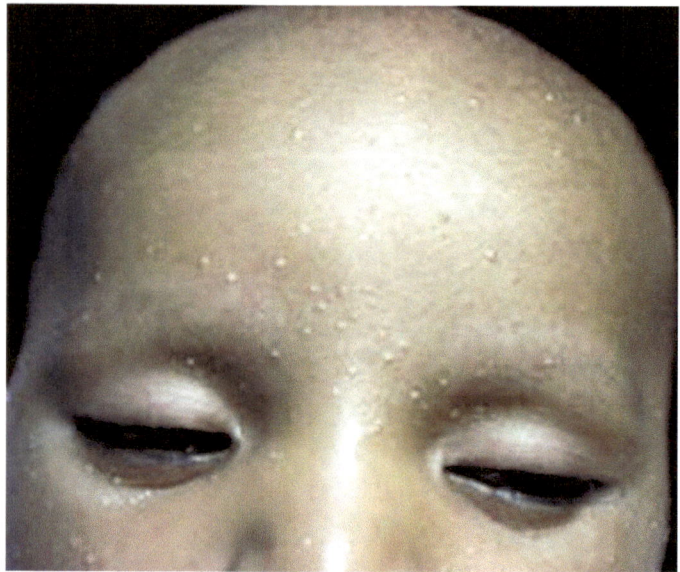

FIGURE 23.3. Milia.

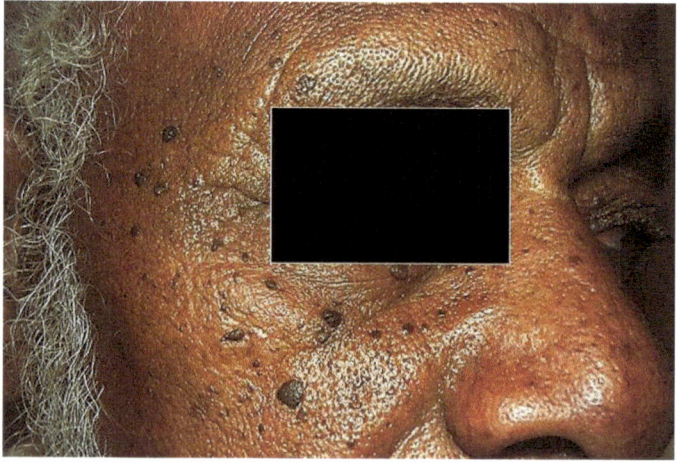

FIGURE 23.4. Dermatosa papulosa nigra.

23.1.4.1 Treatment

These are easily removed by cautery or diathermy. Hyperpigmentation is a common side effect of treatment.

23.1.5 Seborrhoeic Keratosis

The name is a misnomer as it is not related to sebaceous glands. It appears at middle age, as greasy, dry, smooth or rough, brown or black papules or plaques, often with a warty surface. It consists of a mass of basaloid cells with overlying hyperkeratosis and increased pigment production. The surface may show scattered keratin plugs. These horn pearls are easily seen with a magnifying glass. Some may be pedunculated. They have an abrupt edge, which gives the characteristic stuck-on appearance. The lesions occur mainly on the head, neck, and extremities. Sudden appearance of multiple pruritic seborrhoeic keratosis (sign of Leser Trelat), is indicative of internal malignancy usually an adenocarcinoma of the stomach, ovary, uterus, or breast (Fig. 23.5).

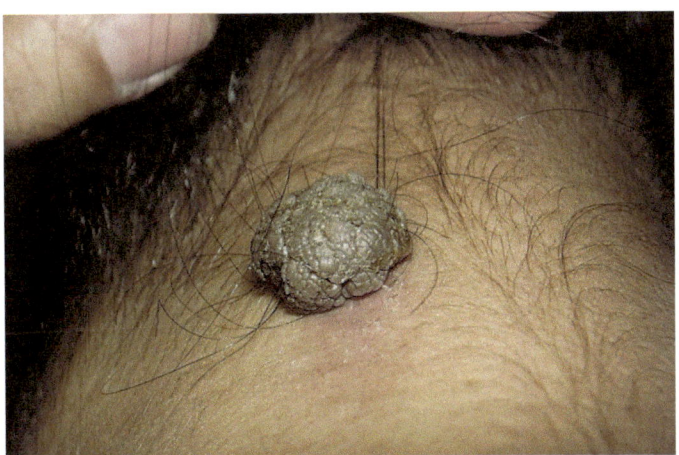

FIGURE 23.5. Seborrhoeic keratosis.

Although easy to diagnose the lesions can sometimes mimic malignant melanoma. Points of differentiation are: melanomas have a smooth surface and variability in elevation, color and pigment density. Seborrhoeic keratosis has a stuck-on appearance, presence of horny cysts on the surface, and a uniform surface.

23.1.5.1 Treatment

Seborrhoeic keratosis are easily removed by curettage or cryotherapy. They can be removed, for cosmetic purpose or if they get irritated by catching on clothing.

23.1.6 Sebaceous Cyst (Epidermoid Cyst)

These are keratinous cysts, common on the scalp, face, and trunk. Sebaceous cysts have a central punctum; when squeezed a cheesy foul-smelling material is expressed. It is thought that they arise from the infundibular portion of the hair follicle. These cysts can get inflamed from time to time (Fig. 23.6).

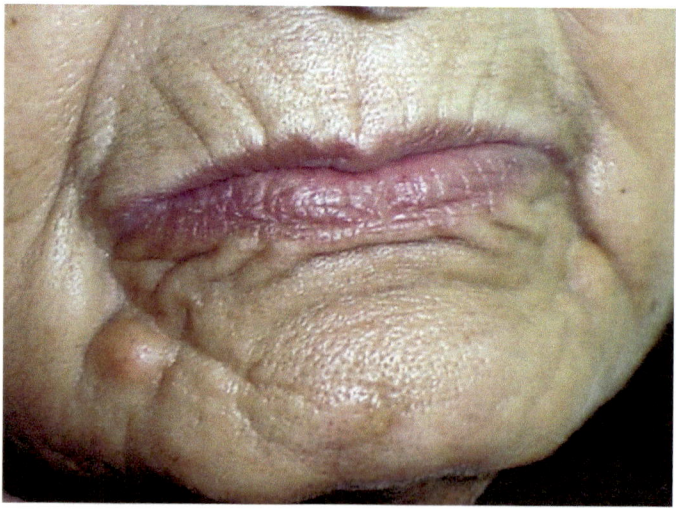

FIGURE 23.6. Sebaceous cyst.

23.1.6.1 Treatment

Surgical removal.

23.1.7 Trichilemmal Cyst

These probably arise from the isthmus of the hair follicle. They are usually seen on the scalp and have no punctum. They are smooth, firm, and skin-colored. When inflamed they become tender. Contents are gelatinous and odorless (Fig. 23.7).

23.1.7.1 Treatment

Surgical removal.

23.1.8 Dermatofibroma

A very common benign tumor of the skin, often brownish in color and firm in consistency. Dermatofibromas probably arise secondary to trauma, which may be very trivial and go unnoticed. The most common site is the lower limb. The most

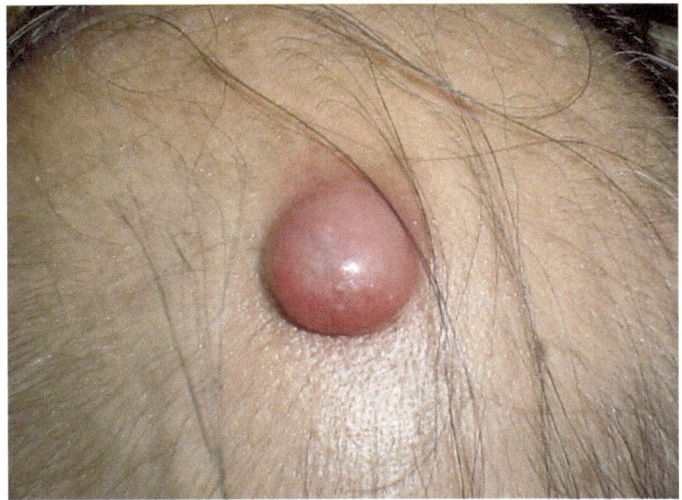

FIGURE 23.7. Tricholemmal cyst.

characteristic sign is the "dimpling sign" – the overlying epidermis dimples when the tumor is squeezed. This sign is seldom found in other tumors. A dermatofibroma is a localized area of dermal fibrosis; if the tumor consists of a number of histiocytes, histologically it is known as histiocytoma. A sclerosing hemangioma shows more of the vascular component, but the result is still dermal fibrosis.

23.1.8.1 Treatment

Surgical removal if desired. The patient should be cautioned that an obvious scar may result.

23.1.9 Lipoma

A soft lobulated tumor of the subcutaneous tissue containing fat cells. It is attached neither to the skin, nor to the underlying tissues. It is a soft, mobile, lobulated growth; it may be single or multiple. It is slightly elevated above the skin, but is easily palpable deep to the skin. It is symptomless. A painful fat tumor is an angiolipoma.

23.1.9.1 Treatment

Surgical removal if required.

23.1.10 Keratoacanthoma

Keratoacanthoma is a tumor of the elderly; its relationship to squamous cell carcinoma is debatable. Some consider it to be a benign tumor which looks malignant. While others consider it to be a relatively benign variant of squamous cell carcinoma, because of its capability of local destruction. It has the histological features of a squamous cell carcinoma, but it shows spontaneous regression.

The tumor occurs on the sun-exposed parts of the body as a solitary lesion usually on the face. It begins as a papule, which grows rapidly within a few weeks to a nodule with a

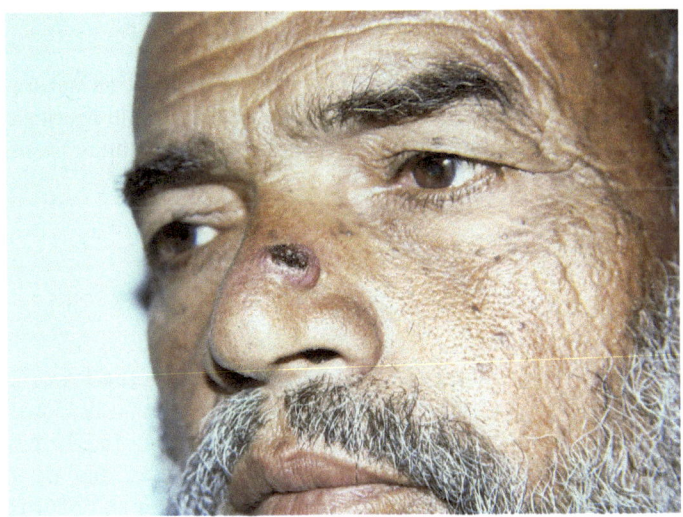

FIGURE 23.8. Keratomacanthoma.

prominent central keratinous plug. The lesion is sharply defined, the surrounding skin is normal. It then involutes in a few months leaving a depressed unsightly scar. In some cases it may be multiple (Fig. 23.8).

Most of the cytological atypia in keratoacanthoma occurs at the dermal-epidermal interface, where many mitoses may be seen. In squamous cell carcinoma the cellular atypia is present at varying levels of the proliferating mass. As the lesion involutes the proliferation at the dermal-epidermal interface ceases and eosinophilic homogeneous hyaline-like cells occur almost throughout the lesion. Keratoacanthomas rarely extend below the level of the sweat glands. When removing keratoacanthomas, efforts should be made to submit the tumor intact for histology. The symmetrical global architecture will assist the histopathologist in making the diagnosis. Fragmented specimens showing cellular atypia are likely to be reported as malignant.

Keratoacanthoma should be differentiated in its early stage from a molluscum contagiosum or a verruca: in the later stages from a squamous cell carcinoma or a basal cell carcinoma.

23.1.10.1 Treatment

The lesion should be excised, due to its destructive nature to avoid an ugly scar. Relapses are common. Multiple lesions can be treated by methotrexate, acitretin or photodynamic therapy.

23.2 Premalignant Tumors

23.2.1 Bowen's Disease

An intraepidermal growth, found commonly on the lower legs of elderly females, but can occur anywhere on the body. Bowen's disease is an intraepidermal squamous cell carcinoma. Bowen's disease presents as erythematous scaly plaques that do not respond to treatment; they are often mistaken for solitary areas of psoriasis, eczema, or dermatophytosis. On close examination, they are seen to have a border, which is sharply defined with notches. Later reniform projections, induration, or ulcers appear which are signs of invasive malignancy as the tumor spreads into the dermis as a true squamous cell carcinoma (Fig. 23.9).

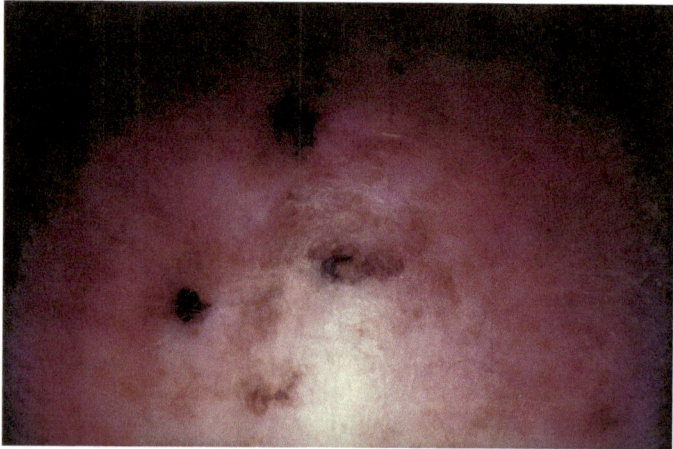

FIGURE 23.9. Bowen's disease.

23.2.1.1 Differential Diagnosis

Bowen's disease should be differentiated from psoriasis, solar keratosis, nummular eczema, tinea corporis, and extramammary Paget's disease.

23.2.1.2 Treatment

- Surgical excision is the best method of treatment.
- Small lesions are treated by electrodessication, curettage, or cryotherapy. In an elderly patient healing can be slow with ulceration.
- Photodynamic therapy is considered for large lesions on the elderly at sites where healing is poor, such as the shins.
- Multiple lesions can be treated by 5-fluorouracil, applied twice a day for 4–6 weeks. Alternatively, imiquimod cream 5% once daily for up to 16 weeks.
- Follow-up of patients is required as recurrences are frequent. Recurrences are due to follicular involvement or due to spread in the lateral margins of the disease.

John T. Bowen (1857–1940)

Bowen was an eminent histopathologist. He first described the pre-cancerous dermatoses. He also described the epitrichial layer of the epidermis. He was the founder of the Boston Dermatological Club.

23.2.2 Solar Keratosis

This is due to photodamage, present predominantly in people with fair skin, and excessive exposure to the sun. The initial lesion is telangiectasia, followed by erythematous scaly plaques. The scales are rough, yellowish brown, and adherent. The margins are ill-defined. They are mainly present in the sun-exposed areas of the body (Fig. 23.10).

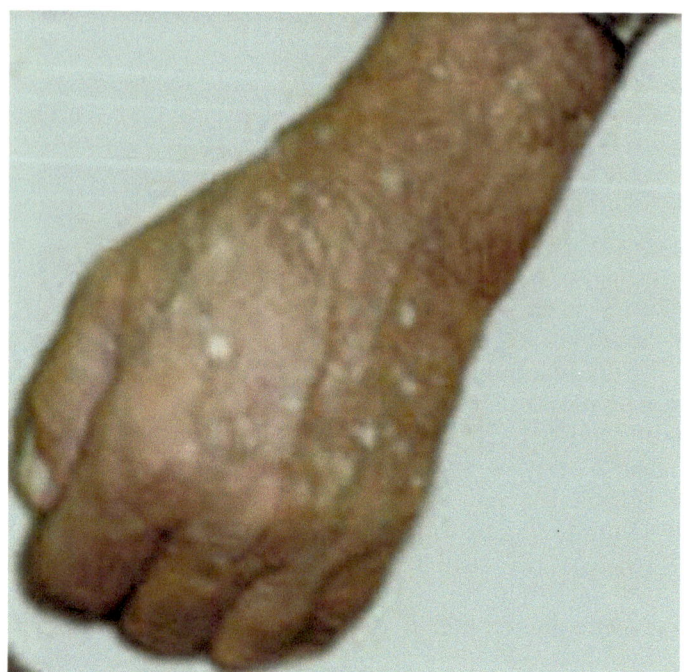

FIGURE 23.10. Actinic keratosis.

23.2.2.1 Treatment

- General: The patients should be advised to reduce sun exposure. Sunscreens should be used on exposed skin. Broad-brim hats and protective clothing should be worn.
- Specific: Cryotherapy.
- Chemotherapy with 5-fluorouracil.
- Photodynamic therapy with topical aminolaevulinic acid.

Leukoplakia is described in Chap. 30

23.3 Malignant Tumors

23.3.1 Basal Cell Carcinoma (BCC)

This is the most common malignant skin tumor; it arises from the basal cells of the epidermis. It is composed of uniform basal cells that invade the dermis as buds, lobules, or strands. Both sexes are equally affected and it is mostly seen in the elderly. The commonest site is the face. People with a fair complexion and those exposed to sunlight are most at risk.

The tumor is most common on the face; the mucous membranes are not involved. Basal cell carcinomas are slow-growing tumors, and locally malignant; they do not metastasize, as they require a vascular fibrous stroma for survival. The tumor grows slowly; it is locally invasive and may destroy the underlying cartilage, bone, and soft tissue structures. As it erodes the local structures, it is given the name "rodent ulcer."

Early tumors present as small, translucent or pearly papules, covered by a thin epidermis, through which a few dilated blood vessels show, or they appear as pearly erythematous lichenoid papules or plaques. In some cases these early tumors present as slight induration or a small ulcer resembling an excoriation. These early presentations should be kept in mind while examining sun-exposed sites in fair-skinned patients in whom BCC is common.

Later presentations of BCC are:

Noduloulcerative. This is the most common type; it begins as a small translucent skin-colored papule, which slowly enlarges. Later central necrosis occurs and an ulcer forms. The ulcer has a rolled pearly edge with telangiectasia. It has the characteristics described above (Fig. 23.11).

Cystic. The nodule becomes tense and translucent; it shows cystic spaces on histology. Telangiectasia is prominent (Fig. 23.12).

Superficial. These are present on the trunk, often multiple, plaque-like with a rolled border. They may grow up to 10 cm in diameter.

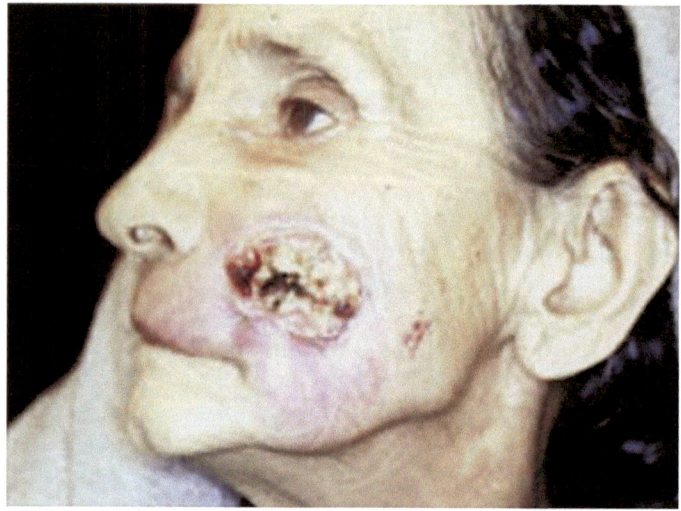

FIGURE 23.11. Basal cell carcinoma – rodent ulcer.

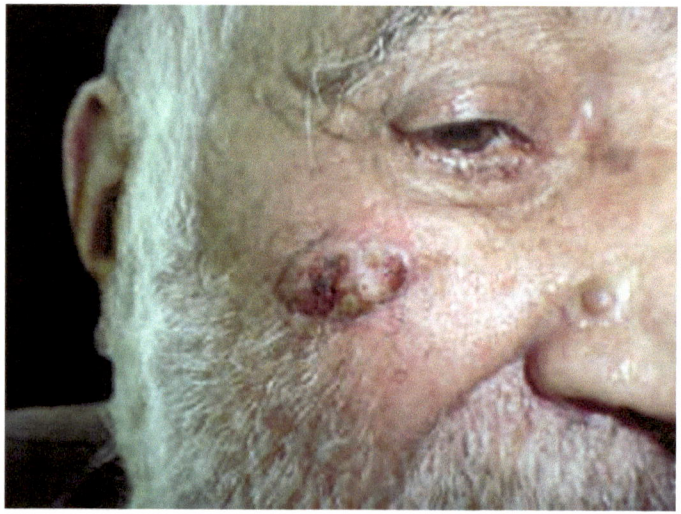

FIGURE 23.12. Basal cell carcinoma – nodulocystic type.

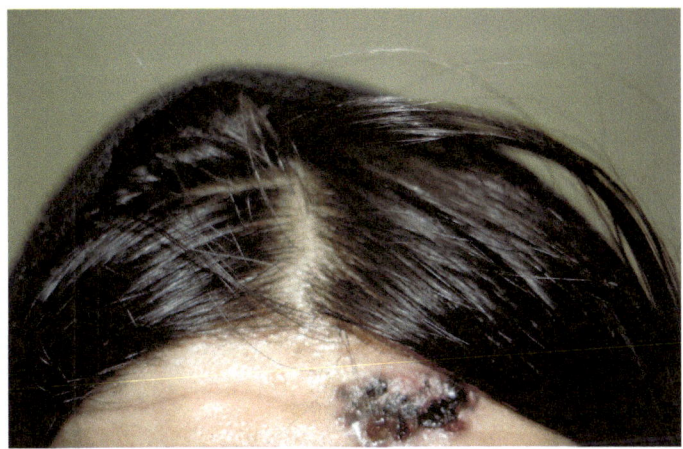

FIGURE 23.13. Pigmented basal cell carcinoma.

Morphoeic. This cicatricial variant is also common on the face; it appears as a white or yellow plaque with an ill-defined edge. Ulceration and fibrosis is common; it may have a central depression.

Pigmented basal cell carcinoma. The ulcerated, superficial, and the cystic type of BCC may have varying amount of melanin present. These tumors should be differentiated from other pigmented lesions particularly malignant melanoma (Fig. 23.13).

23.3.1.1 Differential Diagnosis

Early BCC should be differentiated from a molluscum contagiosum, sebaceous hyperplasia, or an intradermal naevus. The nodular/cystic type should be differentiated from a giant molluscum contagiosum, intradermal naevus, keratoacanthoma, and squamous cell carcinoma. The morphoeic type should be differentiated from morphoea and scars. A pigmented type should be differentiated from malignant melanoma, seborrhoeic wart, and compound naevus. The superficial type should be differentiated from discoid eczema, psoriatic plaque, tinea corporis, and Bowen's disease.

Diagnostic features of BCC are:

- Telangiectasia
- Pearly papules
- Rolled border
- History of bleeding and crusting

23.3.1.2 Treatment

- Surgical excision is the best method of treatment, with removal of 5 mm of the surrounding normal skin.
- In elderly patients small tumors can be removed by photo-dynamic therapy, cryosurgery or curettage and electro-dessication.
- The morphoeic type requires Mohs surgery. Mohs surgery is preferable for BCCs when present in areas where surgical excision is difficult such as near the inner canthus or naso-labial fold. Recurrent BCCs also require Mohs surgery.
- Radiotherapy is for large tumors in the elderly, where surgery is difficult. It should not be used on the dorsum of hands, shin, ears, and skull, due to necrosis of bone and cartilage.
- The skin should be protected from further sun damage.

Try to diagnose and treat cases of BCC early, especially those near the eye before local invasion occurs.

23.3.2 Squamous Cell Carcinoma (SCC)

The tumor arises from moderately well-differentiated kerati-nocytes of the skin. These malignant keratinocytes retain the ability to produce keratin; they destroy the dermo-epidermal junction and invade the dermis.

SCC does not usually arise on normal skin; it is often sec-ondary to chronic ulcers, chronic inflammations, chronic infections, burns, sun damage such as in a solar keratosis, radiation, etc. The first clinical sign is induration. The margins of induration are not sharp; the induration often extends beyond the visible margin of the lesion. The tissue around the

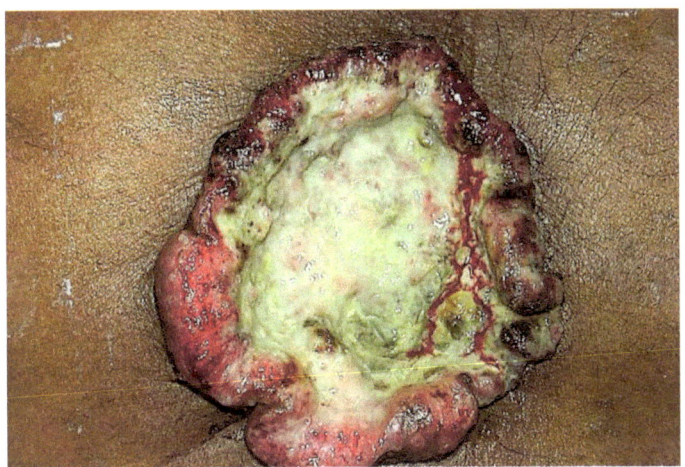

FIGURE 23.14. Squamous cell carcinoma.

tumor is inflamed; the edge is opaque and yellowish in color. Sun exposure is an important cause for the development of SCC as with other malignant skin tumors (Fig. 23.14).

On mobile structures such as the lips and genitals, the presenting sign may be a fissure or small erosion, which fails to heal and bleeds profusely.

The carcinogens that predispose to SCC are X-rays, tar, arsenic, mineral oil, etc. Tumors arising from sun-exposed sites seldom metastasize, but those arising form chronic ulcers, etc. are more likely to metastasize. Larger tumors are more likely to metastasize than smaller tumors.

SCC may be nodular, cauliflower-like, or it may be ulcerated. The characteristic sign is induration. The margins of an ulcerated SCC are firm and the border more raised than in a BCC.

23.3.2.1 Differential Diagnosis

SCC should be differentiated from keratoacanthoma, actinic keratosis, BCC, seborrhoeic keratosis, deep fungal infection, and tertiary syphilis.

Diagnostic features of SCC are:

- Usually solitary.
- Opaque growth not translucent like BCC.
- Indurated nodule or plaque.
- Surface may become crusted or ulcerated.
- Margin of the ulcer is more raised than BCC, often everted and irregular in shape.
- Sun-exposed sites commonly involved, or superimposed on a chronic lesion.

23.3.2.2 Treatment

- Surgical excision with removal of 5 mm of normal skin is the treatment of choice.
- Small tumor in the elderly can be treated by curettage and electrodessication.
- Mohs surgery as for BCC in selected cases.
- Protect the skin from further sun damage.

Percivall Pott (1714–1788)

Percivall Pott was a London surgeon who first gave the description for the fracture of the ankle, commonly known as Pott's fracture. Pott is said to have suffered this fracture himself, when crossing the London Bridge. He also described Pott's disease of the spine, due to tuberculosis.

Pott was the first man to identify an occupational cause of cancer; Chimney sweep's cancer of the scrotum, from repeated contamination with soot.

23.3.3 Malignant Melanoma

This is the most malignant tumor of the skin. It arises from the melanocytes of the epidermis. Like BCC and SCC, it is more common in fair-skinned people with excessive exposure to sun. Short repeated intense exposures to ultraviolet radiation causing burning as seen in sun-seeking holidays are more harmful than chronic sun exposure. The incidence of malignant melanoma has increased over the last 3 decades. The highest incidence is found among white people living in Australia and New Zealand. Ten to fifteen percent of melanomas are familial, molecular defects both in oncogenes and tumor suppressor genes have been linked to these tumors. Melanoma can affect several members of a family in association with familial dysplastic naevus.

The four main types of malignant melanoma are:

Superficial spreading melanoma. About 70% of all melanomas are superficial spreading melanomas, the lower leg and back are common sites in females and the back in males. Its radial growth shows varied colors, when a nodule occurs in such a plaque, it indicates dermal invasion and a poor prognosis.

Nodular melanoma is the most malignant, due to its early vertical growth. The pigmented nodule may grow rapidly and then ulcerate.

Lentigo maligna of the face is seen most often in elderly people; this is an "in situ" melanoma, confined to the epidermis. It often reaches a size of 5–7 mm in diameter before invasion into the dermis occurs when it is termed lentigo maligna melanoma.

Acral melanomas occur on the palms, soles, and distal portion of the fingers and toes. They are most frequent in blacks and Asians. They are often diagnosed late and have a poor prognosis. In their early phase they should be differentiated from "Talon noir" (pigmented petechial area due to trauma) (Fig. 23.15).

Totally, amelanotic melanomas are rare; these usually occur on the sole of feet. Flecks of pigment can be seen with a lens or dermatoscope.

The acronym ABCDE is a useful reminder of some of the clinical features that should raise the suspicion of melanoma in a pigmented lesion: Asymmetry of the lesion, Border irregularity, Color variegation, Diameter greater than 6 mm, and Elevation. The asymmetry of the lesion is the least useful criterion, but the other four criteria have diagnostic significance.

Pigmented naevi usually do not become malignant, those that may develop malignancy are the congenital melanocytic and dysplastic naevi. The signs of malignancy in these naevi are:

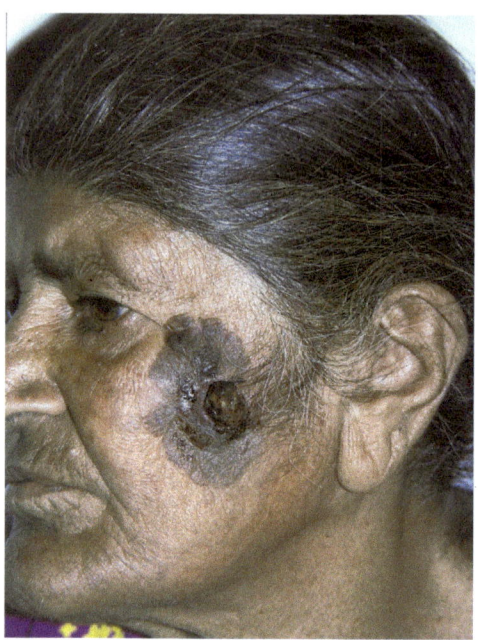

FIGURE 23.15. Lentigo Maligna Melanoma.

- Asymmetry of any mole should be thoroughly evaluated.
- The borders of a pigmented naevi are usually regular, with clear demarcation between the naevi and the surrounding skin. Naevi that develop irregular or ill-defined borders or notching should be evaluated.
- Bleeding from a mole needs assessment.
- The color of a mole is usually an even tan or brown, any variation from the normal should be assessed. Uneven distribution of shades and colors in a naevi should be suspected of malignant change.
- Diameter of a naevus is usually less than 6 mm: most melanomas are over 6 mm in diameter. Sometimes a small lesion may also become malignant.
- Family history of a melanoma, carries a higher risk of malignancy developing

Naevi should be considered as changing into a melanoma if they bleed, crust, itch, increase in size irregularly, or if they becomes inflamed.

23.3.3.1 Prognostic Criteria

Breslow's Prognostic Criteria

This histological method measures with the help of an ocular micrometer, the vertical distance from the granular layer to the deepest part of the tumour. The thicker the penetration, the worse the prognosis.

<0.75 mm 5-year survival 95%
0.76–1.5 mm 5-year survival 85%
1.51–4.0 mm 5-year survival 65%
>4.0 mm 5-year survival 45%

Clark's Prognostic Criteria

This relates to the depth of the tumor spread into the skin layers.

- Level I confined to the epidermis.
- Level II confined up to the papillary dermis.
- Level III confined up to the junction of the papillary and reticular dermis.
- Level IV confined up to the reticular dermis
- Level V infiltration in the subcutaneous tissue.
- Prognosis also depends upon the type of tumor, it is excellent for lentigo maligna, then the superficial spreading and the acral melanomas, and nodular melanoma has the worst prognosis. These differences relate to the depth of invasion of the melanoma at diagnosis. Ulceration in a melanoma is a poor prognostic sign.

Metastatic melanoma is that which has spread to the regional lymph nodes and other organs, it has a 5-year survival rate of less than 10%.

- Increased risk factors for melanoma.
- Individuals with a fair complexion.
- Individuals with numerous atypical-appearing melanocytic naevi or large congenital melanocytic naevi.
- Persons who have had a melanoma previously or have an immediate family member diagnosed with melanoma, 5% of melanomas are familial.
- Excessive exposure to ultraviolet radiation.

23.3.3.2 Differential Diagnosis

Malignant melanoma should be differentiated from pigmented basal cell carcinoma, seborrhoeic wart, dysplastic naevus, talon noir (pigmented petechial area on the heel following trauma) and melanocytic naevus.

23.3.3.3 Treatment

- Early diagnosis and treatment, excision with a measured margin of normal skin should be performed immediately. This margin can be narrow if diagnosis is in doubt, otherwise the following applies. Melanoma < 2 mm in thickness should be excised with a 1 cm margin of clinically normal skin down to the deep fascia. Melanoma > 2 mm thickness should be excised with 2 cm margin down to the fascia (current evidence is insufficient to address the optimal excision for all types of melanomas).
- Radio lymphatic sentinel node mapping and biopsy, is used for melanomas greater than 1 mm thickness and who do not have enlarged nodes on clinical examination. A radioactive dye is injected at the site of the melanoma. The first draining lymph node (sentinel lymph node) is identified by lymphoscintigraphy; this is examined for metastasis after biopsy. Regional lymphadenopathy is performed if the lymph node was involved. This is followed by adjuvant immunotherapy. At present this is primarily a staging procedure and does not improve mortality rates.

- Patients with lymph node metastasis have a poorer prognosis than those who have no metastasis. If metastasis has occurred then chemotherapy with dimethyltriazenyl alone or in combination with other chemotherapeutic agents is preferred.
- Immunotherapy is indicated for disseminated melanomas, with cytokines (interferons and interleukins), monoclonal antibodies, autologous lymphocytes, and specific immunization.
- For facial melanomas, Mohs surgery is preferred.
- In subungual melanomas, amputation of the affected digit is imperative. Involved lymph nodes should be removed.
- Lentigo maligna occurs in the elderly, in areas of actinic damage, surgery may leave unsatisfactory scars. Results with 5% imiquimod cream (aldara) have given satisfactory results when excisional surgery is contraindicated or declined.
- In all cases, follow-up is indicated, as recurrences are common. Once melanomas have spread beyond the skin, prospects for survival are very poor. Chemotherapy and radiation therapies are not very effective in the treatment of malignant melanomas.

Prevention is better than cure, avoid excessive sun exposure.
Patients with many and irregular moles should be taught self-examination.
Any change in a mole such as bleeding, crusting, pain, enlargement, or change of color should be reported immediately.
All doubtful lesions should be completely excised and sent for microscopic examination.

23.3.4 Cutaneous Lymphoma (Mycosis Fungoides)

The name mycosis fungoides is a misnomer; it is not a fungal infection but a cutaneous T cell lymphoma. Early stages of the disease present as premalignant eruptions, which appear as red scaly patches over the body or as a poikilodermatous eruption known as poikiloderma atrophicans vasculare. This is represented by reticular pigmentation, telangiectasia, and atrophy. As the condition progresses, the patches become pruritic with the formation of plaques, eventually bluish purple tumors appear.

The patch form (premycotic form of mycosis fungoides) may last for a number of years. The patches look like psoriasis or eczema. On close examination there is some atrophy with surface wrinkling, the patch is irregular in shape and the distribution is asymmetrical. Less commonly, the patch stage may become poikilodermic. On microscopy T cells (Mycosis fungoides cell) with cerebriform nuclei appear in the upper dermis; these invade the epidermis to give rise to Pautrier's microabscesses. The mycosis fungoides cell is formed by the blast transformation of a lymphocyte. It is a large cell with a cerebriform nucleus, pathognomonic for mycosis fungoides.

Plaque stage – as the lymphoma develops some patches become indurated and palpable.

Tumor stage – some of the plaques develop into tumors, which may become large like a mushroom (hence the name mycosis fungoides); this may then ulcerate.

The first two stages usually last about 20 years or more. The tumor stage is very short, metastasis leads to death within 3 years (Fig. 23.16).

Sezary syndrome – this is the leukemic stage of mycosis fungoides, in which T cells enter the blood stream. It is characterized by erythroderma, pruritus, and edema. Superficial lymphadenopathy and splenomegaly occur.

23.3.4.1 Differential Diagnosis

The patch and the plaque stage should be differentiated from eczema, psoriasis, dermatophytosis, and generalized leishmaniasis. The tumor stage, from lepromatous leprosy and neurofibromatosis.

23.3.4.2 Treatment

- Treatment is aimed to control rather than cure the disease. In the early stages the disease may be kept in check by the

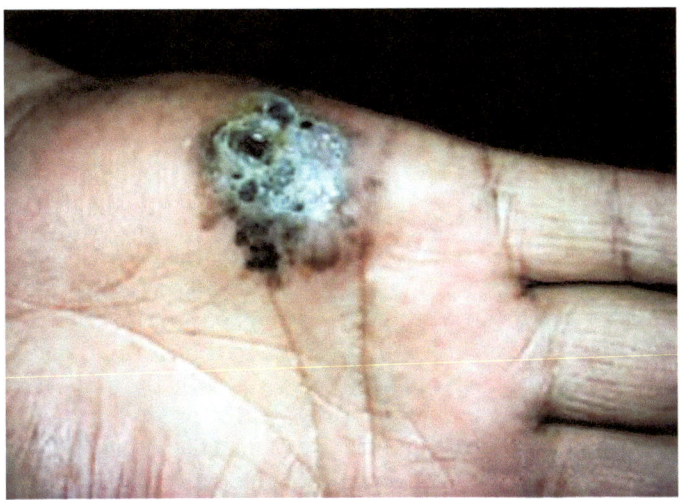

FIGURE 23.16. Acral melanoma.

topical application of corticosteroids some cases may survive up to 20 years before intensive treatment is required.
- In the later stages there are many lines of treatment including PUVA therapy, UVB, localized radiotherapy, whole body electron beam therapy, topical application of nitrogen mustard, and systemic cytotoxic drugs.
- Low-dose methotrexate, isotretinoin, or intramuscular injection of -interferon are used for recalcitrant cases.
- For Sezary syndrome chemotherapy is preferred. Extracorporeal photochemotherapy is also found to be beneficial.
- Systemic chemotherapy is disappointing.

Jean Louis Alibert (1768–1837)

Jean Louis Alibert is called the father of French Dermatology. He brought fame to the St. Louis Hospital as a center for dermatological training. He was the first to describe keloids and mycosis fungoides. His success largely stemmed from the fact that in addition to his ceaseless work with both patients and friends, he was a personification of courtesy and kindness.

Sezary and Bouvrain reported a triad of erythroderma, leukemia, and enlarged peripheral lymph nodes infiltrated with Sezary cells.

23.3.5 Kaposi's Sarcoma

Today the name is associated with AIDS. The disease was first noticed in Jews and East Europeans. Kaposi's sarcoma is a malignant tumor of proliferating capillaries and lymphatics. Two factors are responsible for its occurrence; release of an angiogenetic factor and a malignant transformation via an oncogenic virus. Human herpes virus 8 in the presence of immunosuppression is the primary factor in the development of all forms of Kaposi's sarcoma. Histologically, it consists of spindle-shaped cells and the presence of vascular elements.

The classical Kaposi's sarcoma begins as reddish, blue, or purple macules on the feet and ankles; they are also present on the acral parts of the body. They may develop into verrucous plaques or nodules. Legs may become edematous and lymphadenopathy may occur. These changes are found in Jews and East Europeans.

Endemic Kaposi's sarcoma is the most aggressive type, death usually occurs in a year or two. The tumor occurs on the legs and thigh as nodules or florid infiltrations. Lymphadenopathy is common. This tumor is most prevalent in Africans.

Kaposi's sarcoma associated with immunosuppression. This develops in patients with transplant surgery. The tumor is aggressive; lymph nodes and viscera are involved in most cases. Some tumors regress when immunosuppressive therapy is withdrawn, others respond to radiation and chemotherapy.

Epidemic Kaposi's sarcoma is associated with AIDS and immunodeficiency. The lesions appear as reddish purple papules or plaques, on the head or neck, or any part of the body, they may be single or multiple. Ten percent have erythema nodosum as the sole manifestation. A fulminant and progressive course is expected. It is interesting that HIV positive intravenous drug abusers do not develop Kaposi's sarcoma as often as HIV positive homosexuals.

23.3.5.1 Differential Diagnosis

Kaposi's sarcoma should be differentiated from benign vascular proliferations, sarcoidosis, histiocytosis, and other type of sarcomas.

23.3.5.2 Treatment

- All types are radiosensitive, local radiotherapy is highly effective. Surgical excision for single tumors and cryotherapy (three treatments at 3-week intervals) are alternatives. Cytotoxic therapy is indicated for rapid progressive disease. The Klein regimen of weekly I/V vinblastine 4–6 mg is one of the first lines of treatment. Other drugs used are doxorubin, bleomycin, and vincristine.
- AIDS-related Kaposi's sarcoma responds to local radiotherapy, cryosurgery, I/L injections of vinblastine, interleukin, or interferon. For systemic disease, HAART (highly active antiretroviral therapy) is the treatment of choice.
- Systemic treatment with α-interferon has also been found to be helpful.

Early Kaposi's sarcoma looks subtle, often like a bruise, keep HIV in mind.

Kaposi

Kaposi was Hebra's successor and son-in-law. He was a man of action and gifted with a brilliant mind. He described many skin disorders, best-known are: Kaposi's sarcoma, Kaposi's varicelliform eruption and xeroderma pigmentosa. He contributed to the existing knowledge of herpes zoster, sarcoidosis, lichen planus, and other dermatoses. Kaposi was a master therapist, an excellent teacher and orator with a sparkling temperament.

23.3.6 Paget's Disease of the Nipple

This is due to the extension of an underlying intraduct carcinoma of the breast. It appears as an involuted red scaly eczematous-like patch on the nipple; such cases are often treated for eczema, and fail to respond. An excisional biopsy should be taken to confirm the diagnosis. Eczema of the

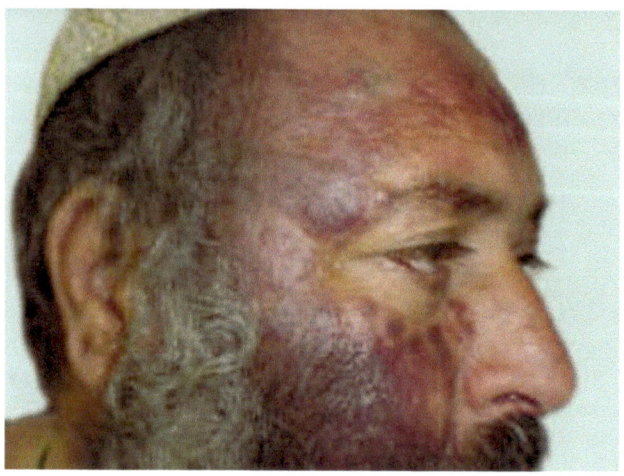

FIGURE 23.17. Mycosis fungoides.

nipple is often bilateral and responds to topical steroids. Over the course of months or years, Paget's disease becomes infiltrated and ulcerated. The plaque of Paget's disease is indurated, has sharp margins, and is fixed to the underlying skin structures. The nipple may or may not retract. The disease is more common in women but carries a worse prognosis in men. Extramammary Paget's disease may involve the anogenital areas due to an underlying apocrine gland tumor (Fig. 23.17).

The disease is characterized by the presence of Paget's cells, these cells are large, round and clear-staining with a large nucleus. They appear singly or in small nests between the keratinocytes. Paget's cells undergoing mitosis are frequent. In the dermis an inflammatory reaction is often present (Fig. 23.18).

23.3.6.1 Treatment

- This is the same as that of breast carcinoma, mastectomy, and removal of the affected axillary glands.

James Paget (1814–1899)

James Paget is best known for the eponym Paget's disease of the nipples and Paget's disease of the bones. He discovered trichinia infestation in

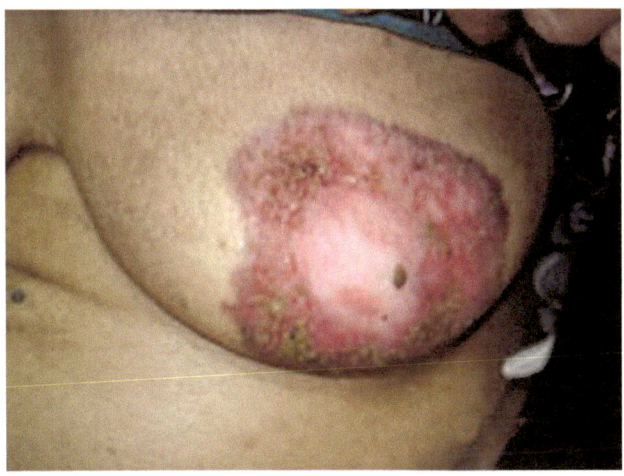

FIGURE 23.18. Paget's disease.

human muscles. He wrote brilliant essays and gave painstakingly prepared eloquent lectures at St. Bartholomew's Hospital. He had the reputation of being the best surgical diagnostician in Britain.

Basal cell carcinoma is the most common and least malignant tumor of the skin.

Malignant melanoma is the most malignant skin tumor.

Exclude AIDS in Kaposi's sarcoma.

All pigmented lesions should be examined to exclude malignant melanoma, especially in the elderly.

Suspect Bowen's disease in an erythematous plaque not responding to treatment. Eczema of the nipples is often bilateral and responds to topical steroids.

Think of Paget's disease in patients with retracted nipples.

When multiple skin tags are present, exclude diabetes and hyperlipidemias

Internal malignancy should be excluded when multiple seborrhoeic warts occur suddenly.

The dimpling sign is characteristic of dermatofibroma.

For painful tumors keep this acronym in mind "BANGLES" Blue rubber bleb naevus, Angiolipoma, Neuroma, Leomyoma, Glioma, Eccrine Spiradenoma.

Cutaneous signs of internal malignancy in Chap. 26

Chapter 24
Naevi and Hereditary Disorders of the Skin

24.1 Naevi

They are uncommon developmental abnormalities of the skin, due to excess or diminution in one or more constituents of the skin. Histologically, the cells are identical or closely resemble normal cells. Naevi can be epidermal, pigmented, follicular, vascular sebaceous, dermal, etc.

24.1.1 Epidermal Naevi

These usually appear as a linear verrucous growth along the length of a limb (Fig. 24.1). Lumbar or sacral regions are common sites for connective tissue naevi. *Sebaceous naevi* are commonly found on the scalp; they appear as yellowish, linear, verrucous growths which are devoid of hair. Sebaceous naevi may be associated with abnormalities of the epidermis and sweat glands. These naevi may develop malignant changes at puberty; they should be excised prior to this. *Becker's epidermal pigmented naevus* is an epidermal pigmented naevus showing hyperpigmentation. The lesion appears in young men at adolescence on the shoulder, upper and lower back and/or submammary areas as a hyperpigmented patch, which slowly enlarges and later becomes hairy; the borders are irregular and sharply demarcated (Fig. 24.2). It may sometimes be associated with other anomalies such as hamartomas of smooth

Z. Zaidi, S. W. Lanigan, *Dermatology in Clinical Practice*,
DOI 10.1007/978-1-84882-862-9_24,
© Springer-Verlag London Limited 2010

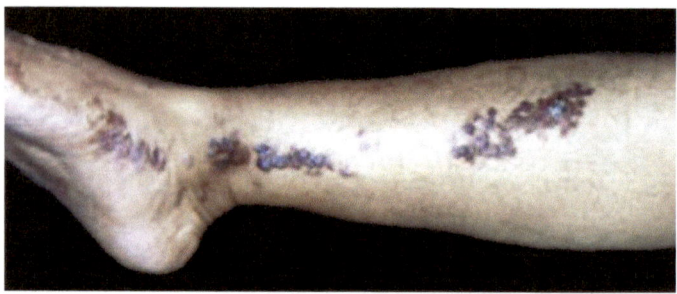

FIGURE 24.1. Linear epidermal naevus.

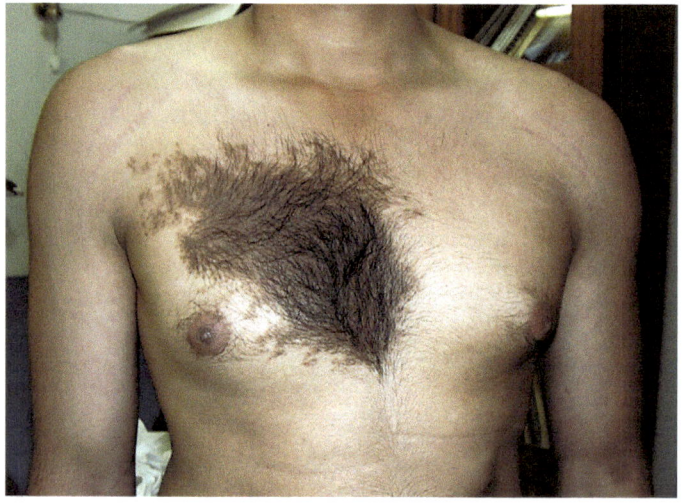

FIGURE 24.2. Beckers naevus.

muscles, hypoplasia of the breast, scoliosis, spina bifida, or hypoplasia of the limbs. The lesions are usually benign.

24.1.2 Vascular Naevi

These naevi are due to dilatation or hyperplasia of the blood vessels. The two common vascular naevi are the Port wine stain and the hemangioma. A *Port wine stain* is due to dilatation of the cutaneous blood vessels. It is present at birth, as a pink or reddish rash on the face of an infant. It usually follows the distribution of a branch of the trigeminal nerve. The condition remains persistent throughout life. It may cause considerable disfigurement to the patient (Fig 24.3). It may be associated with underlying cerebrovascular defects, which may cause epilepsy and hemiplegia. Glaucoma should always be excluded in these cases. Laser therapy is effective but the treatment is slow and expensive. Superficial lesions are treated with the pulsed dye laser. Camouflage is an alternative.

Strawberry hemangioma is a reddish growth that develops soon after birth; it is due to hyperplasia and proliferation of cutaneous blood vessels (Fig. 24.4). It increases in size for about 6–8 months of age, remains static for about 2 years; it then involutes by the fourth year in the majority. It should disappear by the time the child is 4–6 years.

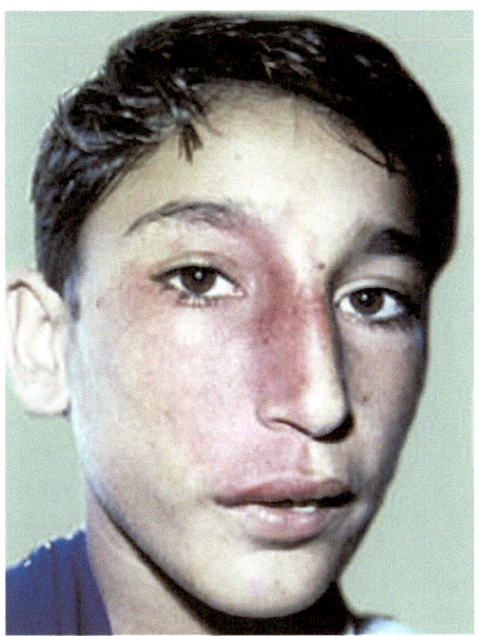

FIGURE 24.3. Port wine stain.

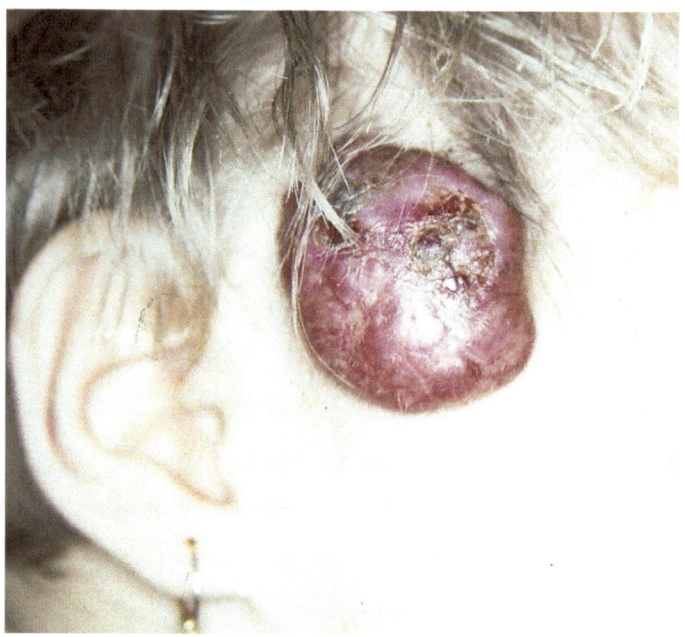

FIGURE 24.4. Hemangioma.

Residual changes including telangiectasia and redundant tissue are not uncommon. Strawberry angiomas should not be treated unless complications occur such as hemorrhage, pressure symptoms, cardiac failure, infection, and purpura secondary to platelet consumption.

24.1.3 Pigmented Naevi (Moles)

Moles are due to proliferation of cells derived from melanocytes. These cells differ from normal melanocytes; they are larger, lack dendrites and have more cytoplasm which has coarse granules. These begin as proliferation from the melanocytes at the basal layer as in *junctional naevus*, the proliferation then extends into the dermis forming the *compound naevus*; when these cells lose their connection with the epidermis the result is the formation of an *intradermal naevus*. A few naevi are present in every individual, these are the most common naevi present in man. Pigmented naevi continue to appear until the fourth to fifth decade and then decline in number. Some naevi may darken and itch during adolescence and pregnancy. Otherwise, symptomatic naevi should alert the attention of the physician for malignancy. The most important fact to remember is that the pigmentation in a benign naevus tends to be uniform. A hand lens and a dermoscope are important instruments to differentiate a benign naevus from a malignant melanoma.

Junctional naevi are flat pigmented lesions; the color varies from light to dark brown, these pigmented naevi are usually less than 6 mm in diameter. They are sharply circumscribed. Compound naevi (Common mole) present as small raised pigmented papules, which have a smooth surface; these may increase in size and pigmentation at puberty, course hair may appear (Fig. 24.5). Intradermal naevi are dome-shaped, verrucous, pedunculated, or sessile, they may be pigmented or nonpigmented.

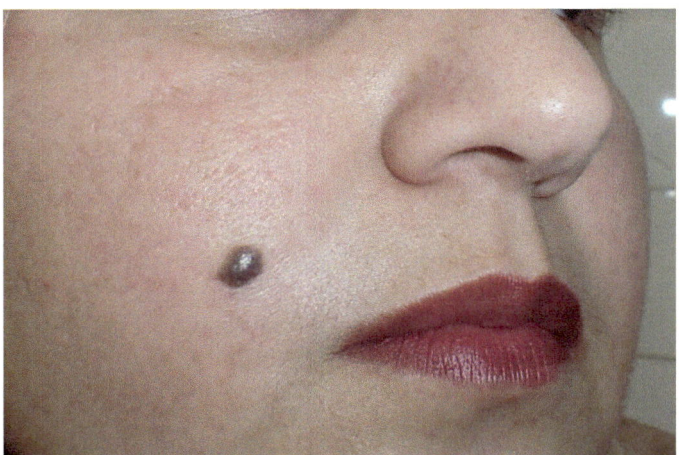

FIGURE 24.5. Common mole.

Other pigmented naevi are congenital melanocytic naevi, naevus spilus, Spitz naevus, blue naevus, halo naevus, and the dysplastic naevi.

Congenital melanocytic naevi are present at birth, they vary in size from a few millimeters to several centimeters in length. Large pigmented naevi on the trunk are known as bathing trunk naevi. Small congenital naevi (size upto 15 mm) have a minor chance of developing malignant melanoma. The medium-sized congenital naevi (size from 15 mm to 20 cm) should be managed conservatively or excised if suspicious of malignancy. Lifelong medical supervision seems a reasonable approach. Chances of malignancy depend upon the histology; if the epidermal element is prominent the chances of malignant change are very low. Large melanocytic naevi may undergo malignant transformation. The incidence ranges from 1.8% to 7.1%. About half of the melanomas occur by the age of 3–5 years. These lesions present a difficult management problem. The treatment of choice is excision, but this is often impossible because of their size in a small infant. Curettage of the superficial dermal component in the first few weeks of life has its advocates both for cosmetic benefit but also to reduce the number of melanocytes in the lesion (Fig. 24.6).

Naevus spilus is a large brown macule, irregular in shape, speckled with hyperpigmented dots. The chances of it developing malignant change are very low. Excision is not necessary.

Spitz naevus (juvenile melanoma) is not a true melanoma, but a naevus. It is a variant of compound naevus; the dermal blood vessels are dilated, giving rise to the red color of the naevus. The naevus cells are larger with abundant cytoplasm; they may be spindle-shaped or epitheloid-like. The naevus occurs on the face of young children. Pink or light brown in color, it is dome-shaped and smooth in its early stages and can become warty later. Lesions vary in size from 3 to 15 mm. The naevus should be removed by local excision, when the diagnosis is in doubt.

Blue naevus. This naevus occurs due to the failure of melanocytes to reach the epidermis. The brown pigment absorbs

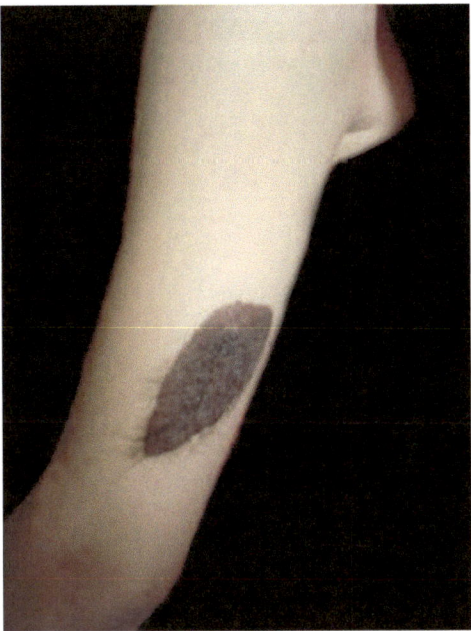

FIGURE 24.6. Congenital melanotic hairy naevus.

longer wavelengths of light and scatters the blue light (Tyndall effect). The naevus appears in childhood; it is most common on the extremities and dorsa of the hands. A variant of cellular blue naevus which is larger and nodular, is frequently located on the buttocks.

The other dermal naevi are the Mongolian spot (around the sacrum), naevus of Ito (affects the shoulder girdle), and naevus of Ota (affects the skin area around the eye, the sclera is also pigmented (Fig. 24.7).

Halo naevus. This is a melanocytic naevus surrounded by hypopigmentation. The hypopigmentation is thought to be due to a prominent host lymphocytic response, which attacks the naevus and may be responsible for its disappearance.

Dysplastic melanocytic naevi. These naevi are often an enigma to clinicians as they have many clinical and histological features of a malignant melanoma. The naevi may occur sporadically or

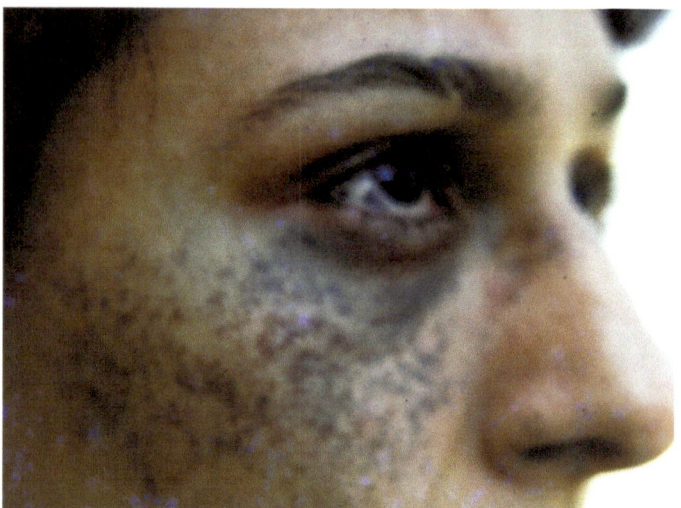

FIGURE 24.7. Naevus of Ota.

are inherited as an autosomal dominant trait. Dysplastic naevi rarely occur before the age of 10 years. They are often multiple, have irregular borders and are unevenly pigmented, commonly found on the trunk. They vary in size from 5 to 15 mm; some have an inflammatory halo around them (Fig. 24.8). They increase in size at puberty. Some may have a fried egg appearance; with a central raised portion surrounded by a flat surface. On microscopy, there is a lengthening and bridging of the rete pegs, presence of melanocytic dysplasia, fibrosis of the papillary dermis, and a lymphocytic inflammatory response. Nests of atypical melanocytes are in elongated nests or singly at the dermo-epidermal interface, oriented parallel to the surface. Atypical melanocytes are found in the upper epidermis, but there is not a distinct pagetoid spread.

Patients with a family history of melanoma are at an increased risk of melanoma. Malignant melanoma may also arise from previously normal skin. Malignancy in a naevus should be considered if the following changes occur:

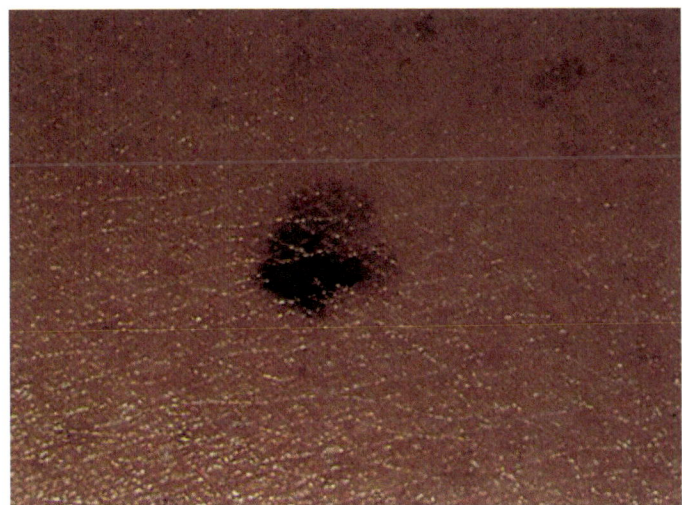

FIGURE 24.8. Dysplastic naevus.

- Increase in size
- Bleeding
- Itching
- Increase or decrease in pigmentation
- Inflammation
- Ulceration
- Alteration in shape
- Alteration in contour
- Irregularity in outline, color, or edge should prompt suspicion

24.1.3.1 Treatment

Patients should take special precautions to reduce sun exposure; sunscreens are necessary. A whole-body photograph of the moles at regular intervals is helpful to detect any change that occurs in them. Patients should also be taught self-assessment of their moles. If any change occurs that is suspicious of a melanoma, the naevus should be excised.

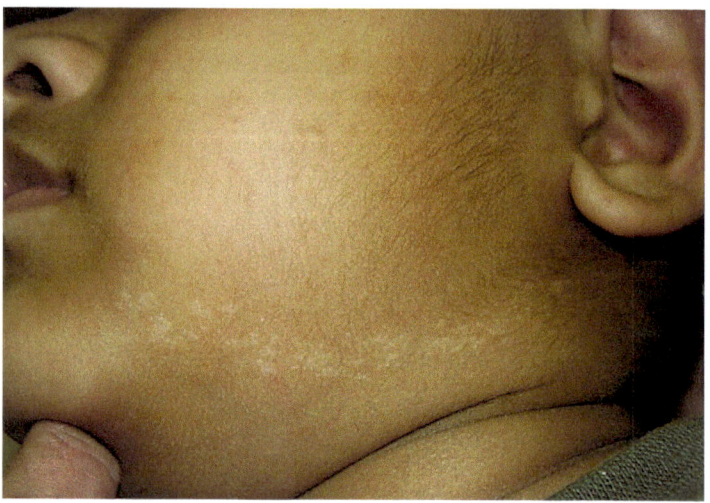

FIGURE 24.9. Nevus achromic.

24.1.4 Naevus Achromicus

Areas of depigmentation are present at birth. The lesions may be single or multiple. These may be round, in a linear distribution or in whorls (Fig. 24.9). The number of melanocytes in naevus achromicus is normal but there is a defect in the transfer of melanasomes from the melanocytes to the keratinocytes.

This should be differentiated from naevus anemicus, in which the pale color of the naevus is due to vasoconstriction. The naevus does not become red with rubbing.

24.1.5 Lymphangioma

This is a naevus of lymphatic vessels. It may be present at any age but is usually noted at birth or appears in childhood. The common sites are the axillary folds, shoulders, neck, proximal parts of a limb, perineum, tongue, and the buccal mucous membrane. It presents as a group of deep-seated vesiculopapules,

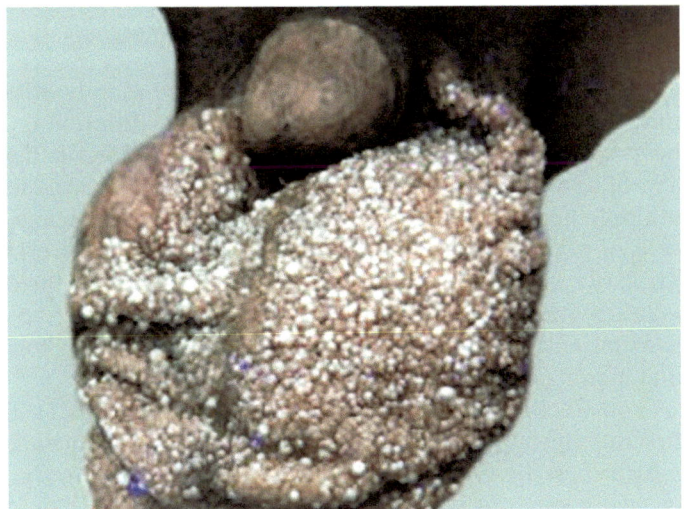

FIGURE 24.10. Lymphangioma.

resembling frogspawn. They are yellowish in color but some may be pink or red in color due to the presence of fresh or altered blood (Fig. 24.10). Lymphangioma circumscriptum may be caused by lymphatic cisterns with muscular walls situated in the subcutaneous tissue.

These naevi should be differentiated from molluscum contagiosum, lymphangioma are compressible with a glass depressor while molluscum are not. Lymphangiomas should only be removed as a last resort for symptomatic lesions, removal of the subcutaneous tissue is necessary or they are likely to recur.

24.1.6 Connective Tissue Naevus

The term is used for cutaneous hamartomas that comprise primarily collagen (collagenomas) and elastic (elastomas) tissue, or it may be a combination of these two. These naevi are produced by fibroblasts. Collagenomas are skin-colored while elastomas may be skin-colored or yellowish.

24.2 Neurofibromatosis

It is an autosomal dominant disorder, which mainly affects
the nervous system, skin, and the bones. Many different types
have been identified; the two most commonly described are
Type 1 and Type 2. Type 1 comprises about 85% of cases, with
multiple neurofibromas; these are derived from the Schawnn
cells of peripheral nerves (Fig. 24.11). Type 2 is characterized
primarily by acoustic neuromas, and few or no cutaneous
manifestations. Leish nodules are absent. There may be an
association with other tumours of the CNS, mainly gliomas
and meningiomas.

Von Recklinghausen's disease (neurofibromatosis 1). The
first manifestation of the disease is the appearance of *café-au-
lait patches*, these are pigmented macules, irregular in shape,
usually present at birth, or they may appear later. Their size
and number increase with age. Six or more cafe-au-lait
patches are diagnostic of neurofibromatosis (0.5 cm or more

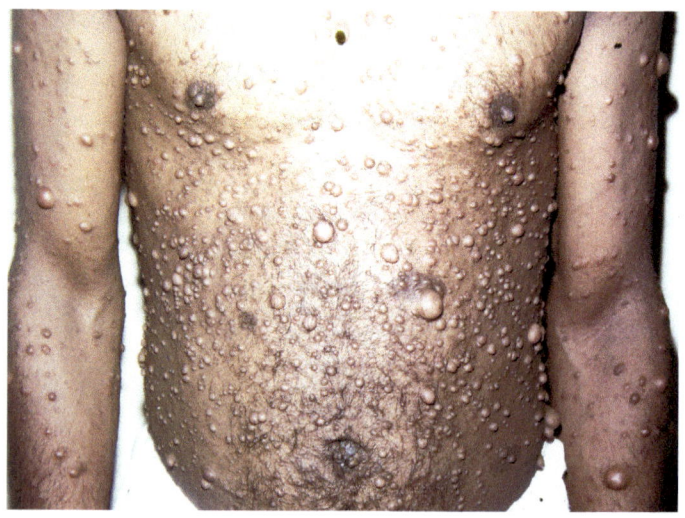

FIGURE 24.11. Neurofibromatosis.

in prepubertal patients and >1.5 cm in postpubertal patients). *Intertriginous freckling* is present in two-thirds of cases. This is pathognomonic of neurofibromatosis; it may occur in the axillae, groin, or inframammary region.

Leish nodules are pigmented, melanocytic iris hamartomas. They increase in number with age, and are asymptomatic. They appear before the neurofibromas, and can help in the diagnosis of neurofibromatosis. These can be more easily seen with the help of a slit lamp.

Neurofibromas are skin-colored, soft tumors, in the form of a papule or nodule, which can be sessile or pedunculated. On compression, they can be invaginated in what seems like a defect of the skin. This is called the buttonhole sign. They are usually present by the age of 8 years; in some cases these may not appear until puberty. A large tumor along the course of a nerve is called a plexiform neuroma. These tumors may become malignant.

The order of appearance of the cutaneous and ocular signs of neurofibromatosis are cafe-au-lait patches, axillary freckling, Leish nodules, and neurofibromas.

The other manifestations of neurofibromatosis 1 are kyphoscoliosis, short stature, macrocephaly, mental retardation, epilepsy, optic glioma, occlusion of the renal artery, pseudoarthrosis of the tibia, and atraumatic fractures. Endocrinal disorders such as phaeochromocytomas, thyroid disorders, acromegaly, and precocious puberty may occur.

24.2.1 Treatment

As the lesions are benign, they need no treatment but should be watched for any change to indicate malignancy, although this is rare. The tumors may be removed for cosmetic reasons. A patient with neuromatosis should be investigated for neurological and other associations when first seen by the physician. An associated hypertension should raise the possibility of pheochromocytoma.

24.3 Adenoma Sebaceum
     (Tuberous Sclerosis)

Also known as Bourneville's disease, this includes the triad of angiofibromas, mental retardation, and epilepsy. It is an autosomal dominant disorder with variable expression. The first sign to appear is the *ash leaf macule* (oval at one end and pointed at the other); these vary in size from 1 to 3 cm, mostly seen on the trunk. Tuberous sclerosis is highly likely if more than three white spots are detected. A tuft of white hair with no depigmentation of the scalp has been reported as an early sign of tuberous sclerosis.

The other cutaneous manifestations are *angiofibromas*. These are usually present by the age of 4, but may appear first at puberty, or they proliferate at puberty. These are firm, red papules, most prominent on the face, at the nasolabial folds, cheeks, and chin (Fig. 24.12). Another cutaneous lesion is the *forehead plaque*; this is a large fibroangioma. *Periungal fibromas* appear at puberty; these are firm, skin-coloured growths

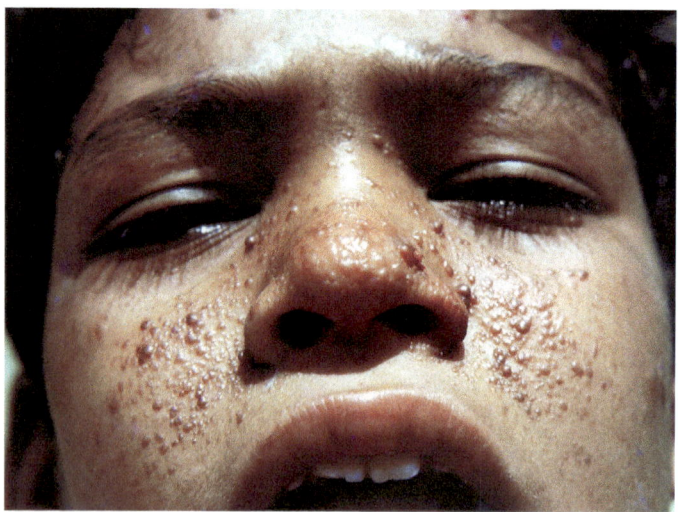

FIGURE 24.12. Adenoma sebaceum.

projecting from the lateral nail folds. A *Shagreen* patch (connective tissue naevus) is a yellowish irregular thickened plaque over the base of the spine. It occurs in early childhood; the lesion may vary from 1 to 10 cm in diameter.

Benign tumors consisting of vascular tissue, fibrous tissue, fat, and smooth muscle are found in numerous organs, including the kidneys, liver, and gastrointestinal tract. Retinal phakomas occur in 25% of cases. Dental enamel pitting is seen in all adult patients. The CNS manifestations of tuberous sclerosis are subependymal nodules, sclerotic patches of astrocytes and giant cells. Calcification of intracranial nodules is common (tubers). Retinal tumors, cardiac rabdomyomas, and bony abnormalities such as cysts and sclerosis may also occur.

24.3.1 Treatment

Dermabrasion, electrodessication, cryosurgery, and laser can remove facial adenomas for cosmetic reasons; but they tend to recur. All cases of adenoma sebaceum should be examined for systemic manifestations on first diagnosis. The investigations should include ophthalmic, abdominal, renal and cardiac assessment, skull X-ray for tubers, and cranial magnetic resonance imaging.

Hereditary disorders of keratinization in Chapter 9.
Hereditary bullous disorders in Chapter 11.
Hereditary disorders of connective tissue in Chapter 10.

Chapter 25
Skin and Malnutrition

Malnutrition is not only seen in developing countries, but it is also prevalent in the West, where it is associated with a variety of diseases. It accompanies any disease that disturbs appetite, digestion, absorption, and utilization of nutrients. Malnutrition can occur secondary to malignancy, malabsorption due to ulcerative colitis or Crohn's disease, after prolonged vomiting, in alcoholism, after resection of a large portion of the small intestine, in old age where adequate nutrition is often neglected, in anorexia nervosa, and atrophic gastritis, which leads to *cyanocobalamin* deficiency. Drugs that cause malabsorption include colchicine, methotrexate, neomycin, cholestyramine, biguanamides, some laxatives, etc. These cases are often missed in clinical practice, as more importance is given to the primary disease that dominates the clinical picture. Generally the skin in malnutrition is dry, pruritic, with symmetrical hyperpigmentation; the nails and hair are brittle.

Malnutrition can be measured in adults by measuring the body mass index (BMI). BMI = weight (kg)/height^2 (m^2).

BMI 20–25	Normal
BMI 18.5–20	Marginal malnutrition
BMI 17–18.5	Mild malnutrition
BMI 16–17	Moderate malnutrition
BMI < 16	Severe malnutrition

Z. Zaidi, S. W. Lanigan, *Dermatology in Clinical Practice*, 447
DOI: 10.1007/978-1-84882-862-9_25,
© Springer-Verlag London Limited 2010

Weight loss of more than 10% in less than 3 months, BMI of less than 19 kg/m², and peripheral edema are indicative of protein calorie malnutrition.

Acute vitamin deficiency is much more frequent with water-soluble vitamins (especially vitamin B1 and vitamin C) than with fat-soluble vitamins, as these have sufficient body stores. Vitamin B1 deficiency is seen in alcoholics and in people with prolonged vomiting. It develops acutely, often in less than 3 weeks, resulting in Wernicke's encephalopathy. Folate stores are small and deficiency can occur quickly giving rise to macrocytic anemia.

Malabsorption of proteins can lead to muscular atrophy and weight loss, while any resulting hypoproteinemia will result in edema.

Malabsorption of fats is characterized by fatty stools (steatorrhea) and weight loss due to lack of these high-caloric components of the diet. Lack of fat-soluble vitamins follows if the cause of fat malabsorption is due to lack of bile salts.

Malabsorption of carbohydrates results in distention and flatulence. If more than 80 g/day of carbohydrates fail to be absorbed, watery diarrhea occurs.

Marasmus and Kwashiokor are common in underdeveloped countries.

Marasmus is derived from a Greek word "marasmos," which means wasting. It is a severe form of starvation. It is often seen in developing countries due to economic problems, improper weaning due to ignorance, poor hygiene, etc. Protein calorie malnutrition leads to suppression of growth, loss of weight, and emaciation results. The skin is dry, loose, and wrinkled due to the loss of subcutaneous fat. The sunken and drawn appearance of the face is due to the loss of buccal fat giving the typical monkey facies appearance. Follicular hyperkeratosis may be prominent in adult persons. The hair is thin and sparse, nails are fissured and cutaneous ulcerations may occur.

Kwashiorkor is characterized by protein malnutrition that impairs growth, produces changes in the skin and hair; there is edema of the feet and a potbelly prominence.

The changes in the skin and hair are striking; they vary from reddish yellow to gray or even white. The hair is dry, scaly, and lusterless; curly hair becomes straight, especially striking is the "flag sign" affecting long dark hair. During periods of poor nutrition, the hair is pale; alternating bands of dark and light hair is this seen, indicating period of good and poor nutrition.

The skin in early stages of kwashiorkor is scaly and erythematous; later these patches become hard, scaly, and distinctively elevated like an "enamel paint" appearance. Other signs of malnutrition are present such as angular stomatitis, glossitis, pallor, etc.

Children affected with kwashiorkor have poor development, their height and weight is below normal and diarrhea is common. There is edema of the feet and face due to hypoalbuminemia. The edema later becomes generalized, subcutaneous fat is lost, and muscles become wasted. The child is irritable and does not smile; smiling is a sign of recovery. The child is prone to bacterial and parasitic infection.

25.1 Vitamin and Mineral Deficiency and Their Effects on the Skin

Vitamins and minerals	Effects on the skin due to deficiency
Vitamin A	Follicular hyperkeratosis, rough and dry skin, night blindness
Vitamin D	Thinning of skin, veins become prominent, diffuse alopecia, rickets in children, and osteomalacia in adults
Vitamin K	Purpura
Vitamin E	Inhibitory effect on hyaluronic acid and cause of wrinkles, infertility
Vitamin C	Clotting defects, poor wound healing, hemorrhage around the hair follicles
Vitamin B1 (thiamine)	Wet and dry beri beri. Skin is edematous and waxy, tongue red with burning sensation

(*continued*)

(continued)

Vitamins and minerals	Effects on the skin due to deficiency
Vitamin B2 (riboflavin)	Oro-genito-ocular syndrome. Stomatitis, cheilitis, corneal vascularization, nasolabial seborrhea, redness, and scaling of the vulva and scrotum
Vitamin B3 (nicotinic acid)	Pellagra - diarrhea, dementia, and dermatitis on sun-exposed parts of the body
Vitamin B6 (pyridoxine)	Cheilitis, glossitis, and seborrhea
Vitamin B12 (cyanocobalamin)	Glossitis, canities, hyperpigmentation especially flexures, anemia
Vitamin H (biotin)	Seborrhoeic dermatitis like lesions, alopecia, conjunctivitis, paraesthesias
Folic acid	Diffuse hyperpigmentation, glossitis, cheilitis, megaloblastic anemia
Iron	Microcytic anemia, glossitis, cheilitis, koilonychia
Selenium	Seborrhoeic dermatitis like lesions
Sulphur	Impaired growth of hair and nails
Calcium	Tetany, proximal myopathy, perioral paraesthesia, mental depression. Cutaneous deposits in hypercalcemia
Zinc	Acrodermatitis enteropathica, alopecia, depression

25.1.1 Treatment

Malnourished patients should be given nutritional support; this can be in the form of oral supplements such as high-caloric diet, protein-rich diet, and vitamin supplements, depending upon the type of deficiency present in the patient. Other forms of intake are by nasogastric tube, percutaneous entrogastostomy, or the total parental route, depending upon the patient's condition. The oral route is preferable due to the decreased risk of infection compared to intubation; it is cheaper and the patient compliance is good.

Remove the cause leading to malnutrition. Many diets are now available for the treatment of specific gastrointestinal conditions and for nonspecific symptoms. Teach the patient how to maintain a well-balanced diet at home.

Chapter 26
Skin and Systemic Disease

Skin is a mirror for the internal organs. A number of systemic disorders have cutaneous manifestations.

26.1 Diabetes Mellitus

Cutaneous manifestations may be vascular, neuropathic, infective, and miscellaneous.

26.1.1 Vascular Manifestations

Both the small and large blood vessels are involved. Microangiopathy leads to the formation of reddish papules on the leg (*diabetic dermopathy*) (Fig. 26.1), that heals by scarring. *Rubeosis* is a reddish discoloration of the face, due to dilatation of the blood vessels; this is related to decreased vascular tone. *Necrobiosis lipoidica diabeticorum* occurs mostly on the shin, less commonly on the forehead. The initial lesion is a reddish papule, which develops into a plaque. The plaque is surrounded by hyperpigmentation, later there is atrophy in the center, which becomes yellowish in color. Ulceration can occur. Stiff skin syndrome (*diabetic scleropathy*) occurs on the fingers and hands. The palm and the fingers of the two hands cannot be opposed properly.

Z. Zaidi, S. W. Lanigan, *Dermatology in Clinical Practice*,
DOI 10.1007/978-1-84882-862-9_26,
© Springer-Verlag London Limited 2010

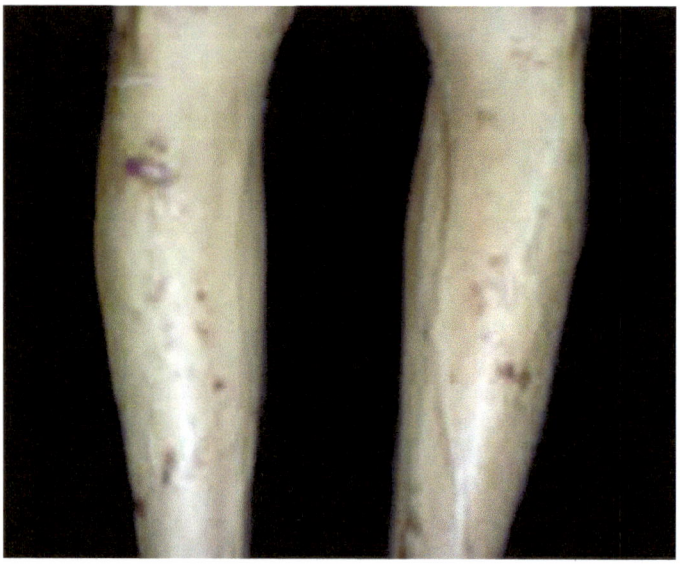

FIGURE 26.1. Diabetic dermopathy.

The involvement of large blood vessels leads to intermittent claudication, the limbs are pale and cold and gangrene of the legs and feet may occur (Fig. 26.2).

26.1.2 Diabetic Neuropathy

This affects the motor, sensory, and autonomic nervous system. Sensory involvement leads to paraesthesias, numbness, and tingling of the hands and feet. Digitally displaced subluxed digits, depressed metatarsal heads, hammertoes and pes cavus characterize motor neuropathy. Autonomic neuropathy leads to decreased sweating in the lower half of the body and increased sweating in the upper half. Painless slowly penetrating ulcers develop on the sole of the foot and pressure points. This is due to both loss of sensations and diabetic vascular lesions.

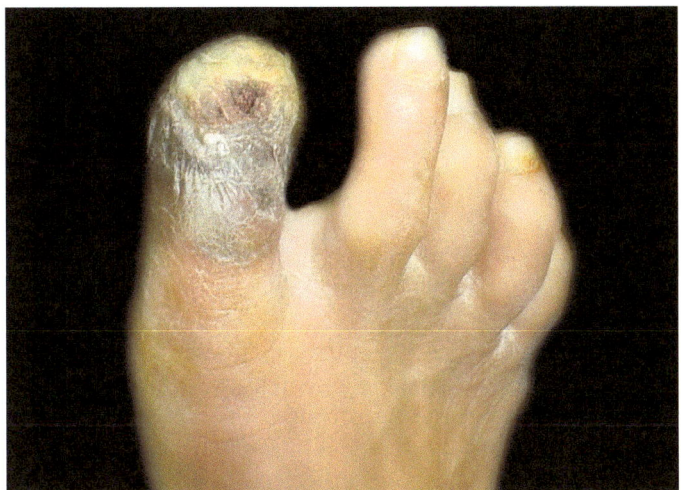

FIGURE 26.2. Diabetic gangrene.

26.1.3 Infections

Diabetic patients are prone to bacterial, fungal, and viral infections, probably due to decrease in neutrophil function. The most serious infection is malignant otitis externa, due to pseudomonas infection. This infection may lead to osteitis, cranial nerve damage, and meningitis.

26.1.4 Miscellaneous

These include generalized granuloma annulare, acanthosis nigricans, skin tags, eruptive xanthomas, Kyrles disease, hemochromatosis, vitiligo, generalized pruritus, carotenemia, and diabetic bullae. These bullae arise on normal skin usually on the hands and feet; they heal in 2–5 weeks.

26.2 Liver Disease

The association between the liver and skin has been known since centuries. Varieties of pigmented lesions were known as liver spots. Barmaids in New York noted spider naevi in customers with advanced liver disease.

Liver diseases are frequently associated with abnormalities of the skin, hair, and the nails. As a general rule the cutaneous findings are nonspecific and may even be absent in severe liver diseases.

26.2.1 Pigmentary Abnormalities

Jaundice is first visible as a yellowish hue of the sclera and the soft palate before it becomes generalized. The commonest cutaneous manifestation is pruritus, which is due to the presence of bile salts in the skin, but other liver products may also be involved. There is no indication of the release of histamine and the use of anti-histamines is therefore limited; oral cholestyramine 8–12 g daily in a diet rich in polyunsaturated fatty acids may produce relief.

Hyperpigmentation is diffuse, or it may be present in the perioral or periorbital region.

Pallor is due to anemia.

26.2.2 Vascular Abnormalities

Urticaria may be due to the presence of circulating immune complexes. Other vascular lesions may present as telangiectasia or hemorrhage.

26.2.2.1 Telangiectasia

Rapid development of multiple spider naevi is seen in chronic liver disease. These are usually found in the distribution of the superior vena cava (above the nipples). Hyperoestrogenemia may be involved; diffuse telangiectasia on the palms occurs as palmar erythema.

Paper Money Skin

Patients with spider angiomata may also show numerous small vessels resembling silk threads as seen in US paper money; these are scattered in random fashion especially over the face, neck, and upper trunk. These may be associated with telangiectatic mats consisting of plaques of telangiectatic vessels.

White Spots

On cooling the skin of cirrhotic patients, especially on exposure to cold air, white spots appear on the arms and buttocks.

26.2.2.2 Hemorrhagic Manifestations

The cause of bleeding in liver disease depends upon the etiology of the underlying disorder. It may be due to a failure of absorption of vitamin K in biliary obstruction, failure of production of coagulative factors or abnormal platelet function. The cutaneous hemorrhage may range from petechiae and ecchymosis to a hematoma.

Dilated abdominal veins, including caput madusae, occur in cirrhosis with portal hypertension.

26.2.3 Hair and Nail

When severe alopecia occurs, zinc deficiency should be suspected. In the nails, there may be clubbing, white flat nails (leukonychia), striations, and white bands. In Wilson's disease, the lunula attain a characteristic azure color.

26.2.4 Miscellaneous Changes

Striae distensae (cutaneous stretch marks) are seen especially on the lower abdomen probably due to hormonal imbalance. Eruptive xanthomas and plain xanthomas may develop on the hands and the fingers. Dupuytren's contracture occurs in alcoholic cirrhosis.

26.3 Kidney Disease

Cutaneous manifestations of renal disease fall into two categories:

- Hereditary or acquired disorders with renal and cutaneous changes.
- Cutaneous changes due to renal insufficiency, these are usually nonspecific.

Generalized pruritus is the most important dermatological finding in renal insufficiency. This may be related to the increase in blood urea, dehydration from the use of diuretics, decrease in the size of the sweat glands, or secondary hyperparathyroidism. Pruritus in secondary hyperparathyroidism is probably due to the deposition of calcium phosphate salts in the skin. Pruritus is reduced as the general condition of the patient improves. Oral antihistamines are usually ineffective apart from their sedative effect. Emollients are given for the dryness of the skin. Oral cholestyramine resin has been reported to decrease pruritus due to absorption of a circulating toxin from the gut. UVA without psoralens has been reported to be effective. Subtotal parathyroidectomy may be very helpful but the problem often recurs. UVB radiation is an effective therapy with reduction of phosphorus levels to normal values.

Anemia with resulting pallor is an early sign of renal failure due to decreased hemopoesis and increased hemolysis. Purpura may occur in the form of scattered ecchymosis and petechiae. Purpura due to mild thrombocytopenia may be corrected by dialysis.

Diffuse hyperpigmentation with accentuation in the sun-exposed areas is characteristic of uremic patients; this is due to retention of chromogens, and deposition of melanin due to impaired renal processing of MSH.

A self-limiting bullous dermatoses similar to that of porphyria cutanea tarda is seen in patients undergoing dialysis; this is due to the high levels of uroporphyrins that do not cross the dialysis membrane.

Premature ageing of the skin and solar keratosis have been described in renal failure, these patients should avoid excessive UVB therapy for their pruritus.

About 40% of the patients undergoing dialysis can develop gynecomastia. A low phosphorus diet and aluminum hydroxide gel may reverse this.

Kyrle's disease occurs in both diabetes and renal failure. The cutaneous lesions consist of hyperpigmented papules up to 1 cm in diameter with a keratin plug. The extensor surface of the limbs is commonly affected.

Half-and-half nails have been emphasized as a marker for uremia, this consists of the proximal nail being white and the distal end reddish brown in color; the pathogenesis is unknown. Cutaneous calcification is uncommon and is seen around the large joints and flexures. Metastatic calcification in the blood vessels may lead to skin necrosis. Uremic frost, a distinctive terminal finding, is seen in patients with severe uremia. Numerous white to tan granules are seen on the nose, beard, arm, and neck; they represent crystallization of urea from the sweat. Oral manifestations of uremia include xerostomia, gingival friability, and ulcerative stomatitis; this is probably an ammonical burn due to bacterial decomposition of salivary urea.

26.4 Rheumatoid Arthritis

Several skin changes are seen in patients with rheumatoid arthritis. These are mainly due to increased deposition of fibrous tissue or secondary to vasculitis.

26.4.1 Rheumatic Nodules

Palpable subcutaneous nodules occur in 20% of patients with rheumatoid arthritis. They are commonly seen on the ulnar border of the forearms, dorsa of the hands, knees, scapula, sacrum, buttocks, heels, and ears. Nodules are associated with severe form of the disease. Rheumatoid nodules may occur in the sclera which then becomes atrophic and can even perforate (scleromalacia perforans), leading to blindness.

26.4.1.1 Linear Subcutaneous Bands

These are elongated bands 3–5 mm wide and about 10 cm or more in length. These are seen in the axilla extending to the iliac crest.

26.4.2 Vascular Lesions

The most characteristic lesions are small infarcts around the nails; these infarcts are transitory and painless, lasting for 2–3 days. Occasionally an infarct may cause grooving of the nail. Digital necrosis similar to that seen in systemic lupus erythematosus may occur; it may be confused with occupational trauma. Small painful purpuric nodules (Bywater lesions) are seen on the pulp of the fingers. Palmar erythema is common. Leg ulcers are seen in 18% of rheumatoid patients most commonly due to venous insufficiency, complicated by vasculitis, ischemia, immobility, and postural factors.

The skin may show necrotic arteritis. Hemorrhage occurs without preceding trauma; it may vary in size from small petechiae to large ecchymosis that may ulcerate. Gangrene may result from changes in the digital vessels; sometimes it may spread to involve a large part of the hand and foot, this may occur in just a few days. Bullae of the finger or toe tips may occur; occasionally they may spread to involve a large part of the body.

Peripheral sensory and motor neuropathy is due to occlusion of the vasa nervosum. Pyoderma gangrenosum is another complication of rheumatoid arthritis. Pressure sores are common because of immobility. Ridging of the nails may occur; the lunula may be red.

26.4.3 Atrophic Skin in Rheumatoid Arthritis

In patients over the age of 60, the skin over the dorsum of the hands becomes loose, thin, inelastic, and transparent, so that the veins and tendons are easily seen. The change is generalized but is seldom conspicuous except on the hands and the forearms. Histologically, the dermis is thinned but shows no distinctive signs.

26.4.4 Rheumatoid Neutrophilic Dermatosis

This is characterized by the appearance of symmetrical erythematous nodules and plaques on the dorsum of the hands, arms, extensor surface of the joints, neck, and the trunk. They are sometimes tender. Histologically, there is a dense infiltration of neutrophils in the dermis.

26.5 Hyperthyroidism

The classical triad of Graves's disease is enlarged toxic goitre, exophthalmos, and dermopathy. The skin is moist, warm, and smooth, due to increased metabolism. Palmar erythema is frequently seen; the hair is thin and has a downy texture. The skin may be diffusely pigmented; sometimes even melasma is seen on the cheeks. Digital clubbing and diaphysial proliferation of the acral and distal long bones characterize thyroid acropathy. Pretibial myxedema is seen on the anterolateral aspects of the shin and is characterized by nodules, which are pink, waxy, yellow, or skin-colored, with prominent hair follicles giving a peau-de-orange appearance. Localized hypertrichosis on the lesions is often noted. Pretibial myxedema is treated with intralesional steroids.

26.6 Hypothyroidism

Mild hypothyroidism results in cold hands and feet in the absence of vascular disease, sensitivity to cold weather, lack of sweating, weight gain, drowsiness, and constipation. Severe hypothyroidism in adults results in myxedema; this condition is characterized by accumulation of mucopolysaccharides in the dermis. The cause of mucin deposition is not known. The skin is dry and rough; in some cases, ichthyosis may be simulated. The facial skin is puffy, expression is dull and flat, and macroglossia may be present. Diffuse hair loss is common and the outer third of the eyebrow is shed. The hair becomes coarse and brittle. The free edges of the nails break easily.

In juvenile hypothyroidism, there is abnormal physical and mental development. Affected children develop hypertrichosis on the upper back and shoulders.

26.7 Cushing's Syndrome

The cutaneous manifestations are similar to those caused by endogenous or iatrogenic hypercortism. The subcutaneous fat is redistributed from the limbs to the trunk, so that the trunk becomes obese with a "buffalo hump," while the limbs remain slim. The plethoric "moon face" is pathognomonic of increased circulating glucocorticoids. Thinning of the skin due to collagen loss may result in large purple striae. Cushing's syndrome increases the susceptibility to cutaneous infection especially to candidiasis and tinea versicolor. The skin is fragile, heals poorly, the blood vessels rupture easily, purpura and bruises are common. Osteoporosis and compression fractures of the vertebrae may occur. If the adrenal androgens are also produced in excess then there may be hirsutism, seborrhea, and acne.

26.8 Addison's Disease

Addison's disease is seen in the skin primarily as hyperpigmentation. The skin becomes darker particularly in light-exposed areas, buccal mucosa, lips, nipples, genitalia, and sites of friction such as the knees, elbows, palms, and soles. Females lose axillary and pubic hair. Acne improves due to decreased levels of adrenal androgen secretion.

26.9 Acromegaly

Excessive growth hormone results in dermatomegaly. All the components of the skin are increased. There is epidermal hyperplasia, hyperpigmentation, increase in the thickness of the dermis, thickness of the hair and nails, increased sweating, and increased growth of the hair. Acanthosis nigricans is another manifestation.

26.10 Hyperlipidemias

Cutaneous xanthomas are signs of hyperlipidemia. A xanthoma is a collection of lipid-filled histiocytes in the skin. Hyperlipidemias may be primary (genetic) or secondary due to diseases such as liver disorders, pancreatic disorders, diabetes mellitus, myxedema, nephritic syndrome, etc. Drugs, for example retinoids, glucocorticoids, and estrogens can also induce hyperlipidemia.

Hyperlipidemias are classified on the basis of fasting blood lipids, electrophoresis of plasma lipid proteins, and ultracentrifugation abnormalities. They are classified into six groups. Xanthomas vary morphologically according to the type of hyperlipidemia. Xanthomas may be localized, generalized, on the palms and soles, over the eyelids, or on tendons. Xanthomas may be in the form of a papule, plaque or nodule; the lesions are yellowish in color. All except type 1 are associated with atherosclerosis. The types are not absolute; one type may change into another and more than one type may be found in an individual.

Type of xanthomas:

Xanthelasma is the commonest form of xanthoma. It may or may not be associated with increased serum lipids. It appears as yellowish plaques on the eyelids (Fig. 26.3).

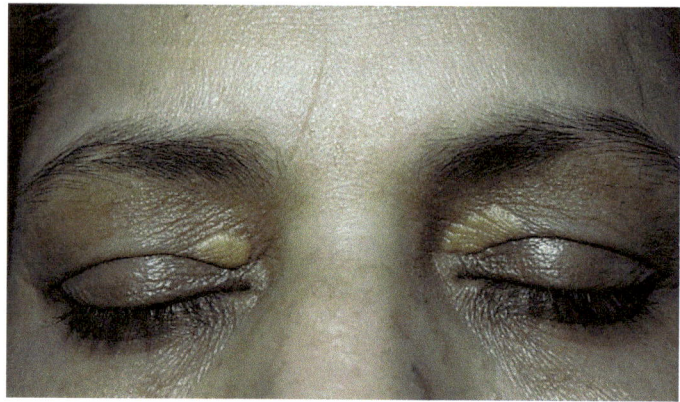

FIGURE 26.3. Xanthelasma.

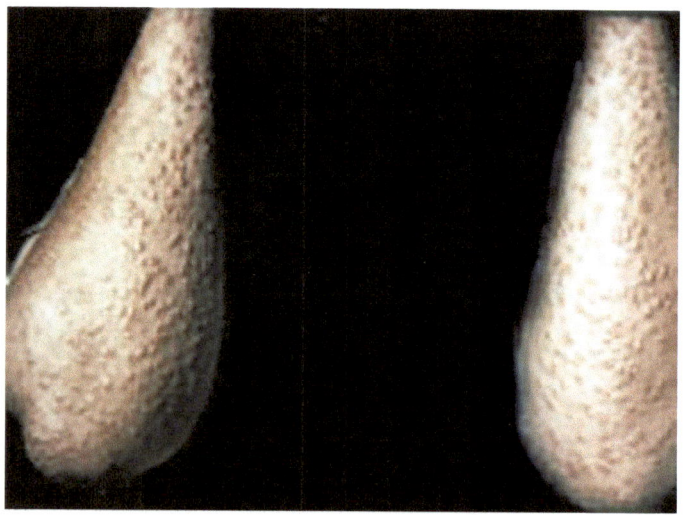

FIGURE 26.4. Eruptive xanthoma.

Eruptive xanthomas are yellowish red papules or plaques; they arise suddenly all over the body, but most frequently on the extensor surfaces (Fig. 26.4). They are seen in patients, with markedly elevated triglycerides.

Tuberous xanthomas are potato-like papules and nodules, often found on the elbow and knees. A corneal arcus may be seen.

Tendonous xanthomas are stony hard nodules on the tendons, mostly found on the Achilles tendon and extensor tendons of the fingers. Because of their depth, their yellow color cannot be appreciated clinically. These are often associated with severe hypercholesterolemia.

Palmar xanthomas are yellow linear xanthomas that appear along the palmar creases.

26.10.1 Treatment

All cases of xanthomas should be investigated to exclude any underlying pathology such as liver, kidney, pancreatic, or thyroid disorders. The patients should be referred to the appropriate physician. Patients with hyperlipidemia should be on a low-fat diet; drugs such as clofibrate, cholestyramine, nicotinic acid, and statins lower blood lipids. Eruptive xanthomas usually resolve when triglyceride levels are lowered; other xanthomas are more persistent.

Xanthelasma can be removed for cosmetic reasons, by chemical cautery, cryosurgery, laser, or surgery, but they can recur.

26.11 Phenylketonuria

This is an autosomal recessive disorder of phenylalanine metabolism, in which phenylalanine is not converted to tyrosine but accumulates in the blood. This results in failure to produce adequate melanin, and CNS manifestations occur due to toxic effects of phenylalanine. Cutaneous lesions occur predominantly in Caucasians. The patients are extremely sensitive to light and 50% have an eczematous eruption similar to atopic dermatitis. Brain damage is seen in early childhood; about 50% of patients have epilepsy and extrapyrimidal tract manifestations.

Phenylalanine levels should be measured in the first week of life. A diet low in phenylalanine brings about normal development if begun shortly after birth.

26.12 Sarcoidosis

This is a multisystem chronic granulomatous disorder. The organs most commonly affected are the lungs, skin, and the eyes. It is also possible to have cutaneous involvement without systemic manifestations. Associated symptoms are malaise, fever, and often a dull ache in the chest. Histology resembles tuberculosis, but does not show the peripheral lymphocytes of the granuloma (naked granuloma) and there is no caseation or bacilli. The disease is more common in cold climates and rarely seen in the tropics.

26.12.1 Cutaneous Manifestations

These may be in the form of papules, plaques, or nodules. The color of the lesion may vary from dull red to purple, brown, or yellow (Figs. 26.5 and 26.6). The lesions are asymptomatic but some may itch. Erythema nodosum is a common manifestation of sarcoidosis.

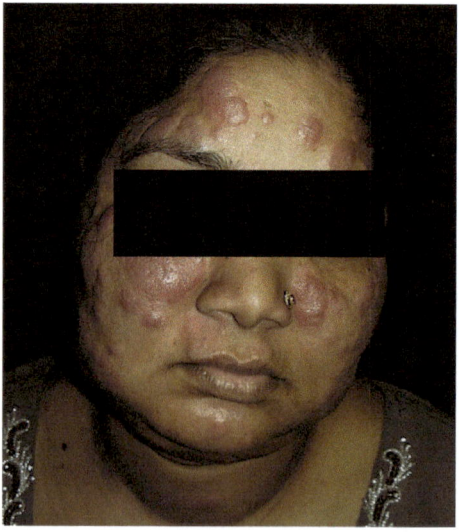

FIGURE 26.5. Sarcoidosis.

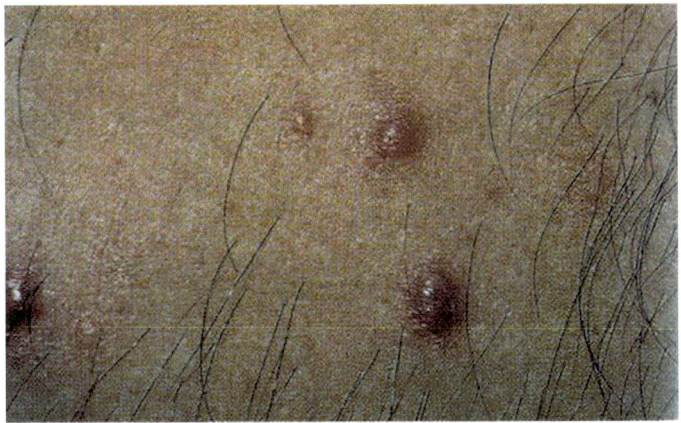

FIGURE 26.6. Sarcoidosis.

Lupus pernio affects poorly perfused areas such as the nose, earlobes, and the fingers. These areas are swollen, indurated, and purplish-red in color; they should be differentiated from chilblains. The nasal bones may erode and the phalangeal bones may have cysts.

Papular lesions are present as crops on the face and extensor surface of the limbs. On the face they are mostly present around the nose and eyelids. They are associated with a good prognosis.

Plaques are common on the buttocks, shoulders, and thigh, and are associated with a poor prognosis.

Annular sarcoid is confined to the head and neck regions; they have a peripheral scaly edge, and a hypopigmented central scarred area. These also have a bad prognosis.

Other cutaneous manifestations are calcium deposition, erythema multiforme, scarring and nonscarring alopecia, dystrophy of the nails, and nodular lesions on the palms and soles.

26.12.2 Pulmonary Manifestations

The most common manifestation is involvement of the hilar lymph nodes, which is asymptomatic. Pulmonary infiltration is more significant, leading to impairment of pulmonary function. Bronchial obstruction and stenosis may occur.

26.12.3 Ocular Manifestations

This is seen as anterior and posterior uvietis, conjunctivitis, and dry eyes.

26.12.4 Treatment

Around 80–90% cases of acute sarcoidosis show spontaneous resolution, so therapy is seldom indicated. Corticosteroids are required in acute sarcoidosis when accompanied by eye lesions, lesion of the central nervous system and cardiovascular system, and patients with pulmonary diseases and functional disability. In chronic sarcoidosis, treatment with oral steroids has to be continued for several years. Alternative therapies such as antimalarials, methotrexate, and azathioprine may also be of value.

Purely cutaneous lesions usually respond better to intralesional steroids, or topical steroids.

26.13 Skin and Immunodeficiency

Immune defects express themselves through frequent, prolonged, often life-threatening infections or through malignancy. Immunosuppression can be due to drugs (steroids, cytotoxics, etc.), congenital diseases (e.g., chronic granulomatous disease, complement deficiency, agammaglobulinaemia, Di George's syndrome, etc.) or acquired immunodeficiency disorders such as AIDS. Long-standing diseases such as liver and renal failure, Crohn's disease, disseminated malignancy, active rheumatoid arthritis, and impaired nutritional status can also lead to immune defects.

Immune deficiency presents with chronic and recurrent infections, particularly with opportunistic infections (candida, cryptococcus, aspergillosis, mucormycosis), viral infections such as warts, molluscum contagiosum, bacterial and fungal infections are common in immunodeficiency. The infections are usually severe; they occur in unusual sites, often with unusual organisms, and are recurrent.

Immunosuppression also leads to increased incidence of malignancy of the skin and internal organs. Squamous cell carcinoma is seen in the sun-exposed areas in renal transplant patients, and Kaposi's sarcoma is seen in patients with AIDS.

26.13.1 Treatment

Long-term treatment with antibiotics, replacement therapy with IgG, every 3–4 weeks to maintain normal IgG levels are required in diseases due to B lymphocyte disorders with IgG abnormalities. Patients with T cell deficiencies should not be vaccinated with live vaccines such as BCG. Success has been reported with daily injections of thymosine.

Bone marrow transfusion should be considered in severe primary disease.

26.14 Skin and Internal Malignancy

Skin involvement in internal malignancy can be due to

- Invasion of the skin by malignant cells, through direct invasion or via the blood and lymphatics
- Exposure to carcinogens
- Physiological changes
- Genetic diseases predisposing to malignancy
- Miscellaneous

26.14.1 Invasion of the Skin by Malignant Cells

Direct involvement of the skin is common in carcinoma of the breast, giving the skin the characteristic peau-de-orange effect, due to lymph stasis. An erythematous plaque, which resembles erysipelas, is called "carcinoma erysipeloides." In Paget's disease of the nipple, there is an eczematous-like eruption on the nipple. Skin metastases are common in terminal tumors due to hematogenous spread.

26.14.2 Exposure to the Carcinogen

Brown staining of the fingers is due to cigarette smoking; patients may have an underlying bronchogenic carcinoma. Arsenic intake with internal malignancy has several cutaneous markers, such as diffuse pigmentation with raindrop areas of normal skin, brownish keratosis on the palms and soles, and Bowen's disease on the covered parts of the body. Chronic radiation dermatitis can progress to squamous cell carcinoma.

26.14.3 Physiological

Some tumors express physiological changes in the skin such as acne in androgenic tumors, flushing in carcinoid syndrome, and jaundice in bile duct carcinoma.

26.14.4 Genetic Disease Predisposing
to Malignancy

Gardner's syndrome has an increased incidence of carcinoma of the colon. These patients present with multiple epidermoid cysts and jaw cysts. Phakomatoses are developmental defects that can involve the skin, eyes, and the central nervous system, e.g., neurofibromatosis and adenoma sebaceum. These disorders may have associated internal malignancies.

26.14.5 Miscellaneous

The three common markers of internal malignancy are:

- Pallor
- Pruritus
- Pigmentation

Pruritus is common in Hodgkin's disease.

The other signs of internal malignancy are acanthosis nigricans, erythema gyratum repens, erythema multiforme (especially bullous), acquired ichthyosis, Bazex syndrome, dermatomyositis, acquired ichthyosis, and Sweet's syndrome. Hypertrichosis lanuginosa, characterized by sudden appearance of fluffy blond hair in an adult is associated with internal malignancy. Glucagonoma syndrome, which is caused by a glucagon-secreting pancreatic tumor, is associated with diabetes, glossitis, diarrhea, and a characteristic blistering rash (necrolytic migratory erythema).

The sorrow that has no vent makes other organs weep.

Chapter 27
Skin and the Psyche

Skin is the largest organ of the body, and is the only organ visible to others and exposed to the external environment. It is, therefore, obvious that any pathology of the skin could have an impact on the psychology of the person. The more extensive the disease and the more chronic it is the greater the psychological effect on the person. Stress can affect any organ of the body such as myocardial infarction, gastric ulcers, irritable bladder, irritable bowel syndrome, etc. The effect of psyche on the skin can be studied under the following two headings:

- The effect of skin disease on the psyche
- The effect of the psyche on the skin

27.1 The Effect of Skin Disease on the Psyche

A number of skin disorders can lead to emotional trauma such as psoriasis, atopic dermatitis, ichthyosis, acne, hair disorders such as alopecia, etc. Acne affects young adults; this can lead to low self-esteem, antisocial behavior, stress, depression, and even suicide. Eczema of the hands can lead to loss of work; this monetary loss leads to its associated problems. A number of skin disorders can be precipitated by stress such as acne, herpes simplex, psoriasis, alopecia areata, discoid eczema, pompholyx, etc.

Z. Zaidi, S. W. Lanigan, *Dermatology in Clinical Practice*,
DOI 10.1007/978-1-84882-862-9_27,
© Springer-Verlag London Limited 2010

It is imperative that a dermatologist should have a very sympathetic approach toward a patient with skin disease. They should take the patient into confidence, explain the problem, and try to act as a liaison between the patients and their family to deal with the skin problem.

27.2 The Effect of the Psyche on the Skin

A number of skin disorders can be due to the emotional trauma suffered by a patient. Patients inflict damage to their skin for complex reasons including to get more attention from the people around them. The skin is the organ to vent out these emotions. These disorders include the following:

27.2.1 Dermatitis Artifacta

This is seen in areas that are accessible to the patients and the lesions do not resemble any known cutaneous disorder, e.g., the ulcers inflicted will be of bizarre shape, they do not heal on treatment, new ones keep on appearing at odd places. The lesions may be in the form of ulcers, burns, blisters, crusting, skin digging, etc. The condition may be difficult to diagnose at times. Lesions will improve with occlusive dressings, but this will not solve the psychiatric problem (Fig. 27.1).

Management aims at building a good rapport with the patient and finding out about any stress to which the patient is subjected. Direct confrontation should be avoided; at times psychiatric help may be required, but the patient frequently rejects this.

27.2.2 Trichotillomania

This is pulling and twisting the hair of the scalp. This leads to a patch of hair loss; the condition is easy to diagnose as the patch is irregular in shape, it is not scaly or inflamed, and

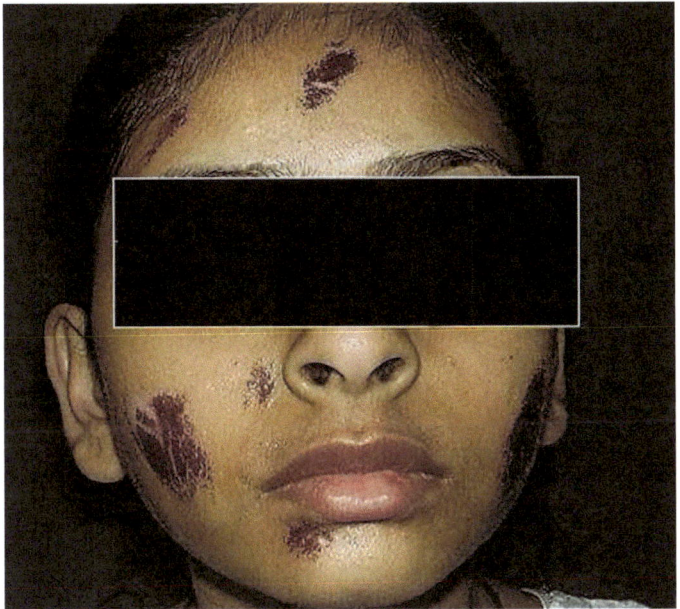

FIGURE 27.1. Dermatitis artifacta.

there are a few hair of varying size in the patch. Occlude the patch and the hair regrows. The condition is common in young children, often unnoticed, and the habit often goes away quickly with appropriate help (Fig. 27.2).

27.2.3 Delusion of Parasitosis

The patient has a feeling that some parasites are crawling or biting on the skin. The patient may even bring some scales, hair, and debris from the skin to show the parasites to the doctor. The skin may show marks of scratching. The condition is seen most commonly in middle-aged people, often women. Delusion of parasitosis is difficult to treat, pimozide is often prescribed. If pimozide is used, an ECG should be performed before starting the treatment and the patient should have periodic ECG

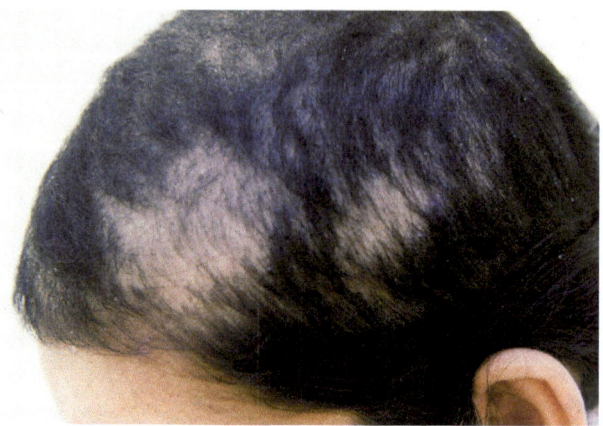

FIGURE 27.2. Trichotillomania.

checks. Pimozide should not be given to patients with prolonged Q–T interval and those with a history of dysrhythmias.

27.2.4 Acne Excoriee

This is seen most commonly in young girls. Although the patients have only minor lesions of acne, they keep on picking at relatively trivial lesions, which leads to scar formation. The scars from picking are far worse than the underlying disorder. This behavioral disorder needs to be identified and addressed. Compliance is poor and sometimes oral isotretinoin is needed to completely eradicate the acne component.

Dysmorphobia is a term applied to a distortion of body image. Minor skin lesions are magnified in the mind to grotesque proportions. Most patients are clinically depressed.

27.2.5 Dermatological Non-disease

In this condition, the dermatologist can find no abnormality of the skin, but the patient keeps on insisting that there is a skin problem such as hair loss, burning, itching, redness of an area, excess of facial hair, etc. It is a form of monosymptomatic hypochondrical psychosis; some patients are depressed and some may show signs of schizophrenia. Psychiatric help is often needed.

Inherent personality difficulties, unsatisfactory interpersonal relationships, and a chronic stressful environment are the basis of psychogenic dermatoses. The majority of dermatological disorders associated with psychological problems fall under the designation of "frictional dermatoses," those that are being manually produced or aggravated. These individuals show evidence of self-harm on their bodies such as dermatitis artifacta. In others, the emotional mental states lead to sweating, or vasolability. Management of the patient's mental state is clearly vital in treating these disorders.

Avoid direct confrontation with the patient in skin disease, due to emotional problems of the patient.

Fully assess a patient's physical and mental state before treating a skin disease due to a psychiatric disorder.

Have a sympathetic approach, try and gain the patient's confidence.

Chapter 28
Erythroderma

Erythroderma is a descriptive term in which about 80–90% of the skin is inflamed. The common causes of erythroderma are drug eruptions, contact dermatitis, atopic dermatitis, psoriasis, malignancy, lichen planus, ichthyosiform erythrodermas, dermatophytosis, pityriasis rubra pilaris, and pemphigus. There is an increase in blood flow to the skin, and the cardiac output increases; this is compensated in a normal healthy adult, but gives rise to cardiac and renal failure in susceptible patients. Patients with erythroderma often develop lymphadenopathy, secondary to cutaneous inflammation (dermatopathic lymphadenopathy).

The clinical effects depend upon whether the erythroderma is acute or chronic. In acute cases the patient feels unwell and shivers from time to time due to hypothermia, as the body is unable to maintain core temperature. There is electrolyte imbalance and dehydration, sudden death has been recorded due to ventricular fibrillation. These patients require hospital admission and management. In chronic cases the body normally compensates to the changes of erythroderma, and the patients can be treated at home, but if signs of decompensation occur, the patient should be hospitalized and treated with particular care (Fig. 28.1).

Z. Zaidi, S. W. Lanigan, *Dermatology in Clinical Practice*, 477
DOI 10.1007/978-1-84882-862-9_28,
© Springer-Verlag London Limited 2010

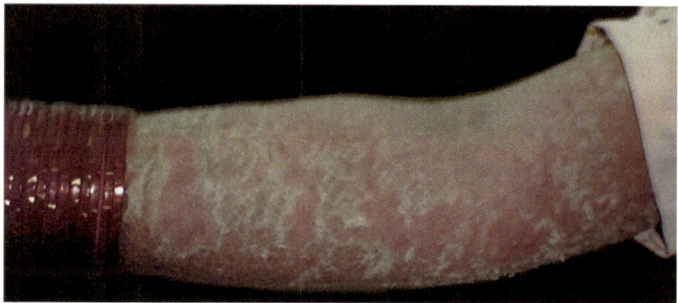

FIGURE 28.1. Erythroderma – most of the body was similarly affected.

The effects of erythroderma on the body are shown in the following table:

Systemic changes	Clinical signs
Hemodynamics. Most of the cardiac output is directed to the skin	Tachycardia, collapsing pulse, heart failure, skin feels hot due to the increased blood flow
Thermoregulation. Hypothalamic thermostat becomes abnormal, perhaps due to a circulating toxin	Patient often complains of hypothermia, due to excessive loss of heat from the skin. Sometimes the patient may become hypohidrotic or anhidrotic due to intraepidermal occlusion of sweat ducts; hyperthermia then becomes a hazard especially in tropical climates
Hematological effects	Increased protein loss and hypoalbuminemia, fall in serum iron and folate levels, hypocalcemia, increased ESR, increase in uric acid level due to increased cell turn over
Fluid balance. There is increased transepidermal water loss	Thirst and oliguria
Prerenal failure (acute)	Hypotension, tachycardia, low venous pressure, decreased skin turgor
Intestinal effects	Malabsorbtion, protein-losing eneteropathy
Lymphadenopathy	Lymph nodes are enlarged, contain lipids and melanin from the skin
Miscellaneous	Gynecomastia

28.1 Diagnosis

Diagnosis of the underlying disease is often difficult in a full-blown case of erythroderma; the diagnosis is based on history of recent drug intake, detailed previous history of the patient and examination of patient's old records looking for evidence of preexisting skin disease, biopsies, etc. A search is carried out to find subtle clues to trace the original disease. Histology is not usually helpful except in cases of malignancy.

28.2 Treatment

The treatment is directed to the cause of the disorder, steroids are generally not indicated, unless the erythroderma is due to drugs or eczema. The fluid and electrolyte imbalance, circulatory status, and body temperature should be monitored. Cooling and overheating should be avoided. Treat cardiac failure if it develops.

Soothing agents are used to treat the cutaneous inflammation. When the erythema resolves, then the primary treatment for the underlying disease should be initiated.

The prognosis depends upon the cause of erythroderma and the age of the patient. Erythroderma due to drugs has a good prognosis. Erythroderma due to psoriasis and eczema continue for months. Prognosis is poor in the elderly. Pneumonia, heart, and kidney failure are the common causes of death.

Chapter 29
Ages of Man and Their Dermatoses

29.1 Neonates and Infants

The skin of neonates and infants differ from adults in the following ways:

- In neonates and during early infancy, the skin defenses are not fully developed, the skin is vulnerable to physical, chemical, and microbial attack.
- The surface area to the weight ratio is higher than at other times of life; there is a greater hazard from increased absorption of topically applied medicaments. Serious toxicity can occur from the application of topical steroids, salicylic acid, neomycin, boric acid, aniline dyes, hexachlorophene, and related antiseptics.
- The rate of transepidermal water loss through intact and non sweating skin of the newborn is high, indicating immaturity of the skin barrier function. Dehydration rapidly develops.
- Hypothermia develops rapidly in widespread skin rashes.
- During early weeks of life, the blood levels of some hormones are similar to that of the mother, e.g., androgens levels are high and these are the cause of neonatal acne.
- Scratching does not seem to develop until around 6 months of age.

Some specific skin diseases of childhood are nappy rash, atopic dermatitis, cradle cap, napkin psoriasis, staphylococcal

Z. Zaidi, S. W. Lanigan, *Dermatology in Clinical Practice*,
DOI 10.1007/978-1-84882-862-9_29,
© Springer-Verlag London Limited 2010

scalded skin syndrome, lip licking, juvenile plantar dermatosis, bullous disease of childhood, acrodermatitis enteropathica, and congenital ichthyosis.

The transient skin lesions are discussed next in this chapter.

29.1.1 Erythema Toxicum Neonatorum (ETN)

Lesions are not present at birth; most cases occur between 24 and 48 hours of birth. ETN occurs in 20–25% of full-term healthy infants, usually in the second or later deliveries. It is rare in premature infants and in those weighing less than 2,500 g.

The rash begins on the face; it spreads to the trunk, proximal extremities, and then to the buttocks. Palms and soles are not affected. Lesions may localize at pressure points. Four types of lesions occur; macules, wheals, papules and pustules. Tiny papules and pustules are superimposed on the macules and wheals. New lesions appear as the old ones resolve. ETN resolves spontaneously without any side effects within a few days. Wright's stain shows numerous eosinophils, peripheral eosinophilia is uncommon.

No treatment is required as the condition resolves spontaneously.

29.1.2 Transient Neonatal Pustular Melanosis

The lesions are present at birth but may be overlooked for a few days. It occurs in full-term infants, more common in black than fair skin. The common sites of involvement are the forehead, behind the ears, under the chin, neck, back, hands, and feet. Palms and soles may be affected. The lesions are vesicopustules with no underlying erythema. These may be isolated or grouped. The lesions are very superficial; they rupture very easily to form a hyperpigmented macule. The pigmentation may last for several weeks.

29.1.3 Miliaria

These appear 1 week after birth. It is common in hot humid climates, it is also seen in babies in incubators, in infants with fever and in neonates wearing warm clothes. The lesion is due to the occlusion of the duct of sweat glands. The level of occlusion indicates the type of miliaria.

29.1.3.1 Miliaria Crystallina

This occurs when the level of occlusion in the duct of sweat glands is in the stratum corneum. The lesions appear as clear dew drops, with little or no erythema. Vesicles may appear individually or in a cluster.

29.1.3.2 Miliaria Rubra

The level of obstruction in the duct of the sweat glands is in the stratum malpighian. Papules and vesicles are surrounded by an erythematous halo, or diffuse erythema develops as an inflammatory reaction.

29.1.3.3 Treatment

Cool water compresses and proper ventilation are all that is necessary.

29.1.4 Neonatal Acne

Lesions appear after 1–2 weeks of birth, in about 20% of newborn infants. Comedones, papules and pustules have the same distribution as that of adults. These are due to maternal androgens in the neonate's blood. They resolve spontaneously.

29.2 Skin and Pregnancy

Physiological changes of pregnancy are:

- Pigmentation. These include melasma (mask of pregnancy); pigmented moles become darker, linea alba changes to linea nigra. There is increased pigmentation of the nipples, areola, axillae and the genitalia.
- Striae gravidarum. These striae occur due to the breakdown of elastic fibers because of increased skin stretching. The striae are prominent on the lower abdomen; they may also be present on the breast, upper arm and thighs.
- Vascular changes. These include spider naevi (face, upper trunk and arms), and palmar erythema.
- Skin tags may increase in number.
- Sebaceous secretion increases, the scalp and the face become greasy.
- Increase deposition of fat and increase in tissue fluids result in coarsening of features.

29.3 Dermatoses of Pregnancy

29.3.1 Pruritus

This usually begins in the third trimester of pregnancy, due to cholestasis of pregnancy; it subsides after childbirth, but may recur in subsequent pregnancies and even when taking contraceptive pills.

29.3.2 Polymorphous Eruption of Pregnancy (Pruritic Urticarial Papules and Plaques of Pregnancy, PUPP)

The lesions begin in the third trimester of the first pregnancy. The patient complains of intense itching. The skin lesions begin within the abdominal striae, later becoming generalized. Cutaneous lesions comprise urticarial papules and plaques, vesicles, target lesions and polycyclic erythematous areas. It rarely recurs in subsequent pregnancies.

29.3.2.1 Treatment

The condition is treated by soothing lotions, such as calamine lotion, and, in resistant cases, topical steroids.

29.3.3 Impetigo Herpetiformis

This is a severe form of pustular psoriasis. It has a febrile onset; grouped pustules appear on an erythematous base. The lesions begin in the flexures such as axillae, groin, and neck. There is a raised peripheral blood count, hypocalcaemia may occur. The condition resolves after delivery, but may recur in subsequent deliveries. Fetal death may occur.

Treatment is with systemic steroids in a dose of 40–60 mg/day.

29.3.4 Herpes Gestationis

This is a rare intensely pruritic blistering disorder of pregnancy. It may appear for the first time in any pregnancy, but once it has occurred it reappears in subsequent pregnancies. It appears in the second or third trimester of pregnancy, resolves within a month or two after delivery. Oedematous plaques appear on the abdomen and extremities, which coalesce to from bizarre polycyclic rings, covering wide areas of the body. Tense blisters form on the initial plaques, these rupture and heal without scarring. Mild recurrences may occur with menstruation and when taking oral contraceptive pills.

29.3.4.1 Treatment

Mild cases respond to topical steroids. Most cases require oral steroids prednisone 0.5–1 mg/kg/day. Newborn babies are at risk of reversible adrenal suppression.

29.4 Skin and the Menopause

Menopause literally means the last menstrual period. Climacteric is a transitional phase lasting for 1–5 years, during which the genital organs involute in response to cessation of gonadal activity.

Skin is a target organ for estrogens and its withdrawal may result in cutaneous changes. The concentration of estrogen receptors in the facial skin are more than in other parts of the body. Some of the cutaneous changes at menopause are dryness of the skin, epithelial thinning, loss of dermal elasticity, some growth of hair on the face, body hair becomes sparse.

29.5 Cutaneous Disease at the Menopause

29.5.1 Menopausal Flushing

This is the most distressing complaint of menopause. There is a sudden feeling of intense heat in the face, neck and chest often accompanied by discomfort and sweating. It lasts for 4–5 min. Visible changes are seen in 50% of cases; this consists of blotchy erythema on the face, neck and chest. Some patients develop palpitations and throbbing in the head and neck. Headache, nausea, and vomiting may occur. Some physiological changes such as increase in temperature, pulse rate, and respiratory rate are also seen.

29.5.1.1 Treatment

Flushes are treated by estrogen therapy which is the most effective treatment for symptomatic hot flushes, alternatives are a mixture of ergotamine, belladonna alkaloids and phenobarbitone.

29.5.2 Keratoderma Climacterum

This is a thickening of the palms and soles especially around the heels. Although most commonly seen in middle aged females, it is also seen in men, and is therefore a nonspecific effect. It is treated by salicylic acid topically and systemic retinoids orally.

29.6 Aging Skin

Aging of skin is both extrinsic and intrinsic. Intrinsic aging is the natural aging, which affects the skin as it affects other organs of the body. Extrinsic aging is due to ultraviolet radiation that affects the skin only. Intrinsic aging is universal and inevitable, while extrinsic aging is neither universal nor inevitable. We can prevent the effects of ultraviolet damage by using protective measures against ultraviolet light, but intrinsic aging is not preventable.

Cutaneous changes of aging are:

- Dry and rough skin
- Thinning of the skin
- Patchy pigmentation
- Wrinkles
- Loss of elasticity
- Decreased tone
- Decreased resistance to mechanical, compressive, and shearing forces acting on the skin
- Easy bruising and purpura
- Facial telangiectasia
- Angulated scars
- Decrease in tactile sensations
- Graying of the hair
- Density of hair decreases
- Increase of terminal hair in the ear and eyebrows of men, slight hirsutism in women
- Rate of nail growth decreases
- Loss of subcutaneous fat

Ultraviolet radiation is damaging to the skin, it exaggerates the process of aging and produces mutations in keratinocytes. Excess of this radiation can result in actinic keratosis, basal cell carcinoma, squamous cell carcinoma, and malignant melanoma. The affect of ultraviolet radiation on the skin can be observed when we see the contrast between the skin of the face and hands to that of the covered parts of the body as the trunk.

29.7 Dermatoses of Old Age

Many dermatoses of the elderly reflect the higher prevalence of systemic diseases such as diabetes mellitus, vascular insufficiency, and various neurological syndromes. Some diseases such as cutaneous infections may be due to reduced local skin care. Reduced tolerance to systematically affected drugs is well documented. Delay in dermal clearance of absorbed substances and possible reduced metabolic capacity may render the elderly susceptible to both beneficial and adverse affects of the topical application of drugs.

Skin diseases of old age include pruritus, senile xerosis, asteotic eczema, peripheral leg ulcers, herpes zoster, and skin tumors. Some benign growths of old age are acrochordon, cherry angiomas, seborrhoeic keratosis, lentigo, and sebaceous hyperplasia.

29.8 Looking Younger

Women have always wanted to look younger; they have used various remedies from time immemorial. Today we have a large armamentarium of remedies for combating old age. These are both surgical and nonsurgical such as; chemical peels, botulinum toxin injections, dermabrasion, skin implants, and lasers.

29.8.1 Nonsurgical Cosmetic Procedures

29.8.1.1 Chemical Peels

There a number of products used for chemical peeling. They penetrate different levels of skin. Peels are thus superficial, medium, and deep depending upon the level of skin to which the peels penetrate. Generally speaking, the superficial peels are used by beauticians and the medium and deep peels by dermatologists and plastic surgeons.

Peeling produces a controlled partial thickness chemical burn of the epidermis and outer dermis. Regeneration of the peeled skin is from the hair follicle and eccrine sweat duct epithelium. The new skin that regenerates is meant to be devoid of the blemishes of the old skin. In the dermis, a narrow band of dense compact orderly collagen is formed, between the epidermis and the underlying dermis. This new band of collagen replaces the old degenerated collagen. New elastic fibers, and ground substance are formed by the fibroblasts. Microdermabrasion acts like a very superficial peel.

29.8.1.2 Botulinum Toxin Injections

This is Botulinum toxin A; it acts by denervating the muscles of facial expression, by inhibiting the release of acetylcholine from the muscle end plate. It relaxes the muscles and thus removes the wrinkles. The drug produces best results when injected in the upper half of the face.

29.8.1.3 Dermal Implants

These are used to remove the wrinkles and filling of lost body contours. Fillers may be injected in the dermis to remove wrinkles, to fill the hollow of the cheeks as seen in old age due to loss of subcutaneous tissue. Different materials are used for temporary and permanent effects. Fillers are of different kinds, depending upon the site to be injected.

Dermabrasion, mid and deep peels, and lasers are used for skin resurfacing, such as removing scars and severe damage of the skin caused by ultra violet light.

Skin protection against ultraviolet light is discussed in Chap. 18

Chapter 30
Diseases of the Oral Cavity

The oral cavity can provide valuable clues to cutaneous disorders, and should be included in every skin examination. A number of skin diseases have oral manifestations, such as pemphigus, erythema multiforme, SLE, lichen planus, psoriasis, viral infections, etc. Most of the lesions are in the form of ulcers or white patches.

The mucous membrane of the oral cavity is covered with stratified squamous epithelium that lacks a stratum corneum; this makes the mucosa more susceptible to infection. Lesions of the mucous membrane are more difficult to diagnose than that of the skin; there is less contrast of color, and greater likelihood of alteration in the original appearance, due to secondary factors such as maceration from moisture, abrasion from teeth and food. Vesicles and bullae rupture easily to form erosions; grouping and distribution is less distinctive in the mouth than on the skin.

30.1 Apthous Ulcer

The most common type of apthous ulcer is apthous minor; these are chronic, recurrent, tender ulcers, usually 3–5 mm in diameter, with a yellowish base and an erythematous halo. The lesions may be single or multiple. The ulcers are commonly found on the buccal or the labial mucosa (Fig. 30.1). It is common in young adults. Minor apthous ulcers usually

Z. Zaidi, S. W. Lanigan, *Dermatology in Clinical Practice*, 491
DOI 10.1007/978-1-84882-862-9_30,

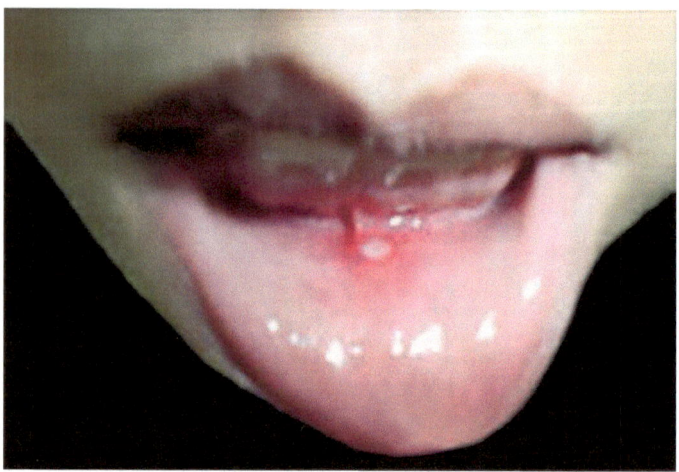

FIGURE 30.1. Apthous ulcer.

heal in about a week. In most cases, the disease remits; the time factor is variable from 5 to 15 years.

The other types are the major apthous ulcer, characterized by large ulcers that heal slowly, and herpetiform ulcers that are small and grouped; they are painful and occur very rapidly.

Factors implicated in the pathogenesis of these ulcers are emotional and physical stress, nutritional deficiency, infection, hormones, and immunological. An immune mechanism is the most likely cause.

30.1.1 Treatment

As the exact cause of apthous ulcer is not yet known, a number of treatment modalities are put forward.

- An underlying folic acid or iron deficiency should be corrected.
- Oral tetracycline mouthwash, by the "swish and swallowed" technique, four times daily helps some patients.
- If tetracycline fails, topical steroids with an adherent base (kenacort in orabase), or a steroid spray solution is applied three times daily.

- I/L steroids may be required for major apthous ulcers.
- Pain relief is obtained by topical anesthetics.

  Consider pemphigus or other bullous disorders if aphthae are persistent.

30.2 Oral Candidiasis (Trush)

Thrush is an infection caused by Candida albicans. It is common in neonates, about one third of infants are affected in the first week after birth. Mothers of infected newborns often have a history of vaginal candidiasis during the late part of their pregnancy. In adults, oral candidiasis is seen complicating diabetes, with steroid therapy, following intake of broad-spectrum antibiotics, with dentures, and complicating imunosuppression from any cause.

The lesions appear as white curd-like patches on the mucosa, which can be scraped off leaving an erythematous base. The tongue and buccal mucosa are frequently involved (Fig. 30.2). In people wearing dentures the angles of the mouth may be affected.

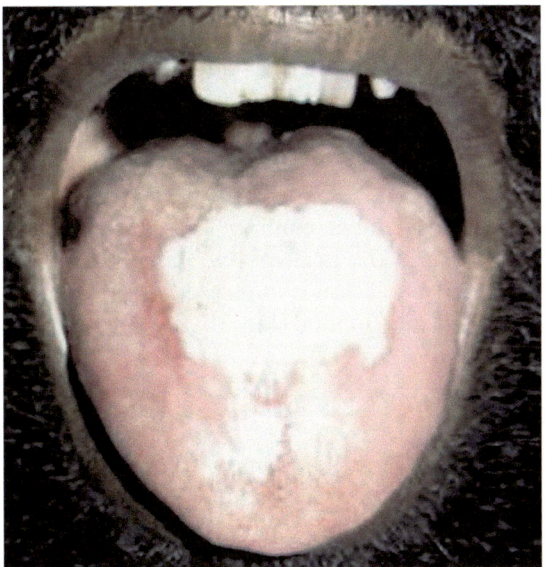

FIGURE 30.2. Oral candidiasis.

30.2.1 Treatment

- Infants are treated by applying nystatin suspension 1 mL (100,000 units) to each side of the mouth, four times daily for a week.
- Adults are treated by a "swish and swallow" nystatin suspension in a dose of 5 mL (500,000 units), four times daily.
- An alternate topical therapy is clotrimazole troches dissolved in the mouth five times daily for 1–2 weeks.
- Sporonox (itraconazole) solution can also be used as a "swish and swallow" regimen.
- Systemic antifungal therapy is required in some cases of immune suppression.

    In denture-wearing patients, candidal colonization of the dentures should also be treated.

30.3 Leukoplakia

Leukoplakia literally means "white plaque," which can be benign or it may show dysplastic changes. The white patch is due to macerated hyperkeratosis. This is usually caused by chronic irritation such as by smoking, chewing paan (betel leaf), dentures, ragged teeth, etc. The disorder is common in the middle-aged or the elderly. The disease is symptomless and is often detected accidentally on a routine examination of the mouth.

Leukoplakia appears as a white patch or plaque, which may be flat or verrucous. The color varies from white to gray. The tongue is the most common site, but leukoplakia can occur anywhere in the oral cavity. Malignant change should be suspected, if the lesion is indurated or ulcerated. A biopsy should rule out malignancy (Fig. 30.3).

30.3.1 Treatment

- The aim of therapy is to remove the cause, and surgically remove the persistent lesions.
- Many cases resolve in the early stages of the disease, when the cause is removed, as in the case of smoking.

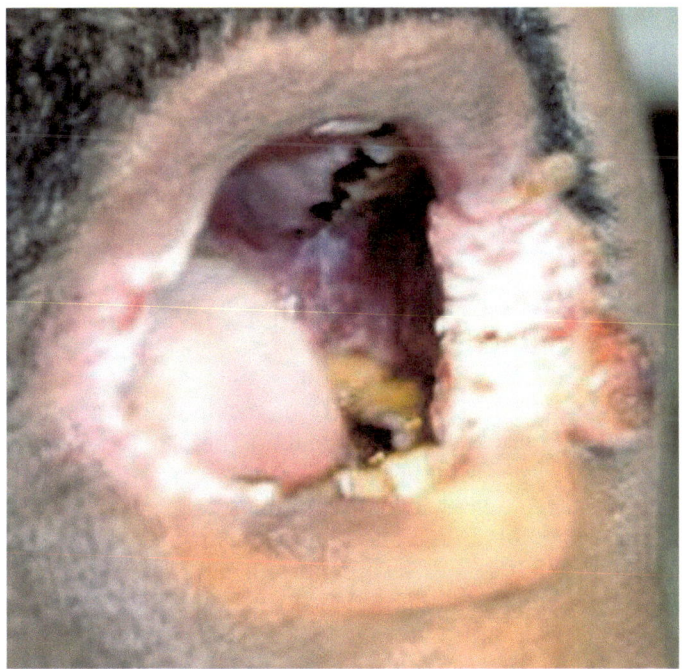

FIGURE 30.3. Oral leukoplakia.

- For persistent lesions that look benign (no induration, ulcer), treatments include cryosurgery, carbon dioxide laser ablation, or shave excision.
- Medical therapy for such lesions include topical bleomycin and systemic retinoids.
- Lesions suggestive of squamous cell carcinoma should be excised.

30.4 White Hairy Leukoplakia

Hairy leukoplakia is seen in patients with immune defects such as HIV infection. It is due to infection with Esptein Barr virus. Candida is usually present in the lesion. The site of predilection is the parakeratinized mucosa of the lateral margin of the tongue.

Clinically the lesion is characterized by a white corrugated or hairy appearance on the lateral surface of the tongue. The condition is asymptomatic.

Hairy leukoplakia needs no treatment, patients infected with HIV infection should be treated with antiretroviral therapy.

30.5 Submucous Fibrosis

Submucous fibrosis is a disease of the Indian subcontinent confined to people using areca nut and betel leaves. The condition develops insidiously, presenting as oral dysaesthesia, and a nonspecific vesicular stomatitis, later there is fibrosis of the tissue, mainly in the buccal mucosa, lip, and palate. When the condition becomes severe, fibrotic bands are seen involving the palatoglossal folds, due to which there is difficulty in opening the mouth and eating (Fig. 30.4). The condition is premalignant and oral cancer can develop in 2–10% of cases.

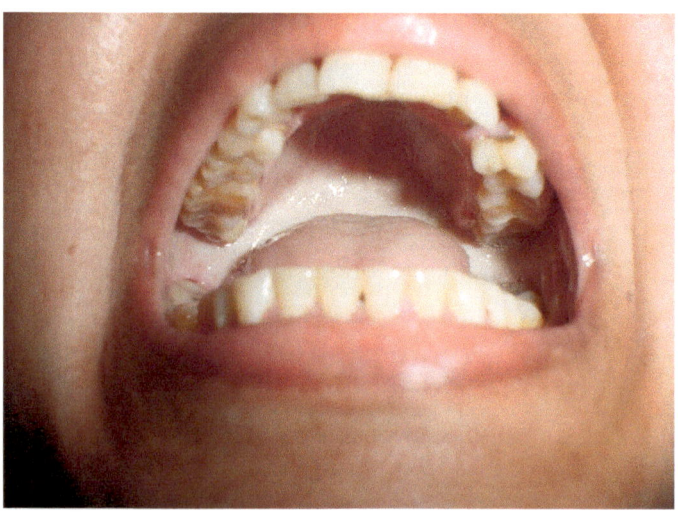

FIGURE 30.4. Submucous fibrosis.

Treatment is difficult, intralesional injections of triamcinolone and jaw exercises are required in the early stages. Surgery to relieve the fibrotic bands is done in the later stages. CO_2 laser provides instant relief but not long-term cure. Vitamin A supplements along with zinc and folic acid relieve the chronicity of the lesion.

30.6 Lichen Planus

The mucous membrane of the mouth is frequently affected. The lesions are usually located on the inner side of the cheeks; these consist of pinhead-sized white papules that form annular lesions, linear patterns, or appear as discrete puncta. More commonly, there is an aggregation of these to form a reticulated or lace-like pattern. Similar lesions occur on the palate, lips, and tongue (Figs. 30.5 and 30.6). On the tongue, plaque-like lesions may appear resembling leukoplakia. On the lips,

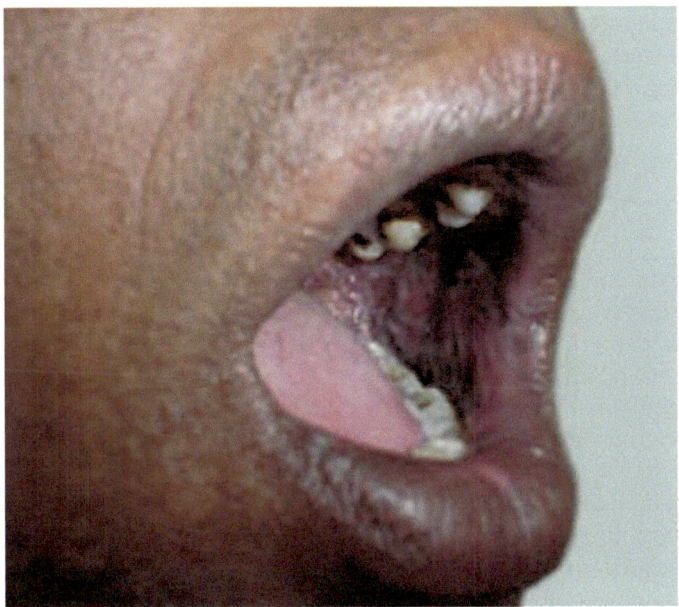

FIGURE 30.5. Lichen planus – oral cavity.

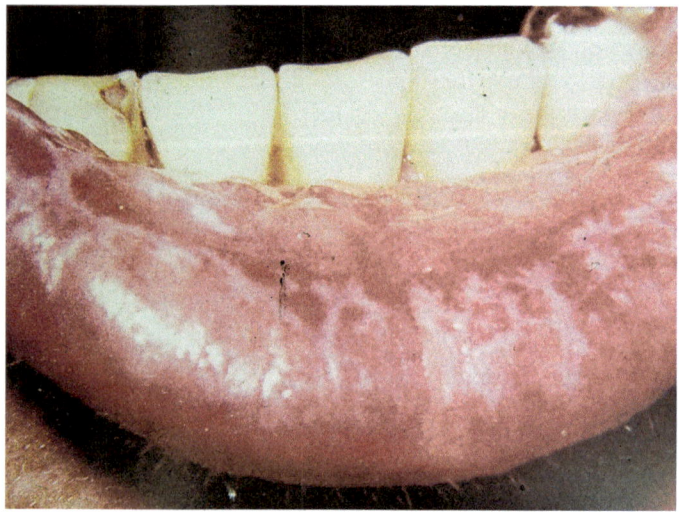

FIGURE 30.6. Lichen planus lips.

papules are often seen in an annular form and there is an adherent scale similar to that of lupus erythematosus. In severe cases, vesicles and bullae appear and these ulcerate; the ulcers are painful and may undergo malignancy. Such lesions need a careful follow-up.

30.7 Betel Leaf Stomatitis

Also called the "paan" mouth, is a common clinical condition seen in the Indo-Pakistan subcontinent. It is merely the outcome of perpetual contact of the oral mucosa with the betel leaf (called "paan" in India and Pakistan) coated with slaked lime and cate-chu (a bark), often retained in the mouth for long hours.

Burgundy-colored, bizarre irregular patches with a some-what corrugated buccal mucosa may look frightening, but is usually benign in nature. However, in rare instances a malig-nant lesion may remain masqueraded underneath. Hence, in suspicious cases thorough removal of the red-pigmented patch should be undertaken, careful follow-up is required.

30.7.1 Treatment

There should be total abstinence from consumption of paan, as in some conditions malignancy may supervene.

> *People of the Indian subcontinent should refrain from paan chewing; it predisposes to malignancy and submucous fibrosis.*

30.8 Lesions on the Tongue

The tongue can also provide valuable clues to a number of disorders. Black hairy tongue is due to the pigmentation and hypertrophy of the filiform papillae due to bacterial overgrowth, as seen after an antibiotic therapy. A smooth tongue is often due to nutritional deficiency, sprue, and malabsorbtion. Fissured tongue may be congenital; it is seen in Down's syndrome, and in the aging process. Geographical tongue may be familial; it can also occur in psoriasis and atopics. White hairy leukoplakia is a characteristic of AIDS. Macroglossia is seen in mucopolysaccharidosis, amyloidosis, growths or tumors; it can also be developmental. Herpes simplex and zoster can manifest on the tongue. Median rhomboidal glossitis can be developmental, due to candidiasis and smoking. Simple furred tongue is due to the hypertrophy of the filiform papillae as seen in infections and fever. Glossodynia or burning-mouth syndrome may be due to trauma, diabetes, menopause, nutritional, candidiasis, dry mouth or it may be psychological.

30.8.1 Treatment

Remove the cause.

30.9 Lesions on the Lips

Lips are a common site for herpes simplex, actinic cheilitis, contact dermatitis, angular cheilitis, and cheilitis exfoliativa.

30.9.1 Actinic Cheilitis

The condition is mostly seen in outdoor workers or athletes due to ultraviolet radiation of the sun. The lower lip is involved is almost all cases; the vermillion border being the most commonly affected site.

30.9.1.1 Clinical Features

In early stages, the lip is red and edematous; it then becomes dry and scaly. In later stages, the lips become thick with small grayish-white plaques. Fissuring, erosion, and crusting may occur. Ulceration is rare; if it does occur it is a sign of malignant change.

30.9.1.2 Treatment

Avoid prolonged exposure to sunlight. Application of sun blocks, 5% flourourocil, topical tretinoin or trichloracetic acid may provide relief in some cases. If malignancy develops, the treatment is vermillectomy or laser ablation.

30.9.2 Angular Cheilitis

This is an inflammation of the angles of the mouth, it can occur at any age. In the young it is due to lip licking and thumb sucking. In adults it may be due to mouth breathing, poorly fitting dentures or aggressive use of dental floss. During old age, it is due to sagging of the skin and weight loss, and an intertriginous space forms at the angle of the mouth. Capillary action draws the fluid from the angle of the mouth into the fold, creating maceration, chapping, fissures, erythema, exudation, and secondary infection. Yeast and bacteria are often involved in the process. Vitamin B deficiency can also cause angular stomatitis.

30.9.2.1 Clinical Features

The infection starts as a sore fissure at the angle of the mouth, followed by erythema, scale, and crust formation.

30.9.2.2 Treatment

Antifungal and steroid creams are applied twice a day. Once healing occurs the steroids should be stopped, the area is then protected by the application of a thick protective film of lip balm. In old age collagen implants can be injected in the depths of the grooves.

30.9.3 Cheilitis Exfoliativa

This is a mild inflammation of the lip; it may be primary, the cause may be unknown, or secondary to atopic dermatitis, psoriasis, retinoid therapy, lip licking, actinic exposure, contact dermatitis, etc. The lower lip is usually involved. Most cases occur in young women, a personality disorder with licking and biting of the lips is frequent.

30.9.3.1 Treatment

Remove the cause; topical steroids and zinc are usually helpful.

White lesions of the oral cavity
Candida
Leukoplakia
Smoker's keratosis
Lichen planus
Koplicks spots
Fordyce spots
Syphilis
Darier's disease
Systemic lupus erythematosus
HIV – white hairy leukoplakia
Submucous fibrosis

Oral ulcers
Apthous ulcers
Herpes simplex
Herpes zoster
Traumatic
Pemphigus
Lichen planus
Erythema multiforme
Systemic lupus erythematosus
Reiter's disease
Syphilis
Tuberculosis
Crohn's disease
Pernicious anaemia
Malignancy-SCC

Chapter 31
Diseases of the External Genitalia

The skin diseases affecting the external genitalia are those that are related to cutaneous disorders, cutaneous manifestations of systemic disease, and sexually transmitted diseases. Almost any cutaneous disorder can manifest on the skin of the external genitalia, the common cutaneous disorders seen on the genital skin are contact dermatitis, seborrhoeic dermatitis, lichen simplex chronicus, fixed drug eruption, intertrigo, candidiasis, lichen planus, psoriasis, herpes simplex, and molluscum contiagiosum. This chapter discusses the diseases specific to the external genitalia.

31.1 Vulval Intraepithelial Dysplasia (VIN)

The term vulval intraepithelial neoplasia (VIN) replaces the previously used terms such as carcinoma in situ, Bowen's disease, Bowenoid papulosis, and leukoplakia.

31.1.1 Clinical Features

An increasing number of women under the age of 40 years are affected. by the disease. Pruritus is most common and 20–45% of the patients are asymptomatic. The lesions appear as plaques with a rough surface. The plaque may be white due to hyperkeratosis, red due to thinness of the epithelium, and brown due to increased melanin deposition. The lesions are

Z. Zaidi, S. W. Lanigan, *Dermatology in Clinical Practice*,
DOI: 10.1007/978-1-84882-862-9_31,
© Springer-Verlag London Limited 2010

often multifocal; in a small number of cases a malignant change can occur.

31.1.2 Treatment

Treatment is difficult; it should be cautious and conservative. If the patient is asymptomatic then it is best to observe the patient at regular intervals to check for any malignant change. Topical steroids are the mainstay of treatment; α-interferon has given promising results in a small number of cases. If the lesion is small then excisional biopsy is the treatment of choice.

31.2 Paget's Disease

This is an uncommon condition, similar to that affecting the breast. Pruritus is the presenting complaint; the lesion is indistinguishable from squamous intraepithelial neoplasms. The lesion appears as red, crusted plaques with a clear margin. The disease is diagnosed by biopsy; one-third of the cases can develop into adenocarcinoma of the apocrine gland.

31.2.1 Treatment

Wide local excision lesion is required, usually involving total vulvectomy.

31.3 Lichen Sclerosus (LS)

This is the commonest condition found in elderly women complaining of pruritus vulvae. LS may also occur in children and less commonly in younger women. The cause is unknown but probably autoimmune.

31.3.1 Clinical Features

The disease can also occur on the upper back, chest, and breast. The lesions begin as white flat-topped papules with an erythematous halo. The papules gradually flatten, coalesce, and become depressed below the surface. The skin, in later stages of LS, looks thin with a crinkled surface. The skin may become lichenified due to itching. Although the risk of malignancy is small (4%), a biopsy should be performed in suspicious cases.

31.3.2 Treatment

If the patient is symptomless then no treatment is required. Mild itching can be treated by 1% hydrocortisone skin ointment; the strength can be increased if required. Although the skin is thin and wrinkled, steroids, even potent ones, can correct itching and some of the pathological changes of LS. I/L steroids can also be used in lichenified cases. Testosterone in bland ointments is also reported to be partially effective in LS. Vulvectomy is required in severe cases.

In men, circumcision relieves the symptoms.

31.4 Erythroplasia of Queyrat

The condition is similar to Bowen's disease of the skin. Single or multiple well-defined, velvety plaques are seen on the glans penis of uncircumcised men over the age of 40. Similar lesions are seen on the vulva in women. Malignant transformation is common (Fig. 31.1).

31.4.1 Treatment

5-flourouracil is the treatment of choice, recurrences are infrequent because the hair follicles that serve as a foci of recurrences are absent on the penile mucosa. Erythroplasia of Queyrat of the distal penis may require Moh's surgery.

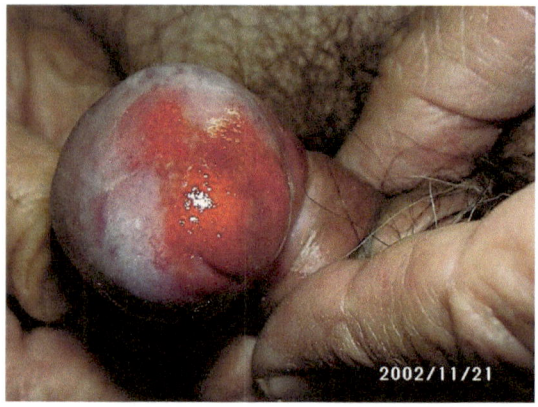

FIGURE 31.1. Erythroplasia of Queyrat.

Syphilis and chancroid discussed in Chap. 4

HIV infection *discussed in Chap. 6*

Chapter 32
Miscellaneous Disorders

32.1 Amyloidosis

This is a disorder of protein metabolism, in which there is an abnormal deposition of insoluble fibrillar protein in the body, which is resistant to proteolysis. The type of amyloid deposits depends upon the precursor proteins that form the fibrillar deposits. Amyloid can be derived from the keratin of the epidermis (amyloid K), from immunoglobulins (amyloid IO), from acute phase proteins (amyloid A), etc. In familial amyloidosis, the amyloid is derived from mutant proteins; the most common is transthyretin.

32.1.1 Cutaneous Amyloidosis

This may be primary or secondary. Secondary amyloidosis is seen in diseases such as psoriasis, hidradenitis suppurativa, dystrophic epidermolysis bullosa, chronic ulcers, burns, basal cell carcinoma, etc.

Primary amyloidosis affects both the sexes, they manifest as macules, papules or nodules. The disease is more common in Orientals. Macular amyloidosis is the most subtle form of the disease. This commonly occurs in the inter-scapular region as brown rippled macules (Fig. 32.1). Lichen amyloidosis is most commonly seen on the shins; the papules are small, brown and discrete (Fig. 32.2). Nodular amyloidosis is the least common form of primary amyloidosis. Single or

Z. Zaidi, S. W. Lanigan, *Dermatology in Clinical Practice*,
DOI 10.1007/978-1-84882-862-9_32,
© Springer-Verlag London Limited 2010

multiple nodules or plaques occur on the trunk, limbs or vulva. The overlying skin is atrophic; petechiae and haemorrhage may be found in the nodules.

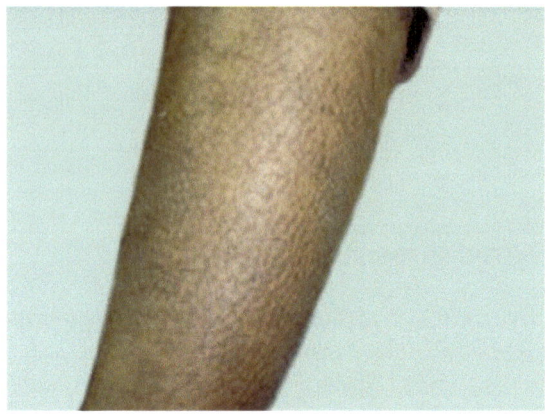

FIGURE 32.1. Macular amyloidosis – note the rippled appearance.

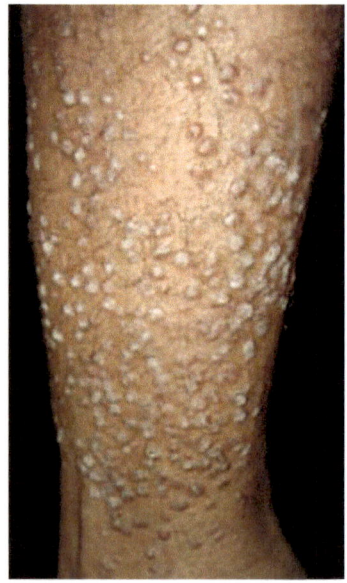

FIGURE 32.2. Lichen amyloidosis.

32.1.2 Systemic Amyloidosis

In primary systemic amyloidosis, cutaneous eruptions appear as shiny, smooth, flat-topped papules of waxy color. These may coalesce to form plaques and nodules. These are commonly found around the mouth, nose, eyes, and mucocutaneous junctions. Alopecia occurs if the lesions are on the scalp. Nails are brittle with long striations.

Secondary systemic amyloidosis does not affect the skin.

In systemic amyloidosis, the clinical features are related to the organs affected, for example, kidney involvement manifests as proteinuria and nephrotic syndrome. Various combinations of carpel tunnel syndrome, macroglossia, and visceral involvement are seen. Amyloid can infiltrate the blood vessels of the skin, these rupture easily, causing purpura. Purpura can occur after minor trauma such as pinching the skin (pinch purpura).

32.1.3 Treatment

The treatment of amyloidosis is disappointing. Mild cases can be helped with a potent topical steroid or intralesional injections of corticosteroids. Topical application of 10% dimethylsulphoxide (DMSO) has been used in the treatment of amyloidosis in Equador where amyloidosis is very common, but evidence for its benefit is conflicting.

Acitretin appears to be helpful in relieving the troublesome pruritus of lichen amyloidosis. The nodular form responds to shave removal or curettage, although recurrences are likely.

Systemic amyloidosis can be treated with melphalan, colchicine, or thymosin. A marked improvement is seen with the long-term use of DMSO, this therapy often results in an obvious odor.

In cardiac and renal failure, cardiac and renal transplantation may benefit.

32.2 Mucinosis

These disorders are characterized by deposition of mucin in the skin. The depositions may be diffuse, focal, or follicular.

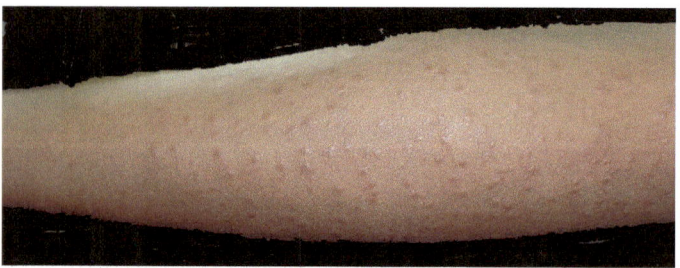

FIGURE 32.3. Lichen mucinosis.

Lichen mucinosis (scleromyxoedema) is seen as generalized papules, nodules, or annular lesions over an erythematous and hardened skin. The skin is thick but is movable over the sub-cutis (Fig. 32.3). Some patients improve with melphalan. *Follicular mucinosis* (alopecia mucinosa) is associated with deposition of excessive mucin in the external root sheath of the hair follicle. On the body, they are seen as plaques of infil-trated skin with follicular prominence, on the scalp it presents as alopecia. Follicular mucinosis may be associated with myco-sis fungoides. *Pretibial myxaedema* is associated with thyroid disorders; it is localized to the front of the shins and feet.

32.3 Langerhans Cell Histiocytosis

The condition was previously known as histiocytosis X, because at that time the nature of the cell infiltration was not confirmed. In these disorders, Langerhans cells accumulate in various tissues and cause damage. A number of these condi-tions are seen in infancy and childhood. Cutaneous involve-ment when present is characterized by a greasy seborrhoeic dermatitis-like eruption on the scalp, chest, and black-brown scaly purpuric papules; and persistent napkin dermatitis. Purpura and petechiae are associated with a poor prognosis.

Treatment includes oral prednisolone, alone or in combi-nation with vinblastine or methotrexate. Radiation is given to those patients who do not respond to chemotherapy. Patients with onset below the age of six, and those with multiple organ involvement have a poor prognosis.

32.4 Benign Lymphocytic Cutaneous Infiltrations

Lymphocytes infiltrate the skin in infective, inflammatory, autoimmune disorders, and in malignancy. However, there are a number of conditions in which the lymphocytes infiltrate the skin, without any known pathology. These are:

32.4.1 Jessener's Lymphocytic Infiltration

The lesions present as pinkish or reddish brown plaques, usually present on the face, neck, and upper trunk. The lesions fluctuate in severity over time and may disappear completely. Some patients complain of exacerbation in sunlight. Treatment is difficult; topical steroids and antimalarials have been used.

32.4.2 Lymphocytoma Cutis

The lesions are usually confined to the head and neck; they appear as red or purple nodules. The lesions do not fluctuate to the same degree as in Jessner's lymphocytic infiltration. The condition is treated by intralesional steroid injections. Penicillin and radiotherapy have also been used.

32.4.3 Pseudolymphoma

Multiple erythematous cutaneous nodules are often seen after systemic therapy with drugs such as beta-blockers and antiscabetic treatment; it is also seen after insect bites. The condition is benign. Pseudolymphoma is a self-limiting condition, once the offending agents are removed.

32.5 Kyrle's Disease

This is a disease caused by areas of abnormal local keratinization. The process of keratinization proceeds faster and at deeper layers than in the adjacent skin. This causes disruption of the epidermis and release of horny material. It is a disease of adults; the lower extremities are commonly affected. The lesions appear as papules with a central keratin plug. The papules may coalesce to form a plaque. This condition is also seen in renal failure. Flattening of the lesion can be achieved by the application of retinoic acid.

32.6 Granuloma Annulare

This is a necrobiotic disorder, which can be localized, generalized, nodular, or perforating. The localized form is the most common, this presents as a ring of small, firm, flesh or red colored papules without scaling. The sites of predilection are the lateral and dorsal surface of the hands and feet (Fig. 32.4). The disease is asymptomatic, other than due to its appearance. The ring may gradually increase in size, many lesions undergo

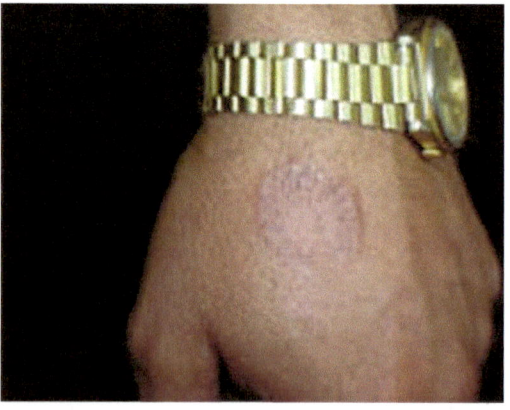

FIGURE 32.4. Granular annulare.

spontaneous resolution. The generalized form is often associated with diabetes mellitus.

32.6.1 Differential Diagnosis

The disease should be differentiated from other annular lesions such as tinea corporis, annular psoriasis, annular lichen planus, and erythema annulare centrifugum.

32.6.2 Treatment

Granuloma annulare can be treated by intralesional injection of 5–10 mg/mL corticosteroids. The solution should be injected into the elevated lesions. Systemic steroids, dapsone, isotretinoin, hydroxychloroquine, or niacinamide are used to treat the generalized form of the disease.

32.7 Reiter's Disease

This is a disease predominantly seen in young men. It is characterized by urethritis, followed by conjunctivitis and arthritis. Other systems of the body can also be involved. The urethritis has the features of nongonococcal urethritis; there is mild to moderate dysuria with transient mucopurulent discharge. Multiple joints of the lower limbs are involved. The joint involvement is nonsuppurative. Nonbacterial conjunctivitis is bilateral. Arthritis is the most serious and disabling feature of Reiter's disease. Chronic deforming arthritis is seen in 10–20% of cases.

Cutaneous involvement is seen in upto 30% of cases, the soles are the commonest sites of involvement, and the lesions present as thick hyperkeratotic plaques, which are psoriasiform with a distinctive circular scaly border. Sometimes the lesions become pustular. Nails are also thick, with subungal hyperkeratosis, but pitting and onycholysis are unusual. The lesions can spread to the palms, scalp, and the limbs similar to psoriasis. Similar lesions appear on the penis.

32.7.1 Differential Diagnosis

The disease should be differentiated from gonorrhea and psoriasis. The cutaneous involvement of the skin in gonorrhea is not significant; with pustules or papules on the extensor surface of the extremities, which heals by scarring. Joint involvement in gonorrhea is purulent; the exudate is rich in gonococci. Psoriasis mainly affects the joints of the upper extremities; pitting and onycholysis are characteristic changes in the nails.

32.7.2 Treatment

Arthritis is treated with nonsteroidal antiinflammatory agents. The skin and joint lesions are best treated with acitretin. When a triggering infection is present tetracycline, 500 mg is given four times daily for 14 days.

Hans Conrad Reiter (1881–1969)

Reiter described the clinical associations of urethritis, conjunctivitis, and arthritis, while in the German army during World War I. In 1932, Hans Reiter signed the oath of allegiance to Hitler and became involved in the infamous studies of eugenics. He was briefly interned in an American prison camp in 1945.

32.8 Poikiloderma

This is a descriptive term characterized by hypopigmentation, hyperpigmentation, atrophy, and telangiectasia. It may appear as a primary disease or secondary to a number of dermatoses such as mycosis fungoides, systemic lupus erythematosus, dermatomyositis, xeroderma pigmentosum, and after radiation. Poikiloderma of Civatte is a reticulate pigmentation limited to the face, neck, and upper chest. It is thought to be due to photosensitive chemicals present in perfumes and other cosmetics. There is no effective treatment. Patients should refrain from the use of such cosmetics, apply sunscreens and avoid exposure to sunlight. Vascular lasers and Intense Pulsed Light can sometimes improve the appearance.

32.9 Cutis Verticis Gyrata

This is a morphological condition in which there is overgrowth of the skin, in relation to the underlying skull. The disease is characterized by the presence of folds and furrows in the skin of the scalp (Fig. 32.5). The condition may be primary or secondary. Primary cutis verticis gyrata is an autosomal recessive disorder, often lethal to females. Secondary cutis verticis gyrata is often found in leukemias, acromegaly, and it is a feature of pachydermoperiostosis. Treatment is surgical.

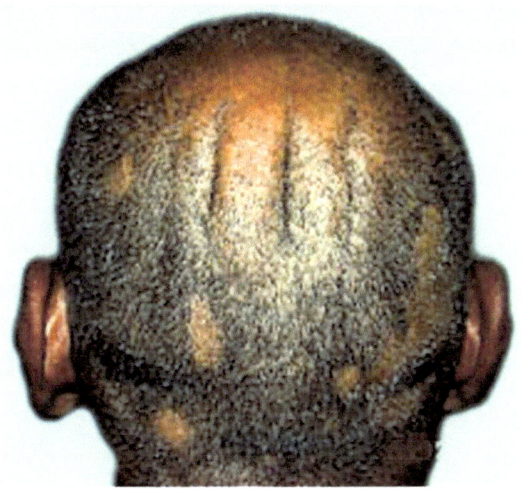

FIGURE 32.5. Cutis verticis gyrate.

Chapter 33
Drug Reactions

A drug can be defined as a chemical substance or a combination of substances administered for investigation, prevention, or treatment of diseases or symptoms. Adverse drug reactions may be the inevitable price we pay for the benefits of modern drug therapy.

33.1 Classification of Drug Reactions

- Pharmacological reactions are due to overdose of the drug, side effects of the drug, accumulation of the drug, delayed toxicity, facilitative effects, metabolic alterations, and teratogenicity.
- Immunological adverse reactions may be mediated by the following mechanisms:

  - Type I, IgE-mediated drug reactions
  - Type II, cytotoxic reactions
  - Type III, arthus or immune-complex-mediated reactions
  - Type IV, delayed hypersensitivity or cell-mediated

- Idiosyncratic reactions; these are peculiar to each individual.
- Miscellaneous

  - Jarish–Herxheimer reaction
  - Infectious mononucleosis ampicillin reaction
  - Lepra reactions in leprosy

Z. Zaidi, S. W. Lanigan, *Dermatology in Clinical Practice*,
DOI: 10.1007/978-1-84882-862-9_33,
© Springer-Verlag London Limited 2010

The two main types of drug reactions are the immunological and non-immunological.

33.1.1 Non-immunological Reactions

These reactions are often predictable, and may affect many patients taking the drug over a period of time. The reactions are studied before marketing and are given in the patient information leaflet of the drug prescribed, e.g., teratogenicity, dryness of the skin, eyes and mucosa in patients taking retinoids; striae in patients taking steroids, etc. Vaginal candidiasis occurs when antibiotics remove the normal flora of the vagina with subsequent overgrowth of yeasts.

33.1.2 Immunological Reactions

These affect a minority of patients, receiving the drug even in low doses. Chemically related drugs may cross-react. These reactions usually occur in the form of urticaria, angioedema, erythema multiforme, morbilliform eruptions, erythroderma, and hypersensitivity syndrome reaction. The syndrome consists of a triad of fever, rash, and internal involvement. The most likely drugs to cause the eruption are antibiotics, analgesics, nonsteroidal antiinflammatory agents, and anticonvulsants.

33.2 Approach to a Patient with a Suspected Drug Reaction

When a patient presents with a rash, and a drug eruption is suspected; a thorough drug history should be taken. An elderly patient often has a history of multiple drug intake. Try and determine which drug is likely to cause the eruption. The drug, which was introduced last, is probably the cause. The majority of drug eruptions fit into a defined category, as shown in the table below. Laboratory tests are often unhelpful. Peripheral blood eosinophilia is sometimes present. Skin biopsy usually shows a nonspecific lymphocytic perivascular infiltrate. The presence of eosinophils in the infiltrate is an indicator of a possible drug eruption.

The offending drug should be stopped immediately. The speed at which the reaction disappears depends upon the type of reaction, and the rapidity with which the drug is eliminated.

Common drugs and the likely pattern of eruption	
Medicament	**Pattern of eruption**
Sulphonamides, penicillin	Morbilliform eruption, erythema, multiforme, systemic lupus, erythematosus, exfoliative dermatitis
Beta-blockers, lithium	Psoriasiform eruption
Barbiturates, sulphonamides	Bullae, fixed drug eruptions
Phenylbutazone	Purpuric eruption
Antimalarials	Lichen planus-like eruption
Iodides and Bromides	Acneform eruption
Phenothiazines, tetracyclines	Light sensitive dermatoses
Salicylates	Urticaria, angioedema
Phenytoin	Gingival hypertrophy, acne
Coumarin anticoagulants, cytotoxics antithyroid drugs	Alopecia

33.2.1 Fixed Drug Eruption

This is a unique form of drug reaction that produces a reaction at the same site, each time the drug is taken. The lesions can be single or multiple. It appears in the form of round erythematous plaques or bullae, the blisters then erode; crusting is followed by pigmentation, which is violaceous or brown in color. Pigmentation persists between the episodes. The genitalia and face are sites of special predilection. The lesions are preceded by itching and burning (Fig. 33.1).

On re-exposure to the drug, the rash usually appears within 30 minutes to 8 hours. Some patients may demonstrate a refractory period of weeks to months during which the offending drug does not activate the lesion.

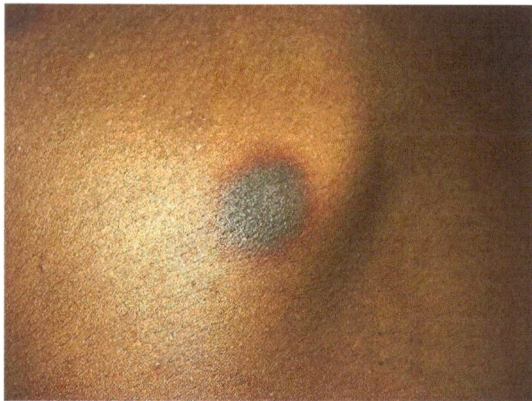

FIGURE 33.1. Fixed Drug Eruption.

Drugs causing this reaction include the sulphonamide, aspirin, ibuprofen, tetracycline, systemic antifungal drugs, psychotropic drugs, hyoscine butylbromide, barbiturates, chlordiazepoxide, dapsone, phenazone, phenophthalein, quinine, benzodiazepines, and paracetamol. Paracetamol is presently the most common offender in the UK.

33.2.2 Exfoliative Dermatitis

Exfoliative dermatitis is a generalized, erythematous scaly eruption and is one of the most dangerous cutaneous reactions to drugs. Sulphonamide, penicillin, antimalarials, phenylbutazone, thiacetazone, topical tar, a variety of homeopathic medicines, and recently captopril and cimetidine have been implicated.

33.2.2.1 Treatment

The offending drug should be discontinued. If a patient is taking many drugs it becomes difficult which drug to exclude. Often, but not always, the latest drug introduced is the likely drug causing the eruption.

Treatment is otherwise symptomatic with antihistamines mostly used for pruritus, or topical lotions such as calamine lotion or calamine cream with 1–2% menthol. Moisturizing lotions may be used if desquamation is prominent.

Patients with bronchospasm or signs of anaphylaxis may require emergency treatment with subcutaneous adrenaline (0.5 mL of 1 in 1,000 solution given slowly in 2–3 min) as well as parental corticosteroids and antihistamines. Intubation may be required.

Systemic steroids may be of value in some cases of severe reactions such as toxic epidermal necrolysis, the hypersensitivity syndrome, sometimes called Drug Reaction with Eosinophilia and Systemic Symptoms (DRESS), which has a mortality rate of about 10% or Steven Johnson syndrome. Steroids may actually have an adverse effect in late cases of Toxic Epidermal Necrolysis (TEN). An initial dose of parental hydrocortisone is followed by oral prednisolone (1 mg/kg body weight) and withdrawn over a period of 7–10 days.

In general the more extensive an eruption, the longer the period required for resolution.

> For any generalized rash think of drug reaction especially in the elderly.
>
> The morbilliform drug eruptions are pruritic, redder, and more confluent than viral exanthems.
>
> Prescribe a drug only if it is necessary; polypharmacy is to be avoided. TEN should be treated in a burns unit.

Chapter 34
Management of Skin Diseases

34.1 Principles of Topical Therapy

Skin is the most accessible organ to treat. There are many therapeutic approaches to skin disease. These are by topical application of drugs, intralesional injections, oral medication, physical therapy, and surgery. The topical approach is time-consuming; a large amount of medication may be required to produce the desired effect and it may not be aesthetical and pleasing to the patient. Patients often complain of the color, smell, and greasiness of ointments. However, this approach has the advantage of delivering the drug to the target organ, and does not have the side effects of systemic toxicity if used within the required limits, and above all the results can be seen by the naked eye.

- The active ingredient should be of low molecular weight, it should be lipid soluble and it should be polar, for easy absorption through the stratum corneum.
- The vehicle to which the active ingredient is added should be nontoxic, nonallergic, nonirritant, chemically stable, bacteriostatic, and cosmetically acceptable. The vehicle can be an ointment, cream, lotion, gel, or aerosol. Ointments are used for dry scaly lesions such as lichenified eczema, psoriasis, etc. Creams and lotions are prescribed for acute and exudative disorders. For weeping eruptions, wet dressings are preferred. The oft-repeated rule while treating skin disease is: "*If it is dry 'wet it', if it is wet 'dry it'.*"

Z. Zaidi, S. W. Lanigan, *Dermatology in Clinical Practice*,
DOI 10.1007/978-1-84882-862-9_34,
© Springer-Verlag London Limited 2010

- Site of application. The drugs move across the stratum corneum by passive diffusion. The higher the concentration, the greater the amount absorbed. The diffusion is slow through the stratum corneum, but rapid through the viable epidermis.

In the palms and soles, where the stratum corneum is thick absorption is poor, while in the eyelids and scrotum, the absorption is rapid as the skin is thinnest in these areas.

A break in the stratum corneum allows the rapid absorption of drugs.

The intertriginous areas act like occlusive dressings because of the apposition of the skin surfaces.

The skin of infants and young children is more receptive to topical medications and respond quickly to weaker creams.

The diaper area also is more absorbent due to the occlusion by diapers.

- The amount of ointment to be dispensed depends upon the surface area of skin affected. It is estimated that 1 g of the drug will cover an area of 10×10 cm of skin. The amount dispensed is as follows:

    - 2 g for the face
    - 2 g for each hand
    - 2 g for each foot
    - 3 g for each arm
    - 4 g for each leg
    - 3 g for the front of the chest
    - 3 g for the back

About 30 g are required for the whole body. The "finger tip unit" (FTU) is used to measure the amount of topical medication required to be dispensed. 1 FTU is the amount of ointment expressed from a tube of a 5 mm diameter nozzle, applied from the distal skin crease to the tip of the index finger. This amount is about 0.5 g.

- Frequency of application. Medicaments can be applied one to four or five times a day depending upon the disease and condition of the skin, e.g., acyclovir is applied after every 3 h during the day: for very dry skin moisturizers can be applied frequently. Generally, for infections the treatments are applied one to three times a day. Stratum corneum acts as a reservoir for topical steroids; it releases the drugs after the initial application. Most steroids are applied once or twice daily.

Topical therapy has the advantage of direct application of the drug to the target organ, and reduced side effects of systemic therapy.

Enough medication to treat all affected areas for 1–2 weeks should be prescribed, to avoid noncompliance on the part of the patient.

34.2 Drugs Commonly Used in the Management of Skin Disorders

34.2.1 Corticosteroids

These can be used topically, by intralesional injections and orally.

Topical steroids are widely used in dermatology; they are used in the treatment of contact dermatitis (this makes up about 30% of patients in a skin clinic), inflammatory disorders such as lupus erythematosus, some bullous disorders, psoriasis, lichen planus, etc. A clinician should have some knowledge of their potency, site of application, side effects, amount to be dispensed, and method of application.

When corticosteroids are applied to the skin, the changes produced are antiinflammatory, immunosuppressive, and antiproliferative.

34.2.2 Potency of Steroids

Steroids are generally graded as follows:

- Weak steroids

    - Hydrocortisone acetate 1.0%
    - Dexamethasone 0.1%

- Moderately potent steroids

    - Fluocinolone acetonide 0.025%
    - Flucortolone hexanoate (ultralanum) 0.1%
    - Clobetasone butyrate (Eumovate) 0.05%

- Potent steroids

    - Betamethasone valerate (Betnovate) 0.1%
    - Betamethasone dipropionate (Diprolene) 0.05%
    - Triamcinolone acetonide 0.1%
    - Hydrocortisone valerate 0.2%
    - Hydrocortisone butyrate 0.1%
    - Flucinalone acetonide (Synalar) 0.05%
    - Diflucortolone valerate (Nerisone) 0.1%

- Very potent steroids

    - Clobetasol propionate (Dermovate) 0.05%
    - Diflucortolone valerate (Nerisone-Forte) 0.3%

34.2.2.1 Vasoconstriction Bioassay

This test is extremely useful to assess the potency and percutaneous absorption of topical steroids. The degree of blanching at the site of application correlates to the antiinflammatory potency of corticosteroids. A solution of corticosteroids is applied to the forearms and the area is occluded for 16 h prior to observation. The assay also measures the penetration and clearance of the steroid.

This effect is especially useful for ranking the efficacy of topical steroids. Hydrocortisone barely vasoconstricts, floucinolone acetonide produces vasoconstriction 100 times that of hydrocortisone. Betamethasone is 360 times and clobetasol propionate is 1,640 times as potent as hydrocortisone.

34.2.2.2 Tachyphylaxis

This refers to the decrease in responsiveness to a drug because of enzyme induction. In dermatology it is used primarily in reference to topical steroids. The decrease in response to a steroid is indicated by the decrease of vasoconstrictive effect on the skin. Experience has shown that the vasoconstrictive effect of the steroid on the skin decreases when a potent steroid is applied on the skin three times a day after about four days of therapy. It is therefore advised that potent steroids should be used on an intermittent basis.

34.2.2.3 Systemic Indications

- Acute allergic contact dermatitis
- Acute autoimmune connective tissue diseases such as systemic lupus erythematosus
- Acute anaphylactic reactions
- Chronic immunobullous disorders such as pemphigus
- Acute generalized exfoliative dermatitis
- Miscellaneous conditions including severe lichen planus, vasculitis, pyoderma gangrenosum, and sarcoidosis. Corticosteroids are often used in other diseases, but the value of such treatment is unproven as in erythema multiforme, toxic epidermal necrolysis, and cutaneous T cell lymphoma

34.2.2.4 Topical Indications

- Eczema
- Lichen planus
- Some forms of psoriasis
- Alopecia areata
- Vitiligo

34.2.2.5 Intralesional Indications

- Keloids
- Granuloma annulare
- Alopecia areata
- Hypertrophic lichen planus
- Nodular prurigo
- Cystic acne
- Lichen simplex chronicus

34.2.2.6 Side Effects of Corticosteroids

These can be grouped under the following headings:

- Side effects of systemic steroids
- Side effects of topical steroids
- Side effects of intralesional steroid injections

Side Effects of Systemic Corticosteroids

Suppression of the pituitary adrenal axis, Cushingoid changes, purpura and ecchymosis, steroid acne, striae, gastritis and peptic ulcer, electrolyte imbalance, hyperglycemia and diabetes mellitus, flare up of latent infection, e.g., tuberculosis, skin and hair become thin and fragile, osteoporosis, and pathological fractures of the bones.

The above changes can also occur by excessive use of potent and moderately potent steroids by cutaneous absorption.

Oral steroids should be given in the morning. This is because the maximum rate of adrenocortisol secretion occurs in the morning, and less adrenocortical suppression will occur at this time, while the therapeutic efficacy is maintained.

If the patient is on a long-term therapy of steroids, it is advisable that he or she should have frequent urine and blood sugar examined, blood pressure and electrolyte levels checked, a potassium supplement administered when serum levels of potassium fall; the patient should be on antacid maintenance to prevent gastric acidity. Bone density should be monitored at regular intervals, osteoporosis prophylaxis should be instituted; this consists of calcium 1.0–1.5 g daily depending on the diet, vitamin D 400 IU daily, and often biphosphonates, as well as weight-bearing exercises.

Side Effects of Topical Steroid

Epidermal effects – epidermal thinning is associated with a decrease in epidermal kinetic activity. The epidermis becomes atrophic; there is a general flattening of the epidermo-dermal convolutions. Melanocytes are inhibited and a vitiligo-like condition has been described.

Dermal effects – collagen synthesis is reduced; this results in the formation of striae. A poor support to the dermal vasculature leads to easy rupture of blood vessels on trauma, leading to blot hemorrhages. This injury results in the formation of a stellate scar.

The skin becomes translucent and yellowish; telangiectasia appear. Cutaneous atrophy and telangiectasia are reversible but striae are permanent.

Vascular effects – corticosteroids first produce vasoconstriction of the superficial blood vessels, followed by a phase of rebound vasodilatation, which in later stages becomes fixed. As the vasoconstriction wears off, the small blood vessels overdilate, allowing edema, enhanced inflammation, and sometimes pustulation.

When corticosteroids are applied close to the eyes, glaucoma can be a hazard. Allergic contact dermatitis to the steroid molecule may also occur.

Potent corticosteroids can also suppress the pituitary adrenal axis when used extensively for long periods. In children, one should be very careful in using corticosteroids; even hydrocortisone when applied topically can suppress the pituitary adrenal axis.

Side Effects of Local Steroid Injections

Good results have been seen in many dermatoses by the intralesional injection of corticosteroids. The injections may produce subcutaneous atrophy at the site of injection. The patients become aware of depression at the site of injection. It may take as much as 6 months for lipid to accumulate and fill the gap; permanent atrophy is not uncommon.

Potent steroids should not be prescribed to infants and young children; who are especially vulnerable to the side effects of steroids.

When potent and very potent steroids are prescribed, discontinue the treatment after 2–3 weeks for a week to prevent tachyphylaxis.

It is unnecessary to learn too many brand names of steroids. It is best to familiarize oneself with a few steroids of each potency, so that the clinician can safely give the right potency steroid at the correct site and for the appropriate disease.

Give the weakest preparation of the steroid that is effective for a particular eruption to the appropriate site.

Always use mild steroids on the face, intertriginous areas, and on infants.

Total dose of potent steroids should not exceed 50 g a week.

Patients who do not respond after 2 weeks of treatment, should be reassessed.

Steroids should be applied once or twice daily, and not more frequently as stratum corneum acts as a reservoir for steroids.

Contact dermatitis to the steroid should be considered when the patient's skin condition becomes worse with steroids.

Glaucoma, cataract, and delayed wound healing of corneal ulcers can occur, when steroids are applied close to the eyes.

Steroids are contraindicated in staphylococcal scalded skin syndrome and toxic shock syndrome.

34.2.3 Methotrexate

This is a folic acid antagonist, a powerful immunosuppressant with a little antiinflammatory activity. It is used for the treatment of psoriasis, bullous disorders, Norwegian scabies, and other uncommon dermatoses. Methotrexate is given on a 1 day a week protocol, either as a single dose or the oral triple dose regimen which is the most common method used. The three doses are given at 12 hourly intervals during a 36-h period, once each week.

Side effects. Methotrexate has a toxic effect on the bone marrow and intestinal epithelium. Mucosal ulceration can occur. Methotrexate is hepatotoxic on long-term use.

Dose. 0.2–0.4 mg/kg/week or 5–25 mg weekly. This is given singly or in three divided doses at 12-hours intervals.

Monitoring. Complete blood picture every week for the first month of treatment, then once a month. Liver function tests should be done every 4–8 weeks and a liver biopsy at a cumulative dose of 1.5 g. Measurement of amino terminal levels of type III procollagen (P3NP) has been advocated as an effective noninvasive test for ongoing hepatic fibrogenesis. This may avoid repeated liver biopsies.

The drug should not be given during pregnancy due to teratogenicity.

34.2.4 Azathioprine

A purine analogue, it inhibits DNA and RNA synthesis. It is an immunosuppressive drug, used as a steroid sparing agent. Azathioprine is used for the treatment of SLE, atopic dermatitis, and other autoimmune disorders such as pemphigus and pemphigoid. It is suitable for older patients as a single therapy for treatment. Younger patients are not generally treated with azathioprine as a single agent, because of the risk of malignancy.

The risk of myelosuppression can be predicted by the thiopurine methyl transferase (TPMT) activity, which should be assessed wherever possible before starting therapy. Patients with a low level of this enzyme are at high risk of myelosuppression.

Dose is 2.5 mg/kg/daily or 150 mg daily, in patients with TPMT levels of 19 or above.

Monitoring. Check blood picture weekly for 4 weeks then every 4–8 weeks.

34.2.5 Cyclosporin

This drug suppresses cell-mediated immunity; it may also have some direct effect of DNA synthesis and proliferation of keratinocytes. Its major toxic effects are nephrotoxicity and hypertension. Hirsutism and gingival hyperplasia may occur in some patients.

It is used in the treatment of psoriasis, lichen planus, bullous disorders, and atopic dermatitis.

Dose. 2–5 mg/kg daily.

Monitoring. Biweekly for serum creatinine levels and blood pressure assessment, for the first 12 weeks of therapy.

34.2.6 Dapsone

This is a long-acting sulphonamide. It acts by increasing lyso-somal activity; it may also act by inhibiting neutrophil chemotaxis. It is bacteriostatic; it also interferes with compliment activation and deposition.

It is used for the treatment of leprosy, dermatitis herpetiformis, chronic bullous disease of childhood, linear IgA dermatosis, pemphigoid, the bullous form of systemic lupus erythematosus, and other dermatoses with a neutrophilic rich cutaneous infiltrate.

Side effects include hemolysis and methemoglobinemia. This is more common in Asians, and people of Mediterranean and African descent, due to the increased incidence of deficiency of glucose 6-phosphate dehydrogenase found in people of these regions. Dapsone hypersensitivity may appear after 4 weeks of therapy. Peripheral motor neuropathy may develop after the first few months of therapy.

Dose. 50–200 mg/day, it is always better to start with the minimum effective dose and then gradually increase the amount.

Monitoring. Blood counts should be done every weekly in the first month, bi-weekly in the second month, then every month for 3 months. LFTs should also be tested periodically.

34.2.7 Psoralens

Available as methoxypsoralen and trimethylpsoralen. Psoralens intercalate with DNA; they react with it on exposure to ultraviolet light A. This method of treatment is called PUVA, where the letter "P" stands for psoralens. Psoralens are taken orally or applied topically. Two hours after oral intake the patient is exposed to ultraviolet light A. Psoralens inhibit DNA replication and increase melanin pigmentation; they may also suppress degradation of mast cells.

Psoralens when taken orally reach all parts of the body, but only those tissues that are exposed to ultraviolet light are affected. The eyes and male external genitals should be protected during treatment. A long-term side effect of PUVA is increased susceptibility to skin cancer. The patients should not sunbathe 24 hours prior treatment and they should avoid sun exposure for 24 hours after taking psoralens. Sunscreens should be used after therapy. Psoralen is a safe therapy, but the patient has to come to the hospital at least twice a week for therapy. Side effects are nausea and dryness of the skin.

Psoralens are used for the treatment of psoriasis, vitiligo, alopecia areata, cutaneous T cell lymphoma, and atopic dermatitis.

Dose. 0.6 mg/kg daily. The treatment is given two to three times a week.

Monitoring. The patients should be assessed after every 20 treatments and not more than 200 treatments should be given in their lifetime, to minimize skin cancer risk.

34.2.8 Retinoids

These are vitamin A derivatives; they affect the differentiation of epithelial cells. There are specific retinoic acid and retinol receptors in the skin. The oral retinoids used thera-peutically are isotretinoin and acitretin.

Isotretinoin is mainly used for the treatment of nodulocys-tic acne. It acts on all the areas of pathogenesis of acne; it decreases the sebum secretion, corrects the altered keratini-zation in the infundibulum of the hair follicle, prevents the formation of comedones and it is antiinflammatory. It can also be used in other disorders such as rosacea, Darier's dis-ease, and hidradenitis suppurativa.

Dose. 0.5–1 mg/kg of body weight/daily

Acitretin. This has replaced etretinate, as it is less bound to body fat than etretinate. It is used in the treatment of psoriasis, especially pustular and erythrodermic psoriasis, ichthyosis, and palmoplantar keratoderma. It is not a potent sebosup-pressive and is therefore not used for the treatment of acne.

Dose. 0.5–1 mg/kg of body weight/daily

Bexarotene, adapalene, and tazarotene are the third gen-eration retinoids. Bexarotene is used in cutaneous T cell lymphoma. Bexarotene has higher chances of metabolic abnormalities, hypothyroidism, and exfoliative dermatitis.

Dose of bexarotene 150–300 mg/m^2 daily

34.2.8.1 Side Effects of Retinoids

The most common side effects are dryness of the skin, cheili-tis, conjunctivitis, hair loss, headaches, skeletal hyperostosis, and depression. There is an increase in serum triglycerides in about 25% of patients. Retinoid should be discontinued if the triglycerides increase to 500 mg/dL, because of the risk of pancreatitis.

Retinoids are teratogenic; pregnancy is an absolute con-traindication to the use of retinoids. The patient should not get pregnant for at least 1 month after isotretinoin, and 2 years after acitretin.

Patients on retinoids should not receive additional vitamin A supplements; they should not wear contact lenses because of dryness of the cornea. Tetracycline should not be given to patients on retinoids because of pseudo tumor cerebri.

Monitoring of retinoids. Pretreatment and follow-up of fasting blood lipids should be done regularly until the lipid response to isotretinoin is established. Thyroxine levels should also be checked when bexarotene is administered.

Children receiving long-term retinoids should have periodic bony skeletal surveys.

34.2.9 Griseofulvin

This was the first antifungal introduced in the 1950s and is still used today. Griseofulvin inhibits fungal cell mitosis. It has low toxicity and it is economical. It is effective only against dermatophytes. The drug is fungistatic; it diffuses well in the stratum corneum, from the extracellular fluid and sweat. Increased sweating leads to increased concentration of the drug in the stratum corneum. Griseofulvin has to be given for longer courses for nail infections as it is not fungicidal.

Griseofulvin is a safe drug; the side effects are headaches and gastrointestinal disturbances. The drug potentiates the intoxicating effects of alcohol.

Dose. Adults: 20 mg/kg/daily
Children: 5–10 mg/kg/daily

34.2.10 Polyenes

These include nystatin and amphotericin B. Nystatin is only used for candidiasis, especially vaginal and oral candidiasis. Nystatin is not absorbed from the gastrointestinal tract, skin or vagina. It acts topically. Oral tablets are used to decrease the gastrointestinal colonization of candida. It is too toxic for systemic use.

Amphotericin B is a naturally occurring polyene macrolide; it is used in the treatment of mucocutaneous candidiasis and for almost all deep fungal infections.

Dose Amphotericin B is given by intravenous infusion in a dose of 0.4–1 mg/kg/day.

Side effects of amphotericin B are anorexia, nausea, vomiting, bronchospasm, and hypotension. Phlebitis is common at the site of infusion. Renal failure is an absolute contraindication for its use.

34.2.11 Azole Antifungals

These are the imidazoles and triazoles. They act by inhibiting the synthesis of ergosterol in the fungal cell wall. These drugs are fungistatic. For skin infections, 2–4 weeks of therapy are required (scalp infections require a little longer treatment), 12 weeks for fingernails, and 16 weeks for toenails. Pulse treatment can also be used for nail infections.

The *imidazoles* consist of a number of topical preparations such as clotrimazole, sulconazole, bifoconazole, oxiconazole, isoconazole, etc. The oral preparation of ketoconazole can be used in the treatment of oral and vaginal candidiasis, tinea versicolor, and seborrhoeic dermatitis. It is also effective against dermatophytes, but due to hepatotoxicity, other drugs are preferred. It is also used to treat deep fungal infections such as histoplasmosis.

Ketoconazole inhibits cytochrome P-450-dependent enzymes. It dissolves in acid gastric contents;food and antacids impair its absorption. It is hepatotoxic which limits its use.

Triazoles. These consist of itraconazole and fluconazole. These are similar to imidazoles in structure and mechanism of action. They are less likely to cause hepatotoxicity, probably due to a lesser effect on cytochrome P-450 dependent enzymes.

Itraconazole is active against dermatophytes, yeast, and deep fungal infections. It is the treatment of choice for blastomycosis. The action in the nails persists for about 6 months after stopping the drug. The drug is still present in the stratum corneum, 4 weeks after stopping the treatment. It is given on a full stomach.

Dose (dermatophytes). Itraconazole <20 kg: 5 mg/kg daily
20–40 kg: 100 mg daily
>40 kg: 200 mg daily
Dose (candida). Itraconazole 200 mg for 3–5 days

Fluconazole is also a broad spectrum antifungal; it is chiefly used for the treatment of candidiasis, cryptococcosis, and coccidioidomycosis. It can be given orally or intravenously. Fluconazole is highly water soluble, and is transported to the skin by sweat and concentrated by evaporation. It achieves high concentration in the stratum corneum and nails and persists for long periods.

Dose (dermatophytes). Fluconazole 150 mg once a week for 2–4 weeks

Dose (Candida). 150 mg only once

Azole antifungal may be teratogenic and should not be given during pregnancy.

34.2.12 Allylamines

These are a group of antifungal agents that inhibit the fungal ergosterol biosynthesis by inhibiting the enzyme squalene epoxidase. They do not inhibit the cytochrome P-450 dependent enzymes. They are fungicidal to dermatophytes, and fungistatic to yeasts. There are few side effects, these being gastrointestinal and loss of taste in some patients. Terbinafine is used both orally and topically; naftidine is available only as a topical preparation.

Terbinafine is keratophilic and lipophilic; it is well-distributed in adipose tissue, dermis, epidermis, and nails. Terbinafine is distributed to the epidermis mainly through sebum. Its action persists in the skin 2–3 weeks after its discontinuation. After 6–12 weeks of oral therapy, terbinafine can be detected in the nail plate for 30–36 weeks. The drug is very effective in onychomycosis due to dermatophytes.

Dose. Terbinafine. <20 kg: 62.5 mg daily

20–40 mg: 125 mg daily

>40 kg: 250 mg daily

34.2.13 Acyclovir

This is an antiviral drug; it requires three phosphorylation steps for its activation. Acyclovir is phosphorylatcd by the herpes virus enzyme, thymidine kinase. The drug is most effective against herpes virus simplex infection; it is less effective against varicella zoster virus and cytomegalovirus. These conditions need an even higher concentration of the drug. Acyclovir acts against the replicating virus; it does not act against the latent virus.

Dose for herpes simplex: 200 mg five times a day for 5–7 days

Herpes zoster: 800 mg five times a day for 7–10 days

Acyclovir is also available for topical applications, and for intravenous injections.

Side effects are few; local irritation and burning occur with topical use. Oral administration is well-tolerated; nausea, vomiting, and headaches are reported in a few cases.

The *other antiviral drugs* used are valaciclovir, famciclovir, and pemciclovir. Foscarnet is used when patients are resistant to acyclovir.

Valaciclovir for herpes simplex: 500 mg b.i.d, for 5 days

Herpes zoster: 1 g t.i.d, for 7 days

Famciclovir for herpes simplex: 125 mg b.i.d, for 5 days

Herpes zoster: 500 mg t.i.d, for 7 days

34.3 Immunobiologicals

Immunobiologicals are biologically active agents that imitate or inhibit naturally occurring proteins; these are useful for the management of immunologically mediated diseases of infectious or noninfectious origin. Principal immunobiologicals are monoclonal antibodies, fusion inhibitors, and interferons. The immunobiologicals used in dermatology are:

- Modifiers of T cell response such as alefacept and efalizumab
- Tumour necrotic factor (TNF) antagonists such as etanercept and infliximab
- Interferons
- Intravenous gamma globulins

34.3.1 Alefacept

This is a fusion protein that binds to CD2 molecules of the T cells and inhibits co-stimulatory signals. It also causes apoptosis of memory T cells. It is used in the treatment of psoriasis. It is given in a dose of 10–15 mg by I/M injection every week for 12 weeks (further courses optional). CD4 levels should be monitored during therapy; levels should be above 250 cells/mm^2.

34.3.2 Efalizumab

This is a humanized monoclonal antibody that binds lymphocytes surface marker CD11a, which binds to intercellular adhesion molecule (ICAM), and therefore inhibits trafficking and activation of T cells. It is used for the treatment of psoriasis. It is given in a dose of 0.7 mg/kg in the first dose by subcutaneous injection and then 1 mg/kg weekly doses. Blood platelets should be monitored before starting therapy, every month for 3 months, and then after every 3 months, as thrombocytopenia can occur during therapy.

34.3.3 Etanercept

This is a fusion protein that inhibits cytokines, tumor necrotic actor (TNF)-α and TNF-β. It is used for the treatment of psoriasis, rheumatoid arthritis, cicatricial pemphigoid, Langerhans cell histiocytosis, Behcet's disease and scleroderma. The drug is given in a dose of 25 mg by subcutaneous injection twice a week; no special monitoring is required.

34.3.4 Infliximab

This is a chimeric monoclonal antibody that inhibits TNF-α and triggers complement mediated lysis of TNF-α expressing cells. It is used in a number of disorders such as psoriasis, rheumatoid arthritis, pyoderma gangrenosum, Behcets disease, graft versus host reaction, toxic epidermal necrolysis, and subcorneal pustular dermatosis. It is given in a dose of 5 mg/kg in an I/V infusion, at 0, 2, and 6 weeks. It can be repeated every 4–6 weeks. Baseline levels of purified protein derivative (PPD) and X-ray of chest should be done, as there is an increased risk of serious infections during therapy.

34.3.5 Denileukin Difitox

This is a fusion protein consisting of diphtheria toxin and interleukin-2, which directs the cytotoxic activity of the diphtheria toxin to cells expressing the interleukin-2 receptor. It is used in the treatment of psoriasis and cutaneous T cell lymphoma. The dose is 9–18 mcg/kg/day for 5 consecutive days, given every 21 days. Complete blood count, liver function, renal function, and serum albumin should be monitored. The drug should not be given if the serum albumin level falls below 3.

34.3.6 Interferons (IFN)

These are a family of glycoproteins, which are synthesized by leukocytes (INF-α), fibroblasts (IFN-β), and immune cells (IFN-γ). IFN-α is mainly used for therapeutic purposes; it has an antiproliferatory and immunoregulatory effect. It can be used in resistant cases of herpes simplex infection, atopic dermatitis, systemic sclerosis, Kaposi's sarcoma, malignant melanoma, etc.

34.3.7 Intravenous Immunoglobulins

These are heterogeneous human gamma-globulins that contain IgG with traces of IgA and IgM. IgG is a safe, therapeutic option in the management of skin diseases when corticosteroids and immunosuppressive agents cannot be used. It acts by suppression of antibody production due to infusions of large doses of IgG, suppresses production of idiopathic antibodies, inhibits formation of cytokines, neutralizes superantigens, etc. It is used in resistant cases of autoimmune bullous disorders, autoimmune connective tissue disorders, Kawasaki's disease, graft versus host reaction, scleromyxoedema, pyoderma gangrenosum, hypersensitivity disorders, etc.

34.4 Topical Immunomodulators

These are topical agents that regulate and modify the immune system. These can be broadly classified as:

- Macrolactams
- Contact sensitizers
- Immunostimulants
- Miscellaneous

34.4.1 Macrolactams

These include tacrolimus, pimecrolimus, and sirolimus. Like cyclosporin they have the structure of a macrolide antibiotic. The drugs inhibit calcineurin, which leads to the deprivation of activated T cells; they also have a potent and prolonged antipruritic effect. Macrolactams are used in the treatment of atopic dermatitis, vitiligo, psoriasis, erosive lichen planus, pyoderma gangrenosum, etc. Side effects include local redness, burning, and irritation. Pimecrolimus is used for mild to moderate atopic dermatitis and tacrolimus for moderate to severe atopic dermatitis.

Preparations. Tacrolimus 0.03%, 0.1% to be applied twice daily
Pimecrolimus1% cream to be applied twice daily

34.4.2 Contact Sensitizers

The drugs include dinitrochlorobenzene (DNCB), diphencyprone, and squaric acid dibutyl ester. These drugs arc mainly used in the treatment of alopecia areata and warts. DNCB is mutagenic; it should be avoided in females of childbearing age. Squaric acid dibutyl ester and diphencyprone are not mutagenic.

34.4.3 Immunostimulants

This includes imiquimod, which is an immunomodulator with antiviral and antitumor properties. It is an inducer of IFN-γ. Imiquimod is used for the treatment of viral infections such as warts and molluscum contagiosum and cutaneous malignancy such as actinic keratosis, Bowen's disease, lentigo maligna, and superficial basal cell carcinoma.

Preparation. 5% cream (aldara) available in sachets

34.4.4 Miscellaneous

These include calcipotriol, topical and intralesional interferon, and anthralin.

Calcipotriol is a vitamin D analogue. It is thought to regulate cell growth and differentiation; it also inhibits the production of cytokines by T cells. Calcipotriol is used in the treatment of psoriasis, morphoea, vitiligo, lichen sclerosis et atrophicus, and disorders of keratinization such as ichthyosis and palmoplantar keratoderma. Side effects include local urticaria, contact dermatitis, photosensitivity, and hypercalcemia. Calcium levels should be monitored prior to and during therapy. To reduce the local side effects, calcipotriol can be combined with topical steroids. It should not be used on the face and intertriginous areas.

Preparations. Calcipotriol 0.005% cream, ointment or lotion
Tacalcitol 0.004% and 0.002%
(In order to prevent hypercalcemia the dose of calciprotriol should be less than 15 g daily and tacalcitriol should be less than 5 g daily.)

Anthralin has an antimitotic and nonspecific immunomodulatory action. It is used for the treatment of psoriasis

(Ingram's regimen), alopecia areata, and vitilgo. Because of the skin irritation caused, it is advised to start the therapy with a low concentration and then gradually build up the therapeutic dose. A higher concentration can be used in short contact therapy. It also causes purplish-brown discoloration of the skin, hair, and clothes. The patients should be warned of this before starting treatment.

34.5 Physical Modalities Used in the Management of Skin Disorders

34.5.1 Cryotherapy

This is generally used for the treatment of warts, seborrhoeic keratosis, actinic keratosis, and molluscum contagiosum in adults. Tissue destruction occurs by intracellular and extracellular ice formation, cell dehydration, and denaturing of lipid-protein complexes.

Liquid nitrogen is the most popular cryogen used; it is inexpensive, the action is rapid, and it is noncombustible. A device supplying a fine spray of liquid nitrogen is used. The frozen skin blanches. The skin lesion and surrounding 2 mm of normal skin should blanch; this is maintained for 15–30 seconds before the tissue destruction is complete. The procedure should take less than 30 seconds. The patients should be told that the lesion might blister and crust, and then heal.

> Be careful while treating lesions on the fingers, as digital nerves can be damaged.

34.5.2 Phototherapy with Psoralens (PUVA)

Dermatologists have used ultraviolet radiation (320–400 nm) from artificial light for over a hundred years; it is still widely used for a number of skin disorders. It is used for the treatment of vitiligo, psoriasis, atopic dermatitis, prurigo, mycosis fungoides, mastocytosis, etc. The principle of treatment is to sensitize the skin first, with a photosensitive substance such as psoralens (oral or topical), and then expose the body to ultraviolet radiation. The radiation is given 2 hours after an oral dose and 15 minutes after local application of psoralen. The treatment is given twice a week, with an interval of 3 days between them. The patients are reviewed after 20 treatments, the maximum number of treatments received should not exceed 200, and the total dose of radiation should not exceed 1,500 J/cm^2 to minimize the side effects of treatment of which skin malignancy is the most important. The amount of radiation given is based on the patient's skin type and disease.

34.5.3 Narrow Band UVB Radiation (311 nm)

This was introduced in 1980; it has now replaced the broadband UVB therapy due to its safety and efficacy. It is used in cases which are not responsive to UVA. Skin type 1 and 2 need particular caution due to the side effect of skin burn. The bulbs used for the source of energy are very expensive and its use is therefore limited to a few centers. It is effective for psoriasis, vitiligo, atopic dermatitis, polymorphous light eruption, etc.

It has the advantage that it can be used without psoralens; therefore, it can be used in children, in pregnancy and lactation, and in the elderly. Narrow band UVB is expensive; it requires close supervision as it is more carcinogenic than PUVA therapy.

34.5.4 Photodynamic Therapy

This includes the therapeutic combination of photosensitizer administered to the patient and its activation by light. The photosensitizer may be topical, such as aminolevulinic acid (ALA), or systemic such as a hematoporphyrin derivative.

5-ALA applied to the skin is metabolized by the epidermal cells to protoporphyrin IX; this is sensitive to a broad range of light starting at the Soret band, 415 nm and through the red region of the visible spectrum. The photochemical reaction between protoporphyrin IX and absorbed photons produce singlet oxygen along with other reactive oxygen combinations and free radicles. The direct effect of these molecules causes localized membrane damage to cellular and mitochondrial membranes. The photosensitivity is lost in 24 hours; another advantage is that there is no systemic accumulation.

This method of treatment is used in the elderly with chronic nonhealing lesions such as Bowen's disease and actinic keratosis, especially on the legs where the results of surgery are poor.

> *The most serious side effect of phototherapy is skin cancer, the maximum dose should not exceed 1,500 J/cm², and the patient should be assessed after every 20 treatments.*
>
> *Eyes and genitals in males should be shielded during treatment.*

34.5.5 Lasers

Laser is an acronym for Light Amplification by Stimulated Emission of Radiation. Lasers are high-intensity, coherent light sources of a particular wavelength. Various media (gas, liquid, and solid) are used to produce these bundles of high-energy light. Lasers are often named after the medium used, method of stimulation, and whether they generate continuous wave or pulsed energy such as argon laser, carbon dioxide laser, flash lamp pulsed dye laser, ruby laser, etc.

The depth of penetration is proportional to the wavelength of the laser. These wavelengths have a particular affinity for different tissues in the skin, which can be targeted accordingly. There are thus different types of lasers for different tissues, e.g., vascular lasers, lasers for pigmented lesions, lasers for skin resurfacing, etc. The effect on the skin is destructive. The effect is influenced by the energy, length of pulse duration, the color, thickness, depth and type of tissue to be targeted. The main side effects of laser therapy are hyperpigmentation, hypopigmentation, and scarring.

Precautions while using lasers. Use protective measures such as goggles, facemasks, gown, and head cap. Do not keep combustible items near laser apparatus. Avoid using mirrors and reflective surfaces in the vicinity of the laser. When lasers are used for tissue ablation an effective smoke removal system should be in operation.

Lasers are mostly used for hair removal (pigmented hair), laser resurfacing such as acne scars, rhinophyma, removal of tattoos, etc., and for vascular lesions such as Port wine stains and telangiectasia. Laser phototherapy by excimer lasers (wavelength 308 nm) is used for treatment of psoriasis and vitiligo; the side effects are similar to UVB therapy.

34.5.6 Electrocautery/Electrosurgery

Cautery in Greek language means hot iron. The electrocautery machine modifies the alternating current to achieve high voltage, high frequency, and low amperage current to generate low oscillating radiowaves referred to as sine waves. Tissue destruction occurs due to passage of oscillating radiowaves through the tissue.

Electrosurgery should not be done on patients who have a cardiac pacemaker, for lesions where the diagnosis is in doubt, patients with a tendency to develop keloids, patients with a history of seizures, and for lesions larger than 1 cm in diameter.

34.5.6.1 Types of Electrosurgery

In electrofulguration, the needle tip is not in contact with the skin, a spark jumps from the needle to the skin; its energy is spread over a larger area of tissue. There is no scarring during healing, as the damage is restricted to the epidermis. It is an effective way of stopping bleeding from the superficial capillaries, and removing lesions such as verruca plana, milia, small molluscum, etc.

In electrodessication, the needle is in contact with the skin, no spark occurs; tissue destruction is slightly deeper than by electrofulguration. Tissue damage occurs up to the level of the papillary dermis, scarring is minimal. Electrodessication is an invaluable way of removing superficial lesions such as warts, seborrhoeic keratosis, pyogenic granuloma, skin tags, spider angiomata, molluscum contagiosum, etc.

Electrocoagulation is used to treat lesions like trichoepithilioma, nail matrix destruction, some BCC; telangiectasia, etc.

34.5.7 Electrolysis

One of the first indications of electrosurgery in dermatology was the use of direct current to destroy hair follicles. In this technique, heat is actually not a factor. A chemical reaction occurs at the electrode tip, with the evolution of sodium hydroxide at the hair root. When the direct current passes through the electrode tip, the sodium hydroxide produced is responsible for hair destruction.

This is a safe technique with minimal pain and risk of scarring. It is a very slow method, requiring a minute or two for each individual hair destruction.

34.5.8 Iontophoresis

This is a method by which ions of soluble salts are introduced into the skin for therapeutic purposes. Basically it is the process of increasing the penetration of electrically charged drugs into the surface tissues by galvanic current. The systemic side effects of the drug are significantly decreased.

Iontophoresis is a method of treating hyperhidrosis of the hands and feet. In this method, a direct current of low voltage can be used to introduce ionized drugs into the skin. Even tap water can be used for the purpose. The electric current selectively damages and blocks the sweat ducts.

34.5.9 Surgical Excision

Surgical excision is used for removal of tissue for biopsy, removal of benign and malignant growths. Surgical incisions should be made parallel to Langer's line, to minimize postoperative scarring. The length of the wound should be three times the width, to ensure easy closure. Facial sutures are removed after 5 days, trunk and extremity after 7–14 days.

34.5.9.1 Mohs Surgery

Frederick Mohs' pioneering work began in late 1930 with removal of accessible forms of cancer under microscopic control. In this method of surgery, the neoplastic tissue is excised, fixed carefully, and marked; sections of the tissue are cut, examined microscopically, and the process repeated until all the cancer tissue is removed. The method is time consuming, but the success rate is high. This is usually in the range of 99% for primary basal cell carcinoma, and 96% for recurrent lesions. Today instead of using fixed tissue technique using zinc chloride paste, a fresh tissue technique is used.

34.5.9.2 Indications

- Mohs surgery is indicated for recurrent basal cell carcinomas, and other cutaneous cancers when other methods have failed.
- Large or deeply invasive carcinomas.
- For lesions on the "H Zone" of the face (the nasolabial fold, nasal alae, periorbital region, and periauricular areas), the region where electrosurgery and radiation cannot be done due to complications.
- In morphoeic and sclerosing basal cell carcinoma.
  The scalp, palms, soles, and nail require systemic therapy for cure, as topical medicines do not penetrate well in the thick stratum corneum.

Phototherapy should be regularly monitored as long-term treatment can give rise to malignancy.

Both topical and systemic steroids, should be gradually tapered to prevent disease rebound.

Always exclude pregnancy before giving retinoids.

Topical fungal treatment should be continued, for 2 weeks after clinical cure to prevent recurrences.

Before any electrosurgical procedure, make sure that the patient does not have a cardiac pacemaker.

Appendix 1
Compression Bandaging for Venous Ulcers

The only effective way of treating ulcers secondary to venous hypertension is by external compression of the leg, by a compression bandage. This compresses the superficial veins so that the blood flows in the deep veins. As the pressure within the veins of a standing subject is largely hydrostatic, it follows that the level of external pressure that is necessary to counteract this effect will reduce progressively up the leg. It is therefore important that the external pressure is applied in a graduated fashion, with the highest pressure at the ankle. It is estimated that an external compression of 20 mmHg could increase the velocity of venous flow in the deep veins of the leg by 45%.

Compression bandage can be four-layer or two-layer. Before applying the bandage, the arterial pulse of the leg should be checked to ensure that there is an adequate blood supply to the limb. This is done by feeling for the pulsation of dorsalis pedis and posterior tibial artery manually or by a Doppler probe. The ratio of arterial pressures in the leg compared to the arm is calculated. A reading >0.9 indicates no arterial disease and a reading <0.7 indicates significant arterial disease.

Z. Zaidi, S. W. Lanigan, *Dermatology in Clinical Practice*,
DOI 10.1007/978-1-84882-862-9_A1,
© Springer-Verlag London Limited 2010

A1.1 Four-Layer Compression Bandage

The ulcer is first cleaned and debrided if necessary; a nonadhesive dressing then covers it. The leg is raised to drain the blood from the superficial veins, assisted by manual massage. The four-layer compression bandage is applied as follows:

- First layer is of orthopaedic wool; it is wound around the leg as a spiral, with 50% overlap, from the toes to below the knee.
- Second layer is of crepe bandage at mid-stretch and with 50% overlap.
- Third layer is of high compression long-stretch bandage. For ankle circumference of <25 cm, a Litepress bandage is used as a figure of 8.
- If the ankle circumference is >25 cm, a Tensopress bandage is used with an overlap of 50%.
- Fourth layer is of cohesive lightweight elastic bandage, with a 50% overlap.

The four-layer compression is very effective; it does not slip down the leg and will remain in place for at least a week. However, it is expensive; normal shoes may be difficult to wear over it and it requires training for safe application.

A1.2 Two-Layer Compression Bandage

This is less expensive and normal footwear can be worn over it. It is applied as follows:

- First layer is of orthopaedic wool; it is applied as a spiral as described above.
- Second layer is of compression bandage; it can be of long stretch (for both mobile and bed rest patients) or short-stretched (for mobile patients), in which case it is pulled to full stretch. The patients can apply the short-stretch bandage themselves.

These bandages should be changed weekly, continuing until the ulcer is healed. This usually takes 12 weeks. The patients should exercise their calf muscles, and should be mobile, to help in venous drainage. While sitting, the foot should be raised on some support, such as a stool and the patient should dorsiflex their feet frequently. When resting, where possible the leg should be positioned higher than the chest. This helps in the flow of blood in only one direction, i.e., back towards the heart.

Once the ulcer heals, compression stockings should be worn for the rest of the patient's life, as the missing or damaged valves in the veins cannot be replaced.

Appendix 2
Patch Testing and Prick Testing

A2.1 Patch Testing

This test is done to establish the diagnosis of allergic contact dermatitis. It is used to identify a type IV hypersensitivity reaction. The allergens are suspended in white soft paraffin or aqueous solution; these are then placed on aluminum discs (Finn chamber). The discs are then applied on the patient's back, and left in place for 48 h. When the tapes are removed, a small circular plaque of eczema at the site of the aluminum disc at 48 or 96 h indicates an allergic response to the antigen.

A patch test should be avoided when the patient's eczema is acute, and if the patient is taking antihistamines, or oral steroids. There should be an interval of at least 2 weeks after stopping these drugs, and for acute eczema to have settled before undertaking the patch test. The back should be free of any inflammation, for the patch test to take place.

A2.1.1 Method

The doctor first decides which allergens are to be tested, taking the patient's history into consideration. A standard battery of 20 or so allergens relevant to the local population is often used. The solid allergens are diluted in petrolatum; they are applied in a line across the diameter of the chamber. This will spread across the chamber when the tests are in place. The allergens in solution are applied on a filter disc, with the help

Z. Zaidi, S. W. Lanigan, *Dermatology in Clinical Practice*,
DOI 10.1007/978-1-84882-862-9_A2,
© Springer-Verlag London Limited 2010

of a pipette. The filter disc is then placed in the chamber. The disc should be completely moistened but not oversaturated.

A2.1.1.1 First Visit

The patient should be seated on a comfortable stool with the back exposed. The back is the most suitable site for the application of allergens. The sites in order of preference are back/upper arm/outer thigh. No special preparation is required, except shaving if required.

The strips of the chamber are fixed on the back with a tape, starting at the bottom end of the tape to avoid dislodging any filter disc. Ensure that the tape is properly fixed. Press each chamber to expel air and to spread the allergen evenly over the area. If several strips are used, place them in line where possible. Number the columns of strips used in order of the allergens applied, so that the doctors know what the allergens in each disc are (the allergen order should be recorded; the doctor will use this when reading the result). Cover the numbers marked on the skin with a hypoallergenic tape. Mark the numbers again on the tape.

The strips should stay in place for 48 h, the test area should be kept dry, and the patient should avoid any strenuous exercise to avoid excessive sweating. If the chambers are exposed, the patient should not try to replace them, as these may not be replaced exactly at the same place, leading to misinterpretation of results. The strip may be removed if any acute and severe reaction occurs.

A2.1.1.2 Revisit at 48 hours

The marker tape should be checked to see if it is secured. The strips applied are now removed. The area is wiped with solvent to remove any remaining allergen or plaster. Allow 20–30 minutes for any plaster reaction to subside.

A positive reaction is manifested by erythema and papules; if the reaction is severe there may be vesicles and bullae.

A2.1.2 Grading of Patch Test

Clinical signs	Reading of test	Interpretation
Faint erythema only	±	Doubtful reaction
Erythema, edema, and papules	+	Weak, nonvesicular reaction
Erythema, edema, papules, and vesicles	+ +	Strong, vesicular reaction
Intense erythema, vesicles, and bullae	+ + +	Extreme bullous reaction

After reading the result, the doctor may order some more tests, for example, rubber ingredients in rubber allergy.

A2.1.2.1 Third Visit at 96 hours

The same procedure is repeated as in the second visit, as some allergens react after a longer time; also to see the results of the new allergens applied on the second visit. When the reading and recording are complete, all the marker tapes are removed and the patient's back is cleaned.

A2.1.2.2 False Positive Reactions

This can occur if there is an active dermatitis; these patients often react to multiple antigens, producing numerous false positive reactions called the angry back syndrome.

- Too much concentration of the allergen may produce an irritant reaction.
- Scratching the area will produce redness, which can be misinterpreted.
- Sensitivity to a vehicle.
- Misreading an irritant reaction as a positive reaction.
- Current or recent dermatitis near the patch test site.
- Adhesive tape reaction.

A2.1.2.3 False Negative Reactions

- Too little concentration of the allergen
- Inappropriate selection of an allergen
- Loosening of the patch
- Systemic steroids or antihistamines taken during the test, or used a few days before the test
- Inappropriate vehicle
- Degraded allergen

A2.1.2.4 Advice to the Patient

The doctor assesses positive patch test reactions, as to whether they are relevant to the patient's current problem. When suspected of allergy to a certain substance, the patient is advised to avoid that allergen. A list of substances, which may contain the offending allergen, are given to the patient, so that they can avoid their use. The patient should be followed up to see if the offending agent was the cause of contact allergy.

A2.2 PhotoPatch Testing

This is done to confirm photoallergic reactions. A standard series of photoallergens are applied in duplicate on each side of the back. After 48 hours the patches are removed and the test is read. One of the sets is then exposed to 5–15 J/m^2 of UVA and further observed after 48 hours. Positive reaction on the photo-exposed test indicates a photoallergic reaction. While positive reactions on both sides indicate allergic contact dermatitis.

A2.3 Prick Testing

Prick test identifies an immediate hypersensitivity reaction, as seen in asthma, contact urticaria, hay fever, etc. It is not useful in the diagnosis of atopic dermatitis or idiopathic urticaria. A prick test is usually done on the flexural aspect of the forearm.

A drop of allergen is placed on the forearm and the skin is then pricked with a lancet or a needle; this breaks the skin and the allergen penetrates into the skin. The results are read after 20 minutes. A saline (negative) and a histamine (positive) control test should also be done. The allergen site is compared with the positive wheal from histamine and negative reaction of saline. Measure the wheal and the peripheral erythema. Positive reactions should be more than 50% of the size of the histamine wheal. The risk of anaphylaxis is low, but appropriate measures for resuscitation should be available.

If the prick test is negative then a 'use test' can be done. If a patient is allergic to latex rubber, then a fingerstall of latex rubber is given to the patient to wear on wet skin for about 15 minutes, and a fingerstall of vinyl glove on another finger. The reaction is seen after 15 minutes. The result is positive if there is a reaction on the finger, similar to that seen in patch test. More extensive exposure can be assessed if necessary.

Oral provocative tests are potentially dangerous and are usually not done; if necessary they should be performed with full resuscitation available.

Appendix 3
Removal of the Nail by Urea

Nails may have to be removed in cases of severe nail dystrophy such as dystrophic nails due to onychogryphosis especially in younger people, onychomycosis, and ingrowing toe nails.

A3.1 Method

The skin around the dystrophic nail is first painted with tincture of benzoin, and then the area around the nails is covered with two elastic adhesive tapes – one around the base of the nail along the proximal nail fold, and the second around the lateral and distal end of the nail. The 40% urea ointment is placed generously on the nail. The nail is then occluded with polythene film. The whole occluded area is secured with elastic adhesive tape.

This dressing is covered with another layer of polythene film to secure it well. Finally, a cotton tubular bandage is placed over the finger or toe is put; which is fixed in place with elastic adhesive tape.

The dressing is kept in situ for 1–2 weeks; it should be kept dry. At the end of this time the nails should be soft enough for removal by the doctor.

Z. Zaidi, S. W. Lanigan, *Dermatology in Clinical Practice*,
DOI 10.1007/978-1-84882-862-9_A3,
© Springer-Verlag London Limited 2010

Appendix 4
Photochemotherapy

A4.1 Ultraviolet Radiation

The sun emits a continuous spectrum of electromagnetic energy, from the short cosmic rays to the long radio waves. This includes ultraviolet light (200–400 nm), visible light (400–700 nm), and infrared rays (700–5,000 nm). The atmosphere absorbs most of the short wavelengths and none shorter than 290 nm reaches the ground level. Ultraviolet radiation spectrum consists of three wavebands – UVC (200–290 nm), UVB (290–320 nm), and UVA (320–400 nm).

Sunburn in the human skin, is produced by a narrow band of radiation that extends from 290 to 320 nm (UVB). Shorter wavelengths UVC (200–290 nm) are more effective in producing sunburn, but these do not reach sea level and are blocked by the ozone layer of the atmosphere. With diminution of the ozone layer, the chances of sunburn and cutaneous malignancy are increased. The radiations of longer wavelength UVA have relatively little effect on normal skin and are invisible to man although they do contribute to skin ageing (photoageing); this wavelength is sometimes called 'black light'. In some diseases such as porphyria and drugs such as psoralens the normal skin is sensitized to UVA. Most window glass absorbs wavelengths less than 320 nm and thus prevents sunburn.

Infrared radiation (700–5,000 nm) generally does not cause biological damage, unless it is of sufficient intensity to generate heat. These are generally used for diathermy. Gamma rays,

Z. Zaidi, S. W. Lanigan, *Dermatology in Clinical Practice*, DOI 10.1007/978-1-84882-862-9_A4, © Springer-Verlag London Limited 2010

X-rays are of very short wavelength (smaller than 200 nm) with high energies that penetrate the skin deeply and pass into the tissues where they can cause extensive damage.

The electromagnetic spectrum

γ and X-rays	UVC 200–290 nm	UVB 290–320 nm	UVA 320–400 nm	Visible light 400–700 nm	Infrared Above 700 nm–10^5	Radio Above 10^5
High energy rays	Ultraviolet rays			Visible rays	Low energy rays	

UV represents ultraviolet

A4.2 Photochemotherapy

Many skin diseases improve in summer, particularly with sun exposure. Sunlight has been used since time immemorial to treat skin disease. Today artificial ultraviolet light is used to treat cutaneous disorders such as vitiligo, atopic dermatitis, psoriasis, urticaria pigmentosum, pityriasis lichenoides chronica, mycosis fungoides, polymorphic light eruption, and itching of chronic renal failure. These disorders are treated by narrow band ultraviolet B or PUVA (psoralens and UVA) therapy.

A4.2.1 PUVA

This combines taking of the drug methoxypsoralen with exposure to UVA. Oral methoxypsoralen tablets are to be taken 2 hours before the exposure to radiation, and the lotion is applied 15 minutes before radiation. The patient is then subjected to radiation; the dose is calculated in terms of light energy (J/cm^2). This is done either by applying a template with 1 cm^2 cut outs to the patient's skin and irradiating it with increasing dose of UV light; the rest of the patient's skin is completely covered. The dose, which produces a pale erythema, is noted. The starting dose is 75% of this minimal erythema dose (MED). MED can also be calculated according to the skin type.

For oral PUVA:

> Skin type 1- 0.5 J/cm^2
> Skin type 2- 1 J/cm^2
> Skin type 3- 1.5 J/cm^2
> Skin type 4- 2 J/cm^2
> Skin type 5- 2.5 J/cm^2

For bath PUVA:

> Skin type 1- 0.2 J/cm^2
> Skin type 2- 0.3 J/cm^2
> Skin type 3- 0.4 J/cm^2
> Skin type 4- 0.5 J/cm^2
> Skin type 5- 0.6 J/cm^2

In vitiligo for all skin types the starting dose is 0.1 J/cm^2. The dose is increased by 0.1 J/cm^2 until a dose of 1.0 J/cm^2 is reached; the dose is then increased by 10% until a pink color is achieved on vitiligo patches. This dose is then maintained.

For full-body treatment the patient stands in a specially designed cabinet; for small areas such as the palms a small UVA unit is used. During PUVA therapy the eyes (to prevent ocular damage) and male genitalia (to reduce the risk of skin cancer) are protected from ultraviolet light. An emollient is applied after treatment to prevent the skin from becoming too dry.

After PUVA therapy the patient is advised to protect the skin (by sunscreens) and eyes (by ultraviolet light protective spectacles) from sunlight for 24 hours. They should avoid any sunbathing or using sunbeds while undergoing treatment. The patient should also avoid any cosmetics or scented toiletries, as these may make the skin sensitive to ultraviolet light.

The individual dose and the cumulative dose is recorded on each visit. The dose is increased at each visit depending upon the response to previous treatment.

Treatment schedule for oral PUVA:

- If there is no response then the dose is increased by 20% of the previous dose.
- If there is mild erythema increase the dose by 10%.

- For well-defined erythema, postpone one treatment, repeat the previous dose at next visit, and then increase by 10% increments.
- If there is marked tenderness and erythema stop treatment until recovery.

Treatment schedule for local PUVA.

- If there is no response, increase the dose by 0.5% J/cm^2 until 5.0 J/cm^2, then increase by 20%.
- If there is mild erythema, repeat previous dose and then increase by 10% increments on each visit.
- For well-defined erythema, postpone one treatment, repeat the previous dose at next visit, and then increase by 10% on each visit.
- If there is marked tenderness and erythema, there should be no treatment until recovery.

The patient should be reviewed after 20 treatments. Max dose 15 J/cm^2.

It is recommended that lifetime exposure to PUVA should be limited to 1,000 J/cm^2 or 200 treatments to reduce the risk of skin cancer. No limit is so far established for UVB therapy, although every effort is made to keep the amount of radiation to a minimum.

A4.2.2 Narrow Band UVB (311 nm)

Introduced in 1980s, it has largely replaced broad band UVB due to efficacy, and has surpassed PUVA as there is no need to take psoralens before therapy. It can therefore be used in pregnancy, lactation, and in children. As it is recently introduced, it will be a decade before we can expect recorded incidence data on phototherapy-induced skin cancer in humans. The number of exposures should be kept to a minimum until epidemiological data is obtained.

Particular caution should be taken with skin type 1 and 2; it is advisable that these patients should have a regular follow-up to check for malignancy. This method of treatment is expensive.

Diseases treated with narrow band UVB include vitiligo, atopic dermatitis, nodular prurigo, mycosis fungoides, pruritus, pityriasis rubra pilaris, pityriasis lichenoides, and some photodermatoses.

Appendix 5
Laser Therapy

Laser is an acronym for Light Amplification by Stimulated Emission of Radiation. Maiman introduced laser in 1960, and Leon Goldman pioneered its dermatological use. It is a device that produces coherent light (all laser light is in phase and focuses to a small area), light is monochromatic (of the same wavelength), and collimated (light that travels in a straight line and does not diffuse).

The laser machine consists of:

- An electromagnetic energy source of high input
- Laser medium, which may be solid, liquid, or gas, e.g., carbon dioxide laser, ruby laser, etc.
- Reflective mirrors – a fully reflective mirror at one end and a partially reflective mirror at the other end

Passing a high electric voltage current stimulates the laser medium. A stimulated molecule of the laser medium emits a photon (light particle), which strikes another stimulated molecule causing it to emit an identical photon (amplification). Emission of photons occurs in all directions, but the light waves are aligned by resonance between the mirrors, and the coherent light exits through the partially reflective mirror. The type of the laser medium determines the wavelength of the coherent light that is produced.

The different wavelengths target different tissues in the skin, e.g., hemoglobin absorption peaks at wavelengths of 532 or 577 nm. The advantage of a laser is that it targets injury to

Z. Zaidi, S. W. Lanigan, *Dermatology in Clinical Practice*,
DOI 10.1007/978-1-84882-862-9_A5,
© Springer-Verlag London Limited 2010

selected sites such as blood vessels, melanin, etc. with minimum damage to the adjacent structures. This effect is called "*selective photothermolysis*." This is achieved if the laser fulfills the following requirements:

- The laser should emit the same wavelength that the target tissue absorbs, e.g., for hemoglobin the wavelength is 532 or 577 nm.
- The laser emits sufficient energy to damage the target tissue.
- The duration of exposure time should be short, to limit damage to the target tissue, without heat diffusing outwards. This is determined by the '*thermal relaxing time*', i.e., how long it takes for the target tissue to dissipate half of its thermal energy. For blood vessels in Port wine stain it is 1–10 ms. The pulse duration of lasers must correspond to the tissues it is targeting. Thermal relaxing time for melanasomes is in nanoseconds.

The penetration of laser in the skin depends upon its wavelength, the longer the wavelength the deeper the penetration. For hair removal, the laser must penetrate to the root of the hair follicle. Lasers are most popular in the following conditions:

- Vascular lasers target hemoglobin, wavelengths are selected around 577 nm to ensure adequate penetration. Pulse duration is selected according to the diameter of the blood vessel being treated. Lasers used include the pulse dye laser, and KTP laser.
- Pigment lasers target melanin and tattoo ink. Between 500 and 1,100 nm there is good penetration and absorption by melanin. Some pigmented lesions (lentigenes and tattoos) are treated by very short pulse durations, which can be achieved by Q switching (this allows very high peak powers to be achieved with pulse durations of 28–40 ns). This generates a shock wave which breaks down melanin and tattoo pigments. The lasers used are Nd: YAG laser, Alexandrite laser, and ruby laser.

- For hair removal, longer pulse widths and long wavelengths are needed to reach and damage the hair follicle. Lasers used are the Nd: YAG laser (skin photo type 4, 5, and 6), alexandrite laser (skin photo type 1, 2, and 3).
- Surfacing and cutting lasers target water and hence all tissue. A short pulse duration and high energy will result in vaporization of tissue with minimal damage to underlying structures. Healing comes from reepithelization from the hair follicles. Lasers used are carbon dioxide and erbium-YAG lasers.
- Excimer lasers are named after the formation of 'excited dimers' in their technology. These lasers have a specific wavelength of 309 nm, which is effective for the treatment of psoriasis and vitiligo. The action is similar to that of narrow band UVB therapy.

Precautions while using lasers:

- Environmental protection. There should be ventilation exhaust systems and prevention of spectral reflectance.
- Specific eye protection is needed for each type of laser, and safety goggles should be used.
- The surrounded skin should be shielded to prevent burning.
- The operator must wear protective gloves.

A test treatment of a small area is advised to test the therapeutic efficacy of the laser on the given tissue, and predict the cosmetic result. A watch period of 4 months is recommended for proper evaluation.

A number of lasers are used in dermatology. To say which is the "best laser" is a question that has no answer; different lasers are used for different purposes. The effect of laser treatment also depends upon the individuals, their color, and type.

Appendix 6
Cryotherapy

The earliest freezing agent used in the treatment of skin disease was salt ice mixture (-20°C) with James Arnott as its pioneer in 1851. Today liquid nitrogen is the most commonly used cryogen; it is used throughout the world, as it is efficient, inexpensive, and noncombustible. Decreasing the temperature also decreases nerve conduction and hence can make a procedure painless.

Cryogens are easy to apply, require no local anesthesia, and usually leave no scars after reepithelialization. The lower the boiling point of the cryogen, the more efficient are its freezing capabilities. The boiling point of Freon 12 is -29.8°C, solid CO_2 is -78.5°C, liquid nitrous oxide is -89.5°C, and liquid nitrogen is -195.6°C.

Freezing produces changes similar to that caused by a burn with erythema, a blister at the site of dermo-epidermal junction, and necrosis of the skin. Cell death is due to intra- and extra-cellular ice formation, osmotic changes in the cell, denaturing of proteins in the cell membrane, and local ischemia due to vasoconstriction.

For most skin lesions cryosurgery produces a blister at the dermo-epidermal junction, so that the abnormal tissue is lifted off the skin in the blister roof. Cryosurgery is usually done for epidermal lesions such as viral warts, molluscum contagiosum, solar keratosis, seborrhoeic warts, etc.

Freezing can easily be performed by liquid nitrogen spray gun. This is a stainless steel insulated vacuum flask with a side

Z. Zaidi, S. W. Lanigan, *Dermatology in Clinical Practice*,
DOI 10.1007/978-1-84882-862-9_A6,
© Springer-Verlag London Limited 2010

arm and a spray tip. Different tips are available depending upon the size of the lesion to be treated. When liquid nitrogen is sprayed at the center of the lesion, a white ball of ice will form and this will gradually expand. Freezing is continued until the ice ball extends to 2 mm outside the margin of the lesion. Repeated freezing thaw cycles are more effective than a single long freeze. The approximate freezing time for common viral warts is about 10 seconds. Do not freeze beyond 30 seconds for epidermal lesions. A little experience will tell us how much freezing time is required for different lesions.

Be very careful while treating lesions of the lower leg; here about half of the freezing time is recommended as excessive freezing over the lower legs can result in ulcer formation. Care should also be taken to avoid excessive freezing of the proximal nail folds as permanent nail dystrophy can arise.

The indications for cryosurgery are limited. It is not a treatment to be used on any skin lesion where the diagnosis is in doubt. It should not be used on dermal lesions; therefore, an accurate diagnosis should be made before performing cryosurgery.

A6.1 Macroscopic Changes After Cryosurgery

During and immediately after cryosurgery, a white ice field develops; a few minutes after thawing a purplish color develops at the periphery of the lesion, which later moves centrally. After about 12–48 hours a hemorrhagic blister develops on an erythematous base in the center of the treated zone; the blister then forms an eschar over a period of a week, which later separates spontaneously. The crusts on the leg take longer to separate.

A6.2 Contraindications to Cryosurgery

These include conditions in which there is an abnormal reaction to cold, such as cryoglobinemia, cryofibrinogenemia, Raynauds disease, cold urticaria, etc.

A6.3 Side Effect of Cryosurgery

- Burning and pain
- Hypopigmentation or hyperpigmentation
- Scarring
- Neural damage
- Headache/pain around the eyes after treatment of lesions on the forehead
- Necrosis of cartilage

Appendix 7
Management and Care of Wounds

Wound care is an essential part of dermatological treatment. Wound healing occurs in three stages:

- Influx of inflammatory cells to the wound, to aid in the reabsorption of necrotic cells and prevent infection. This causes erythema and exudation.
- The formation of granulation tissue and revascularization. At this stage, there is reduction of exudation.
- Migration of epithelial tissue to cover the wound, and growth of new connective tissue underneath.

A disorder of wound healing occurs when the balance between healing and inflammation is disturbed. If the wound healing is delayed for any reason then tissue death may occur, with the formation of a permanent scar. Scarring also occurs when the defect is large and deep. Surgical sutures should be used to close large wounds.

Wound healing takes place rapidly in the following conditions:

- There is a moist environment and any excess fluid is able to evaporate.
- The wound is warm; a drop of temperature of 2°C significantly reduces healing.
- There is good blood perfusion, and any dressing should not affect this.

Z. Zaidi, S. W. Lanigan, *Dermatology in Clinical Practice*,
DOI 10.1007/978-1-84882-862-9_A7,
© Springer-Verlag London Limited 2010

A7.1 Type of Wound and Dressings to Use

Dressings may be open or closed. Open dressings allow for vaporization of fluids. They dry the ulcer or erosions. These dressings are mainly used for wet wounds such as erosions of pemphigus vulgaris, impetigo, small superficial oozing ulcers, etc. Closed dressings are occlusive, they protect the ulcer from external contamination and injury to the wound, these are often used after surgical closure of wounds, venous ulcers, etc.

A7.1.1 Clean Wounds

Wound cleaning for its own sake is not indicated, for the wound bed is disturbed and any new epithelium is ripped off. These wounds should be covered by simple nonadherent dressings, with padding for protection and insulation.

A7.1.2 Removal of Debris

Any excess of necrotic tissue should be removed by scissors, scalpel, saline irrigation, or debriding agents, e.g., hydrogel, hydrocolloid, and maggots. Sterile maggots are available in small container bags; add saline to the maggots and put them in the mesh net provided. Place the maggots next to the ulcer, inside a colloid sheet. Cover the outside of the net with moistened swabs. The maggots, should be left in place for 48–72 h and then washed out with saline. Maggots feed on necrotic tissue without affecting the normal skin.

A7.1.3 Infected Wounds

Wounds are often infected especially in tropical countries due to heat, humidity, and neglect. These wounds have to be cleaned and dressed more often, sometimes even twice a day. Taking a wound swab is not helpful; signs of infection are pain, cellulitis of the surrounding skin, foul odor and exudation of pus, capillary bleeding, and pitted/spongy granulation tissue. Useful preparations include 1–3% cetrimide, chlorhexidine, 0.5% silver nitrate, 0.25% acetic acid, 1% povidine iodine, 1% gentian violet, and potassium permanganate (1 in 10,000 dilution); these are applied as compresses with or without occlusion.

Three percent hydrogen peroxide is frequently used in wound care. The lesion is flushed with hydrogen peroxide and left undisturbed until frothing ceases. If the solution is soaked in gauze then it should be left for about 5 min.

The common organisms that are of concern in wound infection are group A beta hemolytic streptococci and pseudomonas. *Streptococcus* causes cellulitis and is treated with erythromycin or flucloxacillin. Infection with pseudomonas results in a green discoloration and a distinctive foul odor. This infection can be treated with acetic acid, or silver preparations such as flamazine cream; metronidazole cream is also helpful. Systemic ciprofloxacin is indicated in severe cases.

A7.1.4 Absorption of Exudates

Venous ulcers are more likely to produce exudates due to increased hydrostatic pressure. Exudate interferes with healing, soaks through the bandage, and can wet clothing and bedding.

Dressings that absorb exudates are Granuflex, Duoderm extra thin, alignate, hydrofiber, and osmotic absorbents. Iodosorb beads are poured onto the wound and covered by a secondary dressing. They should be changed every 1–2 days, depending upon how much exudate is present. Old beads should be removed before replacing new ones. Dextranomer beads are able to absorb four times their own weight of exudates. Actisorb is a useful charcoal dressing that absorbs exudates and removes odor.

Treatment of venous ulcer in Appendix 1

Bibliography

Arnold LH, Odom RB, James WB. Andrew's diseases of the skin. *Clinical Dermatology*. 8th ed. Philadelphia: S W Saunders; 1990.

Ahsan I. *Textbook of Surgery*. 1st ed. Lahore: Qindeel press; 1991.

Arndt KA. *Manual of Dermatological Therapeutics: With Recent Essentials of Diagnosis*. 4th ed. Boston: Little Brown; 1989.

Baran R, Dawber PR, Tosti A, Haneke E. *A Text Atlas of Nail Disorders*. London: Martin Duntz; 2001.

Brown RG, Burns T. Lecture notes on dermatology. *Diagnosis and Therapy*. 1st ed. New Jersey: Prentice Hall; 1991.

Fitzpatrick JE, Aeling JL. *Dermatological Secrets*. 1st ed. Delhi: Jaypee Brothers Medical Publications; 1997.

Fleischer BA, Feldman RA, Katz SA, Clayton DB. *Twenty Common Problems in Dermatology*. 1st ed. New York: McGraw Hill; 2000.

Goodman and Gilman. *The Pharmacological Basis of Therapeutics*. 8th ed. Oxford: Pergamon Press; 1991.

Gulhric D. *A History of Medicine*. London: Thomas Nelson and Sons; 1960.

Guyton AC. *Textbook of Medical Physiology*. 7th ed. New York: Churchill and Livingstone; 1988.

Habif PT. *Clinical Dermatology*: *A Colour Guide to Diagnosis and Therapy*. 3rd edn. St. Louis: Mosby; 1996.

Z. Zaidi, S. W. Lanigan, *Dermatology in Clinical Practice*,
DOI: 10.1007/978-1-84882-862-9_Bibliography,
© Springer-Verlag London Limited 2010

Irwin M., Freedberg MD, Arthur Z, Klauswolff MD. *Fitzpatrick's Dermatology in General Medicine*. 5th ed. New York: Mcgraw Hill (Health profesional division); 1999.

Kane SK, Ryder BJ, Johnson AR, Baden PH, and Stratigos A. *Colour Atlas of Pediatric Dermatology*. New York: McGraw Hill; 2002.

Kerdel FA, Romanelli P, Trent TJ. *Dermatologic Therapeurtics*. New York: McGraw Hill; 2005.

Khopkar U, Pande S, Nischal KC. *A Handbook of Dermatological Drug Therapy*. Philadelphia: Elsevier; 2007.

Lebwohl M. *Difficult Diagnosis in Dermatology*. 1st ed. New York: Churchill Livingstone; 1988.

Lewis P. *An Illustrated History of Medicine*. Middlesex: Hamlyn; 1968.

Lyons AS, Petrucelli RJ. *Medicine an Illustrated History*. New York: Abrams; 1987.

Marks R, Fry T. *Practical Problems in Dermatology*. 1st ed. London: Martin Dunitz; 1984.

Mackie R. *Eczema and Dermatitis: How to Cope with Inflamed Skin*. 1st ed. New Jersey: Prentice Hall; 1983.

Mehregan AH, Hashimoto K. *Pinkus Guide to Dermatohistopathology*. 5th ed. New Jersey: Prentice Hall; 1984.

Nelson WE, Vaughan VC, Mckay J. *Textbook of Pediatrics*. 9th ed. Philadelphia: WB Saunders; 1969.

Price's *Textbook of the Practice of Medicine*. 10th ed. Oxford: English Language Book Society, Oxford University Press; 1966.

Rook, Wilkinson, Ebling. *Textbook of Dermatology*. 6th ed. In: Champion RH, Burton JL, Burns DA, Breathnach SM (eds). London: Blackwell; 1998.

Sehgal VN, Jain S. *Textbook of Clinical Dermatology*. Delhi: Jaypee Brothers Medical Publishers; 1995.

Sherwood L. *Human Physiology. From Cells to System*. 3rd ed. Wadwont Publishing Company; 1997.

Sterry W, Paus R, Burgdorf W. Theimes clinical companions. *Dermatology*. New Delhi: Saurabh Printers; 2007.

Williams LP, Warwick R, Dyson M, Bannister HL. *Grays Anatomy*. 37th ed. New York: Churchill Livingstone; 1993.

Wojnarowska F, Shahrad P. *Illustrated Encyclopaedia of Dermatology*. 1st ed. Lancaster: MTP; 1981.

Index